Hepatitis C: Choices, 2nd Edition

Authors

Terry Baker
Misha Cohen, OMD, LicAc
Randy Dietrich
Gregory T. Everson, MD
Sylvia Flesner, ND
Robert G. Gish, MD
Douglas R. Labrecque, MD
Lark Lands, PhD
Jo An Lorren
Peggy McCarthy, MBA
Shri K. Misra, MD, MS
Lyn Patrick, ND
Bharathi Ravi, BAMS
Lorren Sandt
Tina M. St. John, MD
Sivaramaprasad Vinjamury, MD
Mark White
Qing Cai Zhang, MD (China), LicAc

Senior Editors

Lorren Sandt
Tina M. St. John, MD

IN LOVING MEMORY

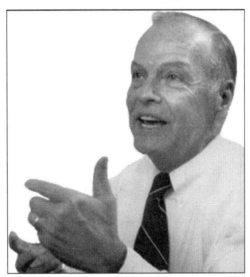

Ken Giddes
July 23, 1937 - January 27, 2001

The Hepatitis C Caring Ambassadors Program dedicates this manual in loving memory of Ken Giddes. As a stage IV lung cancer survivor for over four years, Ken was the first Caring Ambassador. He dedicated the last years of his life to helping others with lung cancer and other forms of cancer. Ken was also our mentor in developing the Hepatitis C Caring Ambassadors Program. He was the epitome of a Caring Ambassador, reaching out to others struggling to survive a life-threatening illness.

Ken was and continues to be our inspiration. He inspires us to research all the options for people living with hepatitis C, and to empower them with knowledge about their disease. He inspired us to write this manual for all of you who are living with hepatitis C.

To Ken and all the patient advocates working tirelessly around the world for the people they represent, we thank you.

ACKNOWLEDGEMENTS

The Hepatitis C Caring Ambassadors Program and this manual would not be possible without the love, generosity, and hard work of the Possehl Family, the Dietrich Family, and all the employees of Republic Financial Corporation. Thank you.

The Hepatitis C Caring Ambassadors Program would like to thank the members of the World Class Brainstorming Team and the other contributors to this manual. We are proud of the way these dedicated professionals from many different disciplines have listened to one another, worked together, and have become a team - a team dedicated to providing better health care to everyone with hepatitis C. Without their willingness to open their minds to treatment possibilities other than their own, this manual would not be possible.

We would also like to thank the first editors, Innovative Medical Education Consortium. We could not have done this without their help. JoAn, thank you for all of your patience. Many thanks to you, Nanette, for your time and effort compiling the glossary.

This second edition of *Hepatitis C: Choices* could not have been possible without the hard work of our new editor, Dr. Tina St. John. Tina, your expertise has been invaluable in the process of making this manual even better.

Joanie Trussel, we greatly appreciate your critical eye towards detail and endless research. Thank you.

The chapter contributors to this manual would like to acknowledge and thank the following people for their support.

Kay Lewis, Jon, and Tara Baker
Linda Bird
Tom Daws
Linda Catherine, Brad, and Todd Everson
Heather French Henry
Jian Gao, MD
Isabelle Lynch
Ken Moore
Gail Rando
Kevin Sandt
Audrey Spolaric
George Webb
Andrew Weil, MD

Table of Content

Title Page

Dedication

Acknowledgements

Table Of Contents   I

An Important Note To The Reader   IV

Purpose Of The Manual   VI

Organization Of The Manual   IX

CHAPTER 1   14
Overview Of Hepatitis C
Robert G. Gish, MD

CHAPTER 2   19
Alcohol And Hepatitis C
Douglas R. LaBrecque, MD and Lorren Sandt

CHAPTER 3   27
Progression Of Liver Disease
Lorren Sandt

CHAPTER 4   37
Signs And Symptoms That May Be Associated With Hepatitis C
Tina M. St. John, MD

CHAPTER 5   46
Laboratory Tests And Procedures
Tina M. St. John, MD

CHAPTER 6   69
Promoting Liver Health
Lorren Sandt

CHAPTER 7   75
Nutrition And Hepatitis C
Lark Lands, PhD

CHAPTER 8
Allopathic (Western) Medicine
   Section 1   87
   Overview Of The Allopathic (Western) Approach To
   The Treatment Of Hepatitis C
Douglas LaBrecque, MD

   Section 2   90
   Treatment Options For Those
   Who Have Never Received Treatment
Douglas LaBrecque, MD

Section 3
Treatment Options For Those Whose Initial Treatment
Failed To Clear The Hepatitis C Virus

Gregory T. Everson, MD

104

Section 4:
The Future Of Allopathic Treatment For Hepatitis C
Robert G. Gish, MD

115

CHAPTER 9
Ayurvedic Medicine
Shri K. Mishra MD, MS, Bharathi Ravi, BAMS (Ayurveda) and
Sivaramaprasad Vinjamury, MD (Ayurveda)

120

CHAPTER 10
Homeopathic Medicine
Sylvia Flesner, ND

132

CHAPTER 11
Mind-Body Medicine And Spiritual Healing
Peggy McCarthy, MBA

140

CHAPTER 12
Modern And Traditional Chinese Medicine
Qing Cai Zhang, MD (China), LicAc

150

CHAPTER 13
Naturopathic Medicine
Lyn Patrick ND

166

CHAPTER 14
Nutritional Supplementation
Lark Lands, PhD and Lyn Patrick, ND

176

CHAPTER 15
Products Marketed To People With Hepatitis C
Lyn Patrick, ND

183

CHAPTER 16
You And Your Healthcare
Mark White, Peggy McCarthy, Jo An Lorren

193

CHAPTER 17
Military Veterans And Hepatitis C
Terry Baker

204

CHAPTER 18:

HCV/HIV Coinfection
Section 1:   **210**
Overview
Misha Cohen, OMD, LAc

Section 2:   **218**
Western Treatment Options
Misha Cohen, OMD, LAc

Section 3:   **221**
Alternative Eastern Treatment Options
Misha Cohen, OMD, LAc

Section 4:   **228**
Naturopathic Treatment Options
Lyn Patrick, ND

CHAPTER 19   **232**

My Journey, My Choices
Randy Dietrich

CHAPTER 20   **269**

A Look To The Future
Lorren Sandt

APPENDICIES

Patient's Bill Of Rights   **APPENDIX I**   **-274**
How To Cut Down On Your Drinking   **APPENDIX II**   **-276**
Western (Allopathic) Medicine   **APPENDIX III**   **-279**
Ayurvedic Medicine   **APPENDIX IV**   **-280**
Modern And Traditional Chinese Medicine **APPENDIX V**   **-289**
You And Your Healthcare   **APPENDIX VI**   **-298**
HCV/HIV Coinfection   **APPENDIX VII**   **-301**

RESOURCE DIRECTORY   **305**

GLOSSARY   **324**

REFERENCES   **327**

ABOUT THE AUTHORS   **380**

ORDER FORM   **—**

MATRIX

Options For Hepatitis C   **—**

AN IMPORTANT NOTE TO THE READER

This manual was created to provide information about a wide variety of approaches to the treatment and management of *chronic hepatitis* C infection. We believe access to good information leads to better decisions. However, this manual is *not* intended to be a substitute for medical advice. It is critical that you consult your health care provider about any matter concerning your health, particularly with regard to new or changing *symptoms* that may require diagnosis and/or medical attention.

Each chapter and section of the manual has been authored independently. Therefore, each chapter reflects the unique approach of its author based on his or her medical discipline and experience. For this reason, an author is responsible only for the accuracy of the information presented in his or her own chapter or section. No author can confirm the accuracy of the information presented in any other chapter or section.

Most of the contributors to the manual are members of the Hepatitis C Caring Ambassadors World Class Brainstorming Team. Others are guest authors invited by the Team to contribute chapters. A unifying characteristic of members of the Team is a willingness to listen and evaluate the diverse points of view and treatment options available to people with chronic hepatitis C. This manual evolved from a consensus within the group that a single resource describing the various modalities of treatment available would be useful to people with hepatitis C. Cooperation and open discussion are key components of the interaction among members of the Brainstorming Team, though individual members remain aligned with their own discipline.

You should be aware that the only treatment proven through controlled *clinical trials* to show sustained clearance of the hepatitis C virus (as detected by HCV RNA testing of the blood) is *interferon-based* antiviral *therapy*. Recent studies of the newest treatment using *pegylated interferon* plus *ribavirin* report sustained responses in 50-60% of those treated. In other words, 50-60% of people receiving this treatment remain virus free for an extended period after treatment has been completed.

We encourage anyone who has significant *fibrosis* on *liver biopsy* to be followed closely for evidence of disease progression. This should include a medical history, physical examination, and laboratory tests. People with *cirrhosis* due to hepatitis C infection need to be monitored for clinical and biochemical deterioration, and considered for referral to a liver transplant center. If *liver failure* occurs, liver transplantation counseling should be sought, and regular screening for the development of liver cancer (*hepatocellular carcinoma*) should be performed.

The choice of treatment for hepatitis C is a personal one. What is right for one person may not be so for another. What is right for you will depend on the status of your disease and the health of your liver as well as your age, lifestyle, and many other factors. We encourage you to carefully assess the information provided here and elsewhere, and to work with your health care providers to choose treatment approaches that meet your individual needs.

The authors, reviewers, and editors of this book have made extensive efforts to ensure that treatments, drugs, and dosage regimens are accurate and conform to the standards accepted at the time of publication. However, constant changes in information resulting from continuing research and clinical experience, reasonable differences in opinions among authorities, unique aspects of individual clinical situations, and the possibility of human error in preparing such an extensive text require that the reader exercise individual judgment when making a clinical decision and, if necessary, consult and compare information from other sources.

With each printing, we have the opportunity to make corrections to this manual. However, because the electronic version is more flexible, we can make changes at any time. Thus, the text in this manual and the internet site at www.hepcchallenge.org may be slightly different.

We created this manual with several purposes in mind:

- to provide information about chronic hepatitis C that might help you make decisions about your treatment options and lifestyle,
- to provide a balanced view of the currently available treatment options from western medicine and *complementary and alternative medicine* (CAM),
- to help you communicate effectively with your health care providers, and
- to provide information to help you become empowered to be the best advocate for your own health care.

MAKING INFORMED DECISIONS

Making potentially life-changing decisions is one aspect of having a serious illness like *chronic hepatitis* C. Each of us is unique in how we make such decisions. Some people want to know everything they possibly can about their disease. They also want to make all of their own treatment decisions. Other people prefer to have health care providers make treatment decisions based on their knowledge and expertise. Some prefer to have a friend or family member seek out and sort through information. Many use a combination of approaches.

Each person with chronic hepatitis C has his or her own treatment goals. Some consider reducing the virus to an undetectable level to be the most important goal. Other people consider enjoying the best quality of life to be the top priority. Many have a list of goals, some being more important than others are. Some people are willing to change their lifestyle, while others know this is not the right choice for them.

We urge you to identify your personal strengths and your limitations. Decide what makes up an acceptable quality of life for you. Knowing these things will help you make health care decisions that best suit your personality.

We hope this manual will help you understand your disease and some of the health care options available to you. This knowledge can empower you to ask the questions you need to have answered to be your own best advocate. When you have asked your questions and had them answered, you and your health care providers will be in the best possible situation to determine the treatment approach that is right for you.

KNOWING YOUR OPTIONS

You have the right to advocate for yourself in order to receive the best possible treatment regardless of whether you are on Medicare, are a member of an HMO, subscribe to an indemnity insurance plan, or are uninsured.

Over the years, many people with chronic hepatitis C found they had few treatment options and little opportunity to participate in their own health care decisions. Increasingly, health care providers and the public are interested in changing this legacy. Being an informed consumer and knowing your rights are particularly important when you are looking for health care that is not only of good quality, but also fits your personal needs. These rights are even more important if you intend to combine or integrate several medical disciplines in your treatment plan. For additional information on your rights as a health care consumer, see *Appendix I: Patient's Bill of Rights*.

REGAINING CONTROL

The day before your hepatitis C diagnosis, you were probably able to say what you hoped to be doing in the near future. The day after your diagnosis, you may have felt that something else had suddenly taken control of your life and your ability to decide your own future. The process of regaining control begins with learning about your disease and your treatment options. Many people newly diagnosed with chronic hepatitis C are relieved to find that it might not be necessary to make an immediate decision about treatment. If your hepatitis C has not progressed significantly and you stop drinking alcohol, you may never have to make a decision about aggressive therapy. However, no matter what your disease status, drinking and hepatitis C infection are a dangerous mix. You should not drink alcohol in any form.

Some people with chronic hepatitis C stay healthy by making lifestyle changes in addition to not drinking alcohol. For some, lifestyle changes such as eating a healthier diet, taking vitamins and/or supplements, and exercising regularly have a profound effect on their health and well-being. Others choose homeopathy, naturopathy, traditional Chinese medicine, and/or other CAM disciplines to maintain their general health and keep the virus in check.

How you go about maintaining your health, and whomever you decide to consult for your health care is up to you. However, we urge you to gather information about the different treatment options you are considering. This will help you make informed decisions about what options are best suited to your treatment goals and personality.

SOME ADDITIONAL THOUGHTS

The decision to begin any treatment is a big step. Only you know if you are ready to take that step. Our purpose in creating this manual was not to advocate for one treatment approach over another, but to encourage you to carefully look at all of your options. Chronic hepatitis C is often a progressive disease, so your options might change over time. The health care provider you choose to see is not nearly as important as having a systematic approach to follow your disease. It is important to realize that unless you have your blood tested and your liver examined periodically, you cannot know if your disease is progressing.

We encourage you to decide on your treatment goals, and discuss all of your options and concerns with your health care providers. It is often helpful to get a second opinion, or even a third. Choosing health care providers you are comfortable speaking with will help you work together as a team. Making decisions that are right for you will make your choices easier to incorporate into your life.

Whatever you decide to do, it is very important to inform each of health care providers about all of the treatment approaches you are using. This is particularly important if you choose an *integrated* medicine approach that involves health care providers or treatments from a number of different medical disciplines.

We created this manual to help you become the best possible advocate for your own health care. We hope it provides some useful information to help you make treatment and lifestyle choices that are right for you. However, this manual is *only* a guide, a collection of reference materials. We strongly encourage you to continue to explore your treatment and lifestyle options, and to gather as much information as you need. Doing so can help you make the best possible decisions for your health care and your life.

ORGANIZATION OF THE MANUAL

We encourage you to read the entire manual to get the most benefit from it. But we realize that for a number of reasons, this may be hard to do. Therefore, we have arranged the chapters in three major parts to help you easily find your way around the manual.

Part One: Information for Everyone with Hepatitis C

These chapters contain information for all people affected by *chronic hepatitis C*. The authors consider this information very important for anyone with chronic hepatitis C, regardless of your treatment goals.

Part Two: Hepatitis C Treatment Approaches

These chapters cover treatment options for chronic hepatitis C. The chapters are arranged alphabetically by treatment approach. Each chapter presents the author's view of the disease, and its treatment and/or management.

Some treatment options have been studied to determine their effectiveness. We have included information about the evidence to support the use of a given treatment if that information is available. Some of this information comes from health care providers' experience (*anecdotal* evidence), and some comes from formal studies such as controlled *clinical trials*.

Part Three: Other Issues for People with Hepatitis C

This part of the manual covers topics of concern to specific populations affected by chronic hepatitis C, and other special issues of interest to people with hepatitis C.

We have included a number of other important documents at the back of the manual, including:

- a matrix showing management options for chronic hepatitis C,
- appendices containing additional information about topics covered in the chapters,
- a directory of resources for people living with chronic hepatitis C, and
- a list of references compiled from the individual chapters.

You might find some medical words in the manual that are new to you. These words are *italicized*. The definitions of these words are in the *Glossary* at the back of the manual. Becoming familiar with these words will probably help you better understand hepatitis C. It might also help you communicate more easily with your health care providers. Foreign words will also appear in italics. These words are explained in the text, but do not appear in the *Glossary*.

Chapter One

OVERVIEW OF HEPATITIS C

Robert G. Gish, MD

INTRODUCTION

Hepatitis C virus (HCV) infection is one of the most common causes of chronic liver disease. HCV is estimated to affect more than four million people in the United States, and 150 million people worldwide.[1, 2] The estimated number of HCV-infected people in the United States is based on population survey, and estimates of the disease in high-risk populations that have not been thoroughly studied. Therefore, many hepatitis C experts believe the actual number of people infected with HCV is higher than the estimates state.

Even ten years after the discovery of HCV, our knowledge about the natural history of chronic hepatitis C is still limited. Studies have provided varying estimates of the risk of disease progression with *chronic hepatitis* C. Usually, the disease is slowly progressive. An estimated 15% of people infected with HCV clear the virus from their body without treatment. Another 25% have no *symptoms*, and have consistently normal levels of *liver enzymes* called aminotransferases. This means that approximately 40% of people infected with HCV either recover or do not develop symptoms.[3] This fact tells us that there are people whose *immune systems* are capable of getting rid of HCV. However, for reasons we do not yet understand, others' immune systems allow the virus to persist, leading to potentially serious consequences.

Several factors have been shown to influence the course of chronic hepatitis C. The most significant of these factors are listed below.

- **Age at infection:** Persons infected past age 35 may have disease that is more rapidly progressive. [4, 5, 6]
- **Alcohol consumption:** Alcohol appears to have a very negative effect on people infected with HCV.[7]
- **Gender:** Overall, women (especially those under age 50) do significantly better than men[7, 8] with less severity of infection.[9] Women also appear to *spontaneously clear* the virus more frequently than men do.[10, 11, 12]
- **Co-infection with hepatitis B virus (HBV) and/or human immunodeficiency virus (HIV):** Co-infection with one or both of these viruses leads to faster disease progression.[13]
- **Fatty liver:** The presence of fat in the liver is associated with higher degrees of *fibrosis*.[14]

Viral characteristics such as HCV type (*genotype*) and *viral load* (the amount of virus present in the blood) do not seem to affect the course of the disease.[4]

HCV was once believed to affect only the liver. We now know it can affect nearly any organ in the body. In other words, hepatitis C is a systemic disease. As you read *Chapter 4: Signs and Symptoms That May Be Associated With Hepatitis C*, you may find some of the symptoms you thought were caused by something else may actually be caused by HCV. This is important because knowing *why* you are having a symptom is often the first step in making it less troublesome.

HOW HEPATITIS C IS DIAGNOSED

You probably learned you are infected with HCV through a blood test. Most likely, the test checked for *HCV antibodies* in your blood. Your immune system produces antibodies to foreign objects such as viruses and bacteria. When someone is infected with HCV, the body begins producing antibodies specifically designed to search out and destroy HCV. An HCV antibody test is sometimes included in a routine physical. It is also done to check for HCV infection in people who have one or more risk factors for hepatitis C.

HCV antibody tests are not always completely accurate. This is especially true in people with weakened immune systems. People with weakened immune systems might not produce enough antibodies to be detected by the antibody test. People with normal immune systems also sometimes have negative antibody tests despite the fact that they are infected with HCV. This is because in some people, HCV antibodies might not be detected for up to one year after the initial infection.[17] If there is any doubt about the results of the HCV antibody test, people are given another test that detects HCV itself in the blood.

There are three methods called molecular tests that are used to detect the hepatitis C virus in the blood. These methods are *polymerase chain reaction (PCR)*, *transcription mediated amplification (TMA)*, and *branched chain deoxyribonucleic acid (bDNA)*.[15] Many physicians believe testing with a molecular method is the most effective way to confirm a diagnosis of HCV. There are other tests, such as the *recombinant immunoblot assay (RIBA)*, that were designed for the blood banking industry, but are also sometimes used to confirm a diagnosis of HCV.[16]

Everyone suspected of having HCV should have *liver enzyme* tests (*ALT* and *AST*) to check for liver damage. Blood tests for liver function should also be performed. Examples of liver function tests include *albumin*, *prothrombin time*, and *bilirubin*.

For more information on laboratory tests, see *Chapter 5, Laboratory Tests and Procedures*.

ACUTE PHASE HEPATITIS C

The first six to nine months after infection with HCV is called *acute* phase *hepatitis* C. After infection, there is an average incubation period of seven to eight weeks before there is a rise in liver enzymes. HCV antibodies are usually detectable in the blood 3-12 weeks after infection. The virus itself is usually detectable in the blood using molecular tests within one to three weeks of infection.[18, 19] After being infected with HCV, most people are *asymptomatic* meaning they do not have any symptoms of disease. However, 25-35% of infected people experience a mild, acute phase illness. The symptoms of this illness are usually vague and *nonspecific*.

Between 15-45% of people infected with HCV appear to clear the virus on their own without developing any *secondary condition* or result from the infection. Experts believe clearing the virus is probably related to the amount of virus in the initial infection.

If your body does not rid itself of HCV within six to nine months after infection, you are considered to be in the chronic phase of hepatitis C.

CHRONIC PHASE HEPATITIS C

The course of chronic phase hepatitis C is usually that of slow disease progression without symptoms. Most people have no physical *signs* or symptoms of HCV infection during the first 10-20 years after infection.

The rate of disease progression in chronic hepatitis C differs from one person to another. The rate at which a person's hepatitis C will progress cannot be accurately determined by liver enzyme levels, viral load, or HCV genotype.[20, 21] It has been noted that people with normal liver enzymes and low viral load usually have mild liver disease with low-grade liver inflammation. However, even these people occasionally develop fibrosis or *cirrhosis*. The inability to predict disease progression makes it difficult for health care providers to identify people who are most likely to benefit from treatment.

Why Liver Biopsies Are Performed and How They Are Used

Many health care providers believe a *liver biopsy* to be the best way to identify people who are most likely to have progressive disease, the group most likely to benefit from treatment.

A biopsy gives your health care provider a great deal of information about your liver including:

- the amount of inflammation present,
- the presence of and amount of fibrosis,
- the presence of and amount of cirrhosis, and
- the need for *liver cancer* screening.

A liver biopsy can also help your health care provider decide if and when an evaluation for a liver transplant is needed.

Your health care provider uses the information from a liver biopsy to help predict the rate of your disease progression, and to determine whether you are likely to benefit from treatment. Studies have shown that hepatitis C progresses slowly in people with mild liver inflammation and no fibrosis. For people with fibrosis, hepatitis C is generally more rapidly progressive.[9]

As treatments become more effective, the role of liver biopsy in the management of hepatitis C may change. Your health care provider will consider a number of factors before suggesting a change from monitoring your disease to treating it. These factors might include your age, general health, likelihood of response to treatment, and other illnesses such as HIV. There are also other considerations to take into account before making the decision to treat chronic hepatitis C. These include such things as the length of therapy, cost, frequency of monitoring, past medical history, side effects, and your ability to take the medication as directed. Your health care provider should discuss all *contraindications* to any therapy he or she recommends to you.

For more information about liver biopsy results, see *Chapter 3: Progression of Liver Disease.*

HCV Genotype

The hepatitis C family of viruses is divided into types called genotypes. To date, six genotypes and more than 90 subtypes have been identified. The types are numbered 1 through 6, and the subtypes are labeled a, b, c, and so on, in order of their discovery. Presently, genotype testing is used primarily to help health care providers advise people about their potential treatment response, and for research purposes.

Genotype testing is considered part of standard, western medical care for people with HCV infection who are being counseled about *interferon-based treatment.* The reason is that researchers have found certain strains of HCV are more likely to respond to interferon-based treatment than others are. Further, some strains respond in a shorter period of time than others do. Therefore, it is very important to know the genotype and subtype of HCV with which you are infected. If you are infected with one of the strains that is hard to treat, your health care provider may advise a longer than normal course of treatment to see if you might eventually respond.

Hopefully, researchers will soon discover why different HCV genotypes respond differently to interferon-based treatment. Currently, subtypes 1a and 1b account for 65-75% of chronic HCV in the United States. Unfortunately, people with subtypes 1a and 1b experience the lowest response rate to conventional western treatment. However, you should not allow your genotype alone to deter you from getting treatment. People with all genotypes have cleared the virus. Remember, your genotype does not determine how your disease will progress. There have been no studies to date to determine if genotype influences response to *complementary and alternative medicine* treatments, but we hope that will soon change.

You may hear the term *quasispecies* in relation to HCV genotype. Quasispecies occur because HCV *mutates* freely, causing diverse genetic strains in each infected person. The longer you have been infected with HCV, the more likely you are to have a number of quasispecies of HCV in your body. One small study found changes in quasispecies were associated with levels of the liver enzyme ALT during the acute phase of infection. This finding suggests that the formation of quasispecies might be related to the severity of HCV infection.[22]

Liver Failure

Liver failure is a common cause of death in the United States, claiming more than 30,000 lives each year. Though some studies indicate that hepatitis C may not be the most common cause of liver failure, hepatitis C is nonetheless a very serious, growing public health problem.[24, 25]

While the number of new HCV infections has recently declined in the United States, it is believed that the number of people who will develop complications of liver disease will increase over the next 10-20 years.[26] Approximately 20-30% of people with chronic hepatitis C will develop cirrhosis over a 20-30 year period. Ten percent of those who develop cirrhosis will eventually progress to end-stage liver disease.[27, 28, 29]

In spite of these statistics, it is important to remember that **a diagnosis of cirrhosis is not a death sentence!** Even if you have a cirrhotic liver, unless you develop complications, you can live a very long life.

Organ and Tissue Transplants

Liver failure due to chronic hepatitis C is the most common reason for liver transplantation in the United States. There are currently more than 20,000 people waiting for a liver transplant in this country, but only about 4,900 livers are available for transplant each year.[23]

Anyone who has an organ transplant has to take medicines called anti-rejection drugs to keep his or her body from rejecting the new organ. Anti-rejection drugs tend to suppress the immune system. This can cause HCV disease to progress faster than it would otherwise. Your health care provider will work closely with you to decide if you should consider using *antivi-*

ral therapy after your liver transplant. It is very important to talk with your health care providers about all treatments and/or supplements you are taking or are considering taking. This information is important in making recommendations regarding liver transplantation.

HOW HEPATITIS C IS TRANSMITTED

Blood-to-Blood Contact

The main way HCV is transmitted from one person to another is through blood-to-blood contact. If you received blood or blood products and/or a tissue or organ transplant prior to 1992, you should be tested for HCV. Other examples of blood-to-blood contact that can lead to HCV transmission are listed below.

- intravenous drug use with unsterile, used needles
- tattoos with unsterile, used equipment or unclean ink pots
- acupuncture treatments with unsterile, used needles
- nasally inhaled drug use with unsterile, used paraphernalia
- accidental needle sticks among health care professionals
- dental work performed with unsterile, used instruments
- other health care procedures that do not adhere to standard sterilization procedures

Pregnancy and Breast Feeding

The risk of transmission of HCV from an infected mother to her infant at birth is 3-6%. Some data suggest delivery by C-section may reduce the risk of mother-to-child transmission.

There is almost no risk of transmitting HCV by breast feeding unless there are breaks in the skin and bleeding.

Sexual Intercourse

The risk of transmitting HCV through sexual intercourse in *monogamous* heterosexuals is less than 3-6%. There is no study data on the risk of sexual transmission in a monogamous homosexual relationship. Things such as the number of sexual partners in a lifetime, sexual practices, and the presence of sexually transmitted diseases can influence the risk of HCV transmission.

SUMMARY

The decision to begin any treatment is a big step. Only you know if you are ready to take that step. Once you have decided on your treatment goals, discuss all of your options and concerns with your health care providers. It is often helpful to get a second opinion, or even a third. Choosing health care providers you are comfortable speaking with will help you work together as a team. Making decisions that are right for you will make your choices easier to incorporate into your life.

Taking steps to enhance your general health by doing things such as eating a low-fat diet, stopping all alcohol consumption, and attaining a normal body weight are important parts of your treatment plan. Exercise, spiritual practices, massage, acupuncture, herbs, and other complementary therapies can all have a role in attaining better health.

We know a great deal about hepatitis C. However, there is even more we do *not* know. Good clinical research is needed in all areas of hepatitis C management including western medicine, naturopathy, traditional Chinese medicine, Ayurveda, homeopathy, nutritional support, and other complementary therapies. This research will lead to the next advances in the care of those living with hepatitis C.

Therapy for hepatitis C is evolving rapidly. As a result, recommendations for therapy will probably change every few years. Hopefully, new approaches will provide therapy that is more effective for people infected with HCV.

Chapter Two

ALCOHOL and HEPATITIS C

Douglas R. LaBrecque, MD and Lorren Sandt

INTRODUCTION

The three most important factors associated with accelerated *chronic hepatitis* C progression are being over 40 years of age, being male, and consuming alcohol.[1, 2] You can't do anything to change your age or sex, but you <u>can</u> eliminate alcohol. **Eliminating alcohol is the single most important lifestyle change you can make to decrease your risk of developing complications from chronic hepatitis C.**

Most people in the United States who drink alcohol do so socially. You may be used to having a glass of wine with dinner, or a mixed drink at a party. Unfortunately, if you have *hepatitis* C, **any** consumption of alcohol can potentially damage your liver. Whether alcohol is consumed in a drink, in cough syrup, or in another nonprescription product, alcohol is an enemy for people with hepatitis C. Alcohol should be <u>completely</u> avoided.

The primary cause of liver damage from alcoholic beverages is the alcohol itself, whether it is contained in beer, wine, or spirits (hard liquor). One 12-ounce can of beer has the same amount of alcohol as a 4-ounce glass of wine, or a 1-ounce 'shot' of whiskey. That means drinking a 6-pack of beer is the same as having six shots or six mixed drinks. 'Doubles' obviously double the amount of alcohol you are consuming. Expensive drinks are just as damaging as cheap ones.

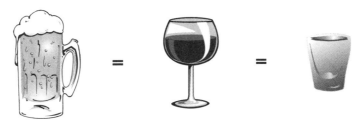

WHAT WE'VE LEARNED ABOUT ALCOHOL AND HCV

A number of studies show that a frighteningly high number of alcoholic people have hepatitis C. The numbers range from 11-36%. Compare this to the 1.8% hepatitis C virus (HCV) infection rate in the general population.[3, 4] Among alcoholics with liver disease, as many as 51% are infected with HCV. This is 4-10 times more frequent than in alcoholics without liver disease.[5-10]

Several studies have shown that alcohol abuse (4-5 drinks per day) accelerates the progression of liver damage and *fibrosis* associated with chronic HCV.[1, 5, 11-18] In one study of 6,664 patients in France, excessive alcohol intake doubled the risk of developing *cirrhosis* and increased the rate of fibrosis progression by 34% per year.[19]

Research has clearly shown that the severity of liver disease in alcoholics increases in the presence of HCV. In one Italian study, the incidence of cirrhosis was ten times higher in alcoholics who had HCV than in alcoholics who did not.[20] Another study found the survival rate for alcoholics who had HCV antibodies was lower than for alcoholics who did not have evidence of HCV infection.[21] In addition, a number of studies have found a significantly increased risk of developing *liver cancer* among heavy alcohol drinkers who also have HCV.[22-25]

The amount of HCV in the blood has been shown to rise in proportion to increasing alcohol consumption, and to drop when alcohol is avoided. This suggests that alcohol has an effect on HCV *replication* (viral reproduction).[26, 27] Alcoholics also have an increase in the number and complexity of HCV *quasispecies*.[28] This finding may explain why alcoholics tend to have a lower response rate to HCV *antiviral* therapy than non-alcoholics. Several studies have shown a decreased rate of *viral clearance* among people who drink alcohol compared to those who do not drink. Studies have shown an even lower frequency of achieving a *durable response*.[29, 30] This decreased response rate to antiviral therapy continues for up to six months after stopping all alcohol intake. Most experts recommend at least six months of *abstinence* from alcohol before attempting *interferon-based therapy*.

There are other effects of alcohol that may contribute to the greater severity of HCV disease in those who consume it. Some of these effects are listed below.

- possible changes in *gene* expression
- reduction in the *immune system's* ability to respond to and fight off viruses
- inhibition of the liver's ability to regenerate and repair itself
- stimulation of fibrosis development in the liver
- increased iron deposition in the liver

Most of the studies discussed above clearly show the increased liver damage suffered by people with HCV who have more than 4-5 drinks of alcohol per day. Other studies show liver damage with as little as **one** drink of alcohol per day. Currently, the amount of alcohol consumption that is considered safe for healthy individuals is one drink per day for women and two for men. However, <u>no</u> amount of alcohol can be considered safe in a person infected with HCV. People with HCV are <u>strongly</u> urged not to drink **any** alcohol.

HOW ALCOHOL DAMAGES THE LIVER

The liver breaks down most of the alcohol a person drinks. However, as the liver breaks down alcohol, byproducts are formed such as *acetaldehyde*. Some of these byproducts are more toxic to the body than alcohol itself.[31]

Inflammation is the body's response to tissue damage or infection. Long term alcohol use abnormally prolongs the inflammatory process. This leads to an overproduction of *free radicals*, molecules that can destroy healthy liver tissue and interfere with some of its important functions such as energy production. Alcohol can also interfere with the production of *antioxidants*. Antioxidants are one of the body's natural defenses against free radical damage. This combination of alcohol effects may lead to liver damage.[32]

Cytokines are produced by liver cells and the immune system in response to infection or cell damage. Alcohol use increases cytokine levels.[33] The development of cirrhosis involves the interaction of certain cytokines and specialized liver cells, such as stellate cells. In a normal liver, stellate cells function as storage depots for vitamin A. When activated by cytokines, stellate cells divide rapidly to increase their numbers. Activated stellate cells lose their vitamin A stores and begin to produce scar tissue. They also constrict blood vessels, reducing the delivery of oxygen to liver cells.[34, 35] Acetaldehyde, a byproduct of alcohol metabolism, may activate stellate cells directly causing liver scarring without *inflammation*.[36, 37]

Normal scar formation is part of the wound healing process. Cell death and inflammation caused by alcohol can result in abnormal liver scarring. Scarring may distort the liver's internal structure and interfere with its function. Scarring in the liver is called fibrosis. Fibrosis that progresses to the point of distorting the structure of the liver is called cirrhosis.

WOMEN, ALCOHOL, AND HEPATITIS C

Studies show that women are more susceptible than men to the damaging effects of alcohol. More alcoholic women die from cirrhosis than do alcoholic men.[38] Why these differences between men and women occur is not entirely clear. However, there appear to be a number of contributing factors.

- Men generally have greater body mass and fluid content than do women. This means women have higher concentrations of alcohol in their blood than men do after consuming the same amount of alcohol.[33, 39-43]

- Women's livers appear to *metabolize* alcohol at a faster rate than men's do, most likely because women's livers are larger (compared to their body size) than those of men.[44, 45]

- Estrogens (female hormones) may add to the effects of alcohol in women's livers.[46]

ABOUT ALCOHOL USE

For most people, drinking alcohol is an occasional social activity. For others, drinking alcohol becomes a chronic often progressive disorder called alcoholism. The symptoms of alcoholism include a strong need to drink despite negative consequences including serious health and/or social problems. Like many diseases, alcoholism has a generally predictable course. It has recognized symptoms and is influenced by both genetic and environmental factors. These factors are being increasingly well defined and understood.

As with chronic hepatitis C, we do not yet have a cure for alcoholism. However, it is a treatable disorder. Alcoholism is a life-long problem. Even an alcoholic who has been sober for a long time may still be at risk of relapsing and should avoid all alcoholic beverages.

Alcoholism has little to do with what kind of alcohol you drink, how long you have been drinking, or even how much alcohol you drink. The defining characteristic of alcoholism is a person's uncontrollable need for alcohol. This description helps us understand why most alcoholics cannot just 'use a little willpower' to stop drinking. He or she is usually in the grip of a powerful craving for alcohol. This craving can feel as strong as the need for food or water. While some people are able to recover on their own, the majority of alcoholics need outside help. With support and treatment, many are able to stop drinking and rebuild their lives.

Cutting down on drinking does not work for an alcoholic. Stopping alcohol use completely is necessary for successful recovery. This is especially important for people living with chronic hepatitis C. Even individuals who are determined to stay sober may suffer one or more slips or *relapses* before achieving longterm sobriety. Relapses are very common and do not mean that a person has failed. Nor do they mean a person cannot eventually recover from alcoholism. Every day a recovering alcoholic stays sober prior to a relapse is extremely valuable time. This time is important for both the individual and his or her family. Sober time gives the liver an opportunity to repair itself. If a relapse occurs, it is very important to try to stop drinking again and to get whatever additional support is needed to *abstain* from drinking.

HELP FOR ALCOHOL ABUSE

Acknowledging that you need help for an alcohol problem is not easy. Many alcoholics do not begin to deal with their alcoholism until a significant life-changing or life-threatening event occurs. Many recovering alcoholics refer to this as 'hitting bottom.' The event that represents hitting bottom is different for each person. It depends on your personality and life circumstances. While it is not necessary for someone to have to hit bottom in order to begin the recovery process, it is often the case. This is because denial is very prevalent in alcoholism. Denial is a coping strategy whereby people avoid dealing with difficult situations by denying that they exist. It is difficult for a person in denial to recognize and understand the effects alcohol has on him or her. This is also true for family members and friends who are frequently in denial with regard to their loved one's alcoholism.

Many people find the following quiz on drinking helpful. It can help you recognize whether alcohol is a problem in your life.

- Do you drink alone when you feel angry or sad?
- Does your drinking ever make you late for work?
- Does your drinking worry your family?
- Do you ever drink after telling yourself you won't?
- Do you ever forget what you did while you were drinking?
- Do you get headaches or have a hangover after you have been drinking?

If you answered yes to one or more of these questions, you may have a problem with alcohol.

Many people feel uncomfortable discussing their drinking habits even with a health care provider or a personal or spiritual advisor. This may stem from common misconceptions in our society about alcoholism. There is a myth in our society that an alcohol problem is a sign of moral weakness. As a result, you may feel that to seek help is to admit a shameful defect in your character. Unfortunately, family and friends may support you in your denial for the same reason. The truth is that alcoholism is a disorder. It is no more a sign of weakness than is asthma or diabetes.

MOVING FORWARD

Even if alcohol is taking a significant and negative toll on your life, it can be very difficult to begin taking steps to address the problem. This is because what lies ahead is unknown. However, eliminating alcohol from your life has an enormous payoff. It is a chance for a healthier, more rewarding life.

Because alcohol has a tremendous impact on the health of people with chronic hepatitis C, your health care provider will probably ask you a number of questions about your alcohol use. If your health care provider determines that you are not alcohol dependent but are involved in a pattern of alcohol abuse, he or she can assist you in the following ways.

- Help you examine the benefits of stopping an unhealthy drinking pattern.
- Help you set a drinking goal for yourself. Some people choose to abstain from alcohol. Others prefer to limit the amount they drink. We have included in Appendix II a worksheet for cutting down on your drinking. Remember, with hepatitis C, the goal is **no alcohol**.
- Help you examine situations that trigger your unhealthy drinking patterns and develop new ways of handling those situations so you can achieve your drinking goal.
- Recommend a specialist and/or treatment program if you are having difficulty eliminating alcohol from your life.

Your health care provider may determine you are dependent on alcohol. He or she may recommend that you see a specialist in diagnosing and treating alcoholism. You will want to have all treatment choices explained to you. Your health care provider may delay treatment of your hepatitis C due to your alcohol problem. Studies have proven that interferon-based therapy is much less effective in people who drink alcohol.[47] For this reason, many health care providers will not offer treatment of any kind for chronic hepatitis C until the person stops all use of alcohol for at least six months.

The nature of treatment for alcohol depends on the severity of a person's alcoholism. It also depends on the resources available in the community. Treatment may include detoxification. Detoxification is the process of safely getting alcohol out of your system. Treatment for alcoholism may involve one or more of the following components: taking prescription medications, individual counseling, and group counseling. There are promising counseling techniques that teach recovering alcoholics to identify situations and feelings that trigger the urge to drink. This can help you find new ways to cope with stressful situations that do not include alcohol use. Treatment for alcoholism may be provided in a hospital, residential treatment setting, or on an outpatient basis.

Involvement of friends and family members is important to the recovery process. Many programs offer brief marital counseling and family therapy as part of the treatment process. Some programs also link individuals with vital community resources such as legal assistance, job training, childcare, and parenting classes.

Treatment for alcoholism may require a combination of social support and drug therapy. When faced with the anxiety and fears associated with hepatitis C, you may feel the urge to turn to alcohol. Remember, you are not alone. Reach out and get help to remain alcohol free.

Several options for eliminating alcohol from your life are outlined below.

Brief Interventions

Many people with alcohol-related problems receive counseling from primary care physicians or nursing staff. This can be done in a few office visits.[48] This form of treatment is known as brief intervention. It generally consists of straightforward information about the negative consequences of alcohol consumption. It also gives practical advice on strategies for eliminating alcohol from your life. Information is provided about community resources to achieve alcohol moderation or abstinence.[49, 50] Most brief interventions are designed to help people at risk for developing alcohol-related problems. They are also used to help reduce alcohol consumption.

Alcohol dependent people are encouraged to enter specialized treatment programs where the goal is complete abstinence.[49]

Couples Therapy

Evidence indicates that involvement of a nonalcoholic partner in a treatment program can improve participation by the alcoholic person. This kind of support increases the likelihood that the alcoholic person will change his or her drinking behavior after treatment ends.[51] There are different approaches to couples therapy. Most of these include shared activities, and teaching communication and conflict evaluation skills. [52]

Motivational Enhancement Therapy

Project MATCH is a national, multi-site, randomized *clinical trial*. It has produced data on the outcomes of specific alcoholism treatment approaches. Motivational enhancement therapy (MET) was developed specifically for Project MATCH. It begins with the assumption that the responsibility and capacity for change lie within the individual.[53, 54] Therapy begins by providing individualized feedback about the effects of the person's drinking. The therapist and client explore the benefits of abstinence. They review treatment options and design a plan to implement treatment goals.

Pharmacotherapy

Medications to block alcohol-brain interactions that might promote alcoholism are available. People with HCV should not take any of these medications before speaking to a health care provider because these medications may be harmful to the liver. Your health care provider will be able to review the drugs available, and can help determine if one of them might be appropriate for you.

Self-Help Programs

Self-help groups are the most commonly used programs for alcohol-related problems.[55] Alcoholics Anonymous (AA) is probably the best known of these self-help groups. AA describes itself as a "worldwide fellowship of men and women who help each other to stay sober." It offers a 12-step program that has been effective for many people seeking to eliminate alcohol from their lives. Alcoholics can become involved with AA before entering professional treatment for alcoholism, as a part of it, or as aftercare. The AA approach is well known, but the program has not been studied in clinical trials.[56] This is due to an essential requirement of the program that people remain anonymous. In AA, only first names are used.

The beneficial effects of AA may in part be due to the replacement of the participant's social network of drinking friends with a fellowship of AA members who can provide motivation and support for maintaining abstinence.[55,57] AA's approach often results in the development of new coping skills. Many of these skills are similar to those taught in more structured treatment settings. These skills can lead to reduction in alcohol consumption. [55,58]

Most treatment programs for alcoholism include AA meetings. AA is generally recognized as an effective support program for recovering alcoholics. However, not everyone responds to AA's style and message. If you do not respond to AA, there are other recovery approaches available. Even those who are helped by AA find that it works best in combination with other forms of treatment. This may include individual counseling and/or medical care.

Treating Alcohol and Nicotine Addiction Together

Nicotine and alcohol interact in the brain. Each drug may affect dependence on the other.[59] Some researchers believe that treating both addictions at the same time may be more effective than treating each one separately. It may even be an essential way to help reduce dependence on both substances. A recent study showed that treatment for nicotine dependence did not interfere with abstinence from alcohol or other drugs.[60]

THE FINAL WORD

No studies have ever determined if there is a safe amount of alcohol to drink. However, if you have HCV, the authors of this manual strongly recommend you eliminate alcohol from your life. You will live better and longer!

RESOURCES

For more information on alcohol abuse and alcoholism, contact the following organizations.

Al-Anon Family Group Headquarters
1600 Corporate Landing Parkway
Virginia Beach, VA 23454-5617
Internet address: http://www.al-anon.alateen.org

> This group provides referrals to local Al-Anon groups, which are support groups for spouses and other significant adults in an alcoholic person's life. They also provide referrals to Alateen groups, which offer support to children of alcoholics.

> Locations of Al-Anon or Alateen meetings worldwide can be obtained by calling the toll-free numbers listed below Monday through Friday, 8 AM.-6 PM (EST).

> U. S.: (800) 344-2666
> Canada: (800) 443-4525

> Free informational materials can be obtained by calling the toll-free numbers listed below. These numbers are available seven days a week, 24 hours per day.

> U. S.: (800) 356-9996
> Canada: (800) 714-7498

Alcoholics Anonymous (AA) World Services
475 Riverside Drive, 11th Floor
New York, NY 10115
Phone: (212) 870-3400
Internet address: http://www.alcoholics-anonymous.org

> Makes referrals to local AA groups and provides informational materials on the AA program. Many cities and towns also have a local AA office listed in the telephone directory.

National Council on Alcoholism and Drug Dependence (NCADD)
12 West 21st Street
New York, NY 10010
Phone: (800) NCA-CALL
Internet address: http://www.ncadd.org

Operators provide phone numbers of local NCADD affiliates that can provide information on local treatment resources. Educational materials on alcoholism are available via the toll-free number above.

National Institute on Alcohol Abuse and Alcoholism
Scientific Communications Branch
6000 Executive Boulevard, Suite 409
Bethesda, MD 20892-7003
Phone: (301) 443-3860
Internet address: http://www.niaaa.nih.gov

Note: Much of the information in this chapter was obtained from the National Institute on Alcohol Abuse and Alcoholism. For more detailed information, visit their internet site at: http://www.niaaa.nih.gov/.

Chapter Three

PROGRESSION OF LIVER DISEASE

Lorren Sandt

INTRODUCTION

Throughout this manual, you will often read that *chronic hepatitis C* and its treatments affect each person differently. This is especially true of disease progression. There is no accurate way to predict how chronic hepatitis C will progress in any one person.

This chapter provides information about possibilities that might happen. Remember, none of the situations discussed in this chapter will necessarily happen to you. However, it is important to be aware of these things so that if any of them do happen, you will be prepared and better able to make good decisions.

ABOUT THE LIVER

The liver is the largest organ in the body. In a normal adult, the liver weighs between 3°-4 pounds (1,300-1,500 grams). It accounts for about 2.5% of the total weight of the body. The liver is wedge-shaped (see below). It measures approximately 7 inches (14 cm) across by 5° inches (18 cm) along its diagonal. The liver is divided into two main lobes, the right and the left. The right lobe is slightly larger than the left and extends down the right side of the rib cage. The left lobe extends from the right lobe to about the middle of the abdomen. There are also two minor lobes of the liver called the caudate and quadrate lobes. *Fibrous* ligaments separate the lobes. All lobes of the liver perform the same functions. The entire liver is enclosed in a fibrous sheath called Glisson's capsule.

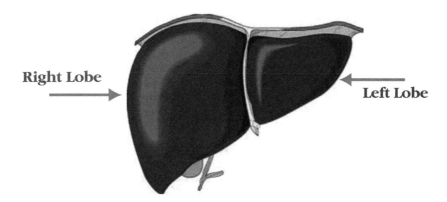

Right Lobe ⟶   ⟵ **Left Lobe**

The liver is located on the right side of the abdominal cavity just below the lungs and diaphragm, the muscle that separates the chest cavity from the abdominal cavity.

The liver is packed so tightly into the abdomen that the right kidney, parts of the large and small intestines, and the stomach actually leave impressions on its surface. Even the ribs and

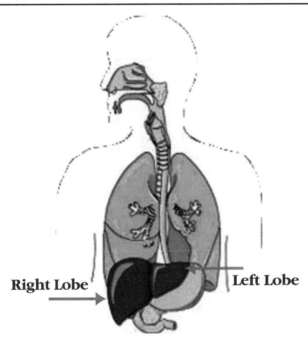

Right Lobe   **Left Lobe**

muscle bands of the diaphragm make indentations on the surface of the liver.

Approximately 25-30% of the blood coming from the heart goes to the liver. Although there are no lymph nodes in the liver itself, it produces over 1/3 of the body's *lymphatic fluid*. The fluid drains into *lymph channels* and lymph nodes in the abdomen.

The hepatitis C virus (HCV) usually enters the body through the blood stream. It is carried by the blood to the liver where it invades and infects liver cells. HCV appears to reproduce itself in liver cells, and in cells of the blood and bone marrow. Although people infected with HCV make *antibodies* against the virus (anti-HCV), these antibodies do not appear to play a significant role in getting rid of the virus.

Once you are infected with HCV, chances are you will have many tests to determine the status of your disease. For detailed information on the tests you may have and why, see *Chapter 5: Laboratory Tests and Procedures*.

Testing the level of the *liver enzymes alanine aminotransferase (ALT)* and *aspartate aminotransferase (AST)* in the blood is one way to tell if liver cells are dying. When liver cells die, ALT and AST are released into the blood. After an abnormal amount of liver cell death, ALT and AST levels rise over a period of 7-12 days and then slowly return to normal. If liver cells continue to die, ALT and AST levels will stay elevated. ALT and AST levels tell your health care provider how much damage is happening in your liver. However, having elevated ALT and AST levels does *not* necessarily mean your disease is getting worse. Although these tests can detect liver damage, they cannot determine how much liver repair is taking place. Studies show that liver enzyme levels are good markers of disease progression, but they do not necessarily predict disease outcome. Liver enzymes also provide no information about how well your liver is functioning.[1,2] Your liver can maintain its many functions despite a remarkable amount of damage. Therefore, it is important to look at the results of other test such as *albumin, bilirubin, prothrombin time*, and *platelet* count to determine how well your liver is functioning.

STAGES OF DISEASE PROGRESSION

Like other liver diseases, HCV disease progresses in stages. The usual progression is from *inflammation* to *fibrosis* to *cirrhosis*. Cirrhosis can progress to end-stage liver disease and/or can give rise to *liver cancer*. Normally, when the liver is damaged, liver cells die but the organ regenerates itself without scarring.

Inflammation

Liver inflammation refers to the presence of special cells called inflammatory cells in the liver. Chronic inflammation is inflammation that persists over a long period of time. It leads to changes in liver structure, slowed blood circulation, and the death of liver cells *(necrosis)*. Chronic inflammation eventually causes scar tissue to form, a condition known as fibrosis. By controlling liver inflammation, you can control progression to fibrosis.

Fibrosis

Fibrosis is the harmful outcome of chronic inflammation. Fibrosis is scar tissue that forms as a result of chronic inflammation and/or extensive liver cell death. Your health care provider uses the amount of fibrosis in your liver as one way of evaluating how quickly your disease appears to be progressing. Having knowledge of approximately when you were initially infected with HCV is a great help in determining your rate of disease progression.

The only way to determine the amount of fibrosis in your liver is to have a *liver biopsy*. No other available test is able to give you and your health care providers this important piece of information.

Cirrhosis

When fibrosis becomes widespread and has progressed to the point where the internal structure of the liver has become abnormal, fibrosis has progressed to cirrhosis. Cirrhosis is the result of longterm liver damage caused by chronic inflammation and liver cell death. The causes of cirrhosis include viral hepatitis, excessive intake of alcohol, inherited diseases, and *hemochromatosis* (abnormal handling of iron by the body).

Cirrhosis is accompanied by a reduction in blood supply to the liver. The loss of healthy liver tissue and the reduced blood supply can lead to abnormalities in liver function. Even when liver disease has progressed to cirrhosis, it may still be possible for the damage to be at least partially reversed if the underlying cause can be eliminated. Cirrhosis progression can usually be slowed or even stopped with treatment.

The onset of cirrhosis is usually silent, with few specific *symptoms* to identify this development in the liver. As scarring (fibrosis) and destruction continue, some of the following *signs* and symptoms may occur: loss of appetite, nausea and/or vomiting, weight loss, change in liver size, gallstones, itching, and *jaundice*. However, a large number of people live many, many years with cirrhosis without any *decompensation* or symptoms.

It is important to know that once cirrhosis develops, it is critical to avoid further progression of the disease. The consumption of alcohol in any form, including such things as certain mouthwashes and cough medicines, must be completely avoided by people with cirrhosis.

If you have cirrhosis, this may be a time to reevaluate your treatment goals. If you have not had *interferon-based therapy*, you may want to consider it or other available treatments that aim to eradicate the virus. It may also be time to look into other means of improving the health of your liver.

Liver Cancer

Though most people with HCV never develop liver cancer, it is a risk associated with chronic hepatitis C. The presence of cirrhosis and/or having been infected with HCV for more than 20 years further increase the risk. For this reason, frequent liver cancer screening is advisable for people who have cirrhosis.

Liver cancer is life-threatening, so it is important to know the warning signs. For information on warning signs and symptoms, see *Chapter 4: Signs and Symptoms That May Be Associated With Hepatitis C*. Do not delay telling your health care provider about any changes in your symptoms. Symptom changes may indicate a change in your liver *histology*.

There are effective therapies for liver cancer if it is detected early. If you have developed cirrhosis from HCV, you need to be closely followed by a health care provider who can monitor you with the appropriate liver cancer screening tests.

DETERMINING DISEASE PROGRESSION WITH LIVER BIOPSY

The most accurate way to check the severity of liver disease is with a biopsy. A *liver biopsy* is a test in which small pieces of liver tissue are removed so they can be examined under a microscope. The three main things that will be looked for are inflammation, fibrosis, and cirrhosis. The biopsy report may also reveal other histological and *pathological* findings such as the presence of lymphoid nodules, damage to small *bile ducts*, and/or the presence of fat.

Scoring and Grading Liver Biopsies

When you receive the results of your liver biopsy, you will hear the terms inflammatory *grade* and fibrotic *stage*. Health care providers use these terms to indicate the amount of injury to the liver. There are three different methods used for scoring liver biopsies. This can cause confusion for both patients and health care providers. Be aware that the scoring systems are also subject to interpretation by the pathologist who examines your biopsy.

The three scoring and grading systems for liver biopsies are the Original HAI (Histology Activity Index), the Modified HAI, and the Metavir. There are important things to know about how biopsies are scored in order to understand what your score means.

- A score for a given biopsy characteristic in one system does **not** mean the same thing in the other systems.
- The scores for **all** of the characteristics of the tissue sample are added together for a final score, except as specified in the notes under the table for that system (see Tables 1-5).
- A final score from one biopsy may have the same score as that of a follow-up biopsy, but the scores for individual characteristics may have changed. This means your situation could actually be better or worse depending on the individual characteristic scores.

Until there is a single biopsy scoring system, there are things you need to know and track regarding your liver biopsy results.

- What system did the pathologist use to grade each of your biopsies?
- If you have had more than one biopsy, you need to look at changes in both the individual characteristics and the overall score.

Make sure your health care provider completely explains the results of your biopsy to you. Ask for an explanation of the individual scores as well as the overall score. You should be given a description of the inflammatory grade and fibrotic stage. Ask to speak with the pathologist who evaluated your biopsy if your health care provider is unable to provide this information.

Biopsies are invasive and therefore, you are not likely to have one done often. For this reason, it is very important that you understand the results of your liver biopsy so you can use this information to help you make decisions about your health care.

The following tables comparing the three systems used to score liver biopsies are courtesy of David Kleiner, MD of the National Cancer Institute.

Table 1. Comparison of Scoring Systems: Periportal Necroinflammatory Changes

Score	Original HAI[a] [3]	Modified HAI[4]	Metavir[b] [5]
0	None	Absent	Absent
1	Mild piecemeal necrosis	Mild (focal, few portal areas)	Focal alteration of the periportal plate in some portal tracts
2		Mild/Moderate (focal, most portal areas)	Diffuse alteration of the periportal tract in some portal tracts or focal
3	Moderate piecemeal necrosis (involves less than 50% of the circumference of most portal tracts	Moderate (continuous around <50% of tracts or septae)	Diffuse alteration of the periportal plate in all portal tracts
4	Marked piecemeal necrosis (involves more than 50% of the circumference of most portal tracts	Severe (continuous around >50% of tracts or septae)	

The periportal component of the Knodell HAI has been split into a periportal piecemeal necrosis and a bridging/confluent necrosis component for better comparison to the other scoring systems. In order to recreate the original scale, the bridging/confluent necrosis component should be added to the periportal piecemeal necrosis component.

The periportal component of the METAVIR score is used with the focal necrosis score to determine overall inflammatory activity.

Table 2. Comparison of Scoring Systems: Bridging and Confluent Necrosis

Score	Original HAI[a(3)]	Modified HAI[(4)]	Metavir[b(5)]
0	Absent	Absent	Absent
1		Focal confluent necrosis	Present
2	Bridging necrosis (more than two such bridges)	Zone 3 necrosis in some areas	
3		Zone 3 necrosis in most areas	
4		Zone 3 necrosis + occasional portal-central bridging necrosis	
5		Zone 3 necrosis + multiple portal-central bridging necrosis	
6	Multilobular necrosis	Panacinar or multiacinar necrosis	

The periportal component of the Knodell HAI has been split into a periportal piecemeal necrosis and a bridging/confluent necrosis component for better comparison to the other scoring systems. In order to recreate the original scale, the bridging/confluent necrosis component should be added to the periportal piecemeal necrosis component.

The METAVIR score for bridging necrosis is not used in the overall activity determination by this system and is provided only for comparison with other scales.

Table 3. Comparison of Scoring Systems: Focal (Spotty) Lobular Necrosis and Hepatocellular Apoptosis

Score	Original HAI[(3)]	Modified HAI[(4)]	Metavir[(5)]
0	None	Absent	Less than one necroinflammatory focus per lobule
1	Mild (acidophilic bodies, ballooning degeneration, and/or scattered foci of hepatocellular necrosis in less than 1/3 of lobules/nodules)	One focus or less per 10x field	At least one necroinflammatory focus per lobule
2		2-4 foci per 10x field	Several necroinflammatory foci per lobule or confluent/bridging
3	Moderate (involvement of 1/3 to 2/3 of lobules/nodules)	5-10 foci per 10x field	
4	Marked (involvement of more than 2/3 of lobules/nodules)	More than 10 foci per 10x field	

Table 4. Comparison of Scoring Systems: Portal Inflammation

Score	Original HAI[3]	Modified HAI[4]	Metavir[a(5)]
0	No portal inflammation	None	Absent
1	Mild (sprinkling of inflammatory cells in less than 1/3 of portal tracts)	Mild, some or all portal areas	Presence of mononuclear aggregates in some portal tracts
2		Moderate, some or all portal areas	Mononuclear aggregates in all portal tracts
3	Moderate (increased inflammation in 1/3-2/3 of portal tracts)	Moderate/marked, all portal areas	Large and dense mononuclear aggregates in all portal tracts
4	Marked(dense packing of inflammatory cells in more than 2/3 of portal tracts)	Marked, all portal areas	

The METAVIR score for bridging necrosis is not used in the overall activity determination by this system and is provided only for comparison with other scales.

Table 5. Comparison of Scoring Systems: Fibrosis

Score	Original HAI[a (3)]	Modified HAI[4]	Metavir[b (5)]
0	No fibrosis	No fibrosis	No fibrosis
1	Fibrosis portal expansion	Fibrosis expansion of some portal areas, with or without short fibrous septa	Stellate enlargement of portal tracts without septae formation
2		Fibrosis expansion of most portal areas, with or without short fibrous septa	Enlargement of portal tracts with rare septae formation
3	Bridging fibrosis (portal-portal or portal-central linkage)	Fibrosis expansion of most portal areas, with occasional portal to portal bridging	Numerous septae without fibrosis
4	Cirrhosis	Fibrosis expansion of portal areas, with marked bridging (portal to portal as well as portal to central)	Cirrhosis
5		Marked bridging with occasional nodules (incomplete cirrhosis)	
6		Cirrhosis, probable or definite	

Table 6 shows how the HAI inflammation scores relate to the grade of histological injury. In the HAI system, the various inflammation scores are added together. These numbers are directly related to the descriptive grade of inflammation.

Table 6. Relationship of Aggregate Inflammation Scores to grade of Activity

Sum of inflammation scores in HAI or modified HAI systems	Description of activity
0	None
1-4	Minimal
5-8	Mild
9-12	Moderate
13-18	Marked

OTHER LIVER BIOPSY FINDINGS

Fatty Liver (Steatosis or Steatohepatitis)

Fatty liver is the accumulation of fat in liver cells. *Steatosis* is the presence of fat in liver cells without inflammation. *Steatohepatitis* is the presence of fat in liver cells with inflammation. You may hear other terms to describe fatty liver, depending on your medical condition.

- *NAFL* – nonalcoholic fatty liver
- *NAFLD* – nonalcoholic fatty liver disease
- *NASH* – nonalcoholic steatohepatitis

Fatty liver is emerging as a major medical problem. Obesity effects up to 40% of the U.S. population, half of whom have fatty livers. The risk of cirrhosis for those with fatty livers ranges from 7-15%. It is important to know if you have a fatty liver so you can understand your risk of developing cirrhosis and make lifestyle changes to decrease this risk. A liver biopsy can determine both the presence of fat in the liver and the level of fibrosis. This information will allow your health care provider to counsel you about your risk of progressive liver disease.

Alcohol can increase the amount of fat in the liver and is the most common cause of fatty liver. The association between fatty liver and alcohol is another very important reason for you to refrain from drinking alcohol. However, not all cases of fatty liver are caused by alcohol use. Diabetes and high *triglycerides* are also associated with fatty liver and should be managed closely by your health care provider.

The liver must *metabolize* any fat that is not eliminated through the intestinal tract. If you eat excessive amounts of fat, the amount that goes to your liver may be too much for it to metabolize. The excess fat that is not metabolized will begin to accumulate in the liver. This accumulation of fat can cause inflammation. Inflammation can lead to scarring, which may eventually lead to decreased liver function. Therefore, it is very important not to have excessive amounts of fat in your diet. It is particularly important to limit your intake of animal fat because animal fat is especially difficult for the liver to metabolize. For suggested dietary guidelines, see *Chapter 7: Nutrition and Hepatitis C.*

Achieving or maintaining your ideal body weight (a *body mass index* BMI of approximately 25) and limiting the amount of fat in your diet are important for the health of your liver. Your BMI is calculated by taking your weight (in kilograms) and dividing by your height (in meters) squared. A free BMI calculator is available on the Internet at http://www.nhlbisupport.com/bmi/ bmicalc.htm. Normal body weight not only helps your liver but can also improve your energy level, reduce hypertension, and lower your risk of a heart attack. Regular exercise can help you maintain a normal body weight and avoid the development of fatty liver.

If you are considering interferon-based therapy, obesity may play a role in your response. Health care providers have recently begun to advocate for individualized weight-based dosing of interferon/ribavirin to improve the chance for response to treatment.

People with fatty liver often have high blood sugar and *lipids* such as cholesterol and triglycerides. If you have a fatty liver, your health care provider should monitor you for the development of these problems.

Some medications and other substances can cause fatty liver. Be sure to review all of your medications with your health care provider and avoid the following, if possible.
- alcohol
- amiodarone (an antidepressant medicine)
- methotrexate (an arthritis medicine)
- high doses of vitamin A
- tetracycline (an antibiotic)
- cortisone (a steroid medicine)
- prednisone (a steroid medicine)

OTHER COMPLICATIONS OF HEPATITIS C

Although the effects of HCV on the liver are most visible, the virus can affect other body systems and organs. This results in *extrahepatic* (outside the liver) conditions or manifestations of chronic hepatitis C.

Many autoimmune diseases occur as secondary diagnoses after a primary diagnosis of chronic hepatitis C, or in association with hepatitis C. Some examples of these diseases include type 2 diabetes, mixed *cryoglobulinemia, thyroiditis, erythema nodosum, erythema multiforme, glomerulonephritis, hypothyroidism, lichen planus, polyarteritis, urticaria, porphyria cutanea tarda, polymyalgia, B-cell lymphoma,* and *Mooren corneal ulcers.*

There is much controversy regarding the true cause of the many HCV-related conditions that have been reported. Some of them probably are related to hepatitis C. Others probably are not, and have occurred by chance in a few individuals unrelated to their HCV. Many studies on this topic come from clinics that treat only specific diseases, which may skew the study findings. The way HCV produces extrahepatic conditions is the subject of ongoing research. In some HCV-related extrahepatic conditions, HCV stimulates the *immune system* to produce autoimmune antibodies, antibodies against the body's own tissues. This appears to be the mechanism for HCV-related *thyroid* and blood disorders.

SUMMARY

The question of whether it is the virus or the person infected by the virus that determines how HCV disease will progress is an active area of research. At this point, we know of several person factors and several virus factors that may influence the rate of HCV disease progression.

Factors related to the person include some variables you can control. The consumption of alcohol can markedly affect disease progression. The amount of fat in one's diet and body weight can also influence disease progression.

In terms of viral characteristics, we know that the existence of multiple *quasispecies* can accelerate disease progression. We also know that HCV *genotype* is a factor in whether or not someone responds to therapy and is therefore able to arrest his or her disease progression.

Based on our current knowledge, it seems that both the person and the virus affect disease progression. Therefore, your environment, diet, exercise plan, lifestyle, and support system may all be important factors that could affect the course of your HCV.

Progression of chronic hepatitis C in any given person cannot be predicted. However, the seriousness of this disease for people with advanced cirrhosis is beyond question. If you follow the progression of your disease with all the tests available to you, you will be in a better position to make informed decisions about your treatment options.

It is hoped that ongoing research will improve our ability to predict disease progression and to intervene more effectively.

Chapter Four

SIGNS AND SYMPTOMS THAT MAY BE ASSOCIATED WITH HEPATITIS C
Tina M. St. John, MD

INTRODUCTION

Hepatitis C affects different people in different ways. Your personal experience with hepatitis C will be as unique as you are. This chapter reviews the most common *signs* and *symptoms* experienced by people with chronic hepatitis C. At first glance, the mere length of the chapter may appear overwhelming, but keep in mind, this is just a list of possibilities. If you have any of the signs or symptoms described in this chapter, it is important that you do not assume they are a result of having hepatitis C. Your health care provider can determine if they are associated with your hepatitis C. Very few people experience all of these signs and symptoms. Many of them will come and go on their own. For troublesome and/or persistent problems, there are things you and your health care provider can do to either make them go away, or make them easier to live with.

You may be wondering what the difference is between a sign and a symptom. A sign is an abnormality that is detected by your health care provider during an examination. A symptom is something you, as a person with hepatitis C, experience as a result of the disease. Signs and symptoms are discussed together because sometimes a sign is also a symptom. Fever is a good example of something that is both a sign and a symptom. Your health care provider can take your temperature and find out that you have a fever, so it is a sign. But if you have a fever, you can tell you have a fever because your skin is warm, so fever is also a symptom.

There are three sections following this introduction. The first section briefly explains how the hepatitis C virus causes disease. The second section reviews possible signs and symptoms that people with hepatitis C who do not have cirrhosis may experience. The last section reviews additional signs and symptoms that people with hepatitis C who have cirrhosis may experience.

HOW THE HEPATITIS C VIRUS CAUSES DISEASE

According to current understanding, the hepatitis C virus (HCV) causes disease in two general ways. The first is by infecting cells. Once inside the cell, the virus directly damages or kills the cell. This mechanism is called cytopathic damage. The second way the hepatitis C virus causes damage is by provoking an immune response. The *immune system* is your body's way of protecting itself from invading agents such as viruses and bacteria. An overactive or misdirected immune response can damage infected cells and the normal surrounding tissue. This mechanism is called immunopathic damage.

When HCV was first discovered, experts thought the virus infected only liver cells. However, more recent research has revealed that HCV also infects parts of the immune system, specifically the lymphatic system and *peripheral blood mononuclear cells*. Experts now understand that hepatitis C is not just a liver disease but is a systemic disease, meaning it can affect nearly any organ of the body. As you read through the list of possible signs and symptoms associated with hepatitis C infection, you may find some of the symptoms you have been experiencing that you thought were caused by something else may actually be caused by hepatitis C. This is important because knowing why you are having a symptom is often the first step in alleviating the symptom, or making it less troublesome.

SIGNS AND SYMPTOMS OF HEPATITIS C WITHOUT CIRRHOSIS

The possible signs and symptoms of hepatitis C without cirrhosis involve every organ system of the body. Although some of these symptoms can be quite uncomfortable, most of them do not indicate that your liver disease is getting worse. New symptoms should always be discussed with your health care provider so you can work together to keep your life with hepatitis C as active, productive, and enjoyable as possible.

Arthralgia

Arthralgia is pain in the joints. Frequent sites of joint pain are the hips, knees, fingers, and spine, although any joint can be a source of pain. Arthralgia associated with hepatitis C can be migratory, meaning it moves around. You may have pain in your hip one day and in your knee the next. This symptom usually comes and goes, and is rarely present all the time. If you experience joint pain, it is important to talk with your health care provider before taking anything to treat the pain because some over-the-counter pain medicines (such as acetaminophen) are potentially harmful to the liver.

Fever, Chills, and Night Sweats

Many people with HCV periodically experience fevers. The fevers are usually low, typically less than 101 degrees Fahrenheit. As the fever comes down, you may experience chills and sweating. You may have fevers only at night. If this happens, you may wake up with your bedclothes and/or your sheets wet with sweat. This experience is called night sweats.

Fatigue

Fatigue is feeling tired, and nearly all people with hepatitis C experience fatigue at one time or another. The fatigue may be mild and relieved by naps or going to bed earlier. However, the fatigue can be severe at times, feeling like near exhaustion even after a full night of sleep. Fatigue experienced by people with hepatitis C may also be accompanied by increased feelings of anger, hostility, and depression.[1] These feelings may persist even after the fatigue has passed.

Fluid Retention

Fluid retention occurs when your body holds on to more water than it needs. The extra water leaks into the tissues. If you have fluid retention, you may notice swelling of your feet, ankles, fingers, and/or face. People with fluid retention often have frequent urination, especially at night.

Flu-like Syndrome

People with hepatitis C can experience periodic flu-like syndromes. These episodes usually last a few days, rarely more than a week. The most common symptoms are fever, chills, headache, fatigue, and muscle aches.

Lymphadenopathy

Lymphadenopathy is swelling of the lymph nodes. Lymph nodes are normally about the size of a pea or a kidney bean. Because HCV infects the lymphatic system, it frequently causes the lymph nodes to swell. The lymph nodes of the armpits, groin, and neck are relatively close to the skin surface, and are usually examined to see if you have lymphadenopathy. If you have lymphadenopathy, it may or may not be painful when you press on the swollen lymph nodes.

Myalgia

Myalgia is muscle pain or aching. People with hepatitis C may experience myalgia. Usually, if you have this symptom, you will experience it as a generalized feeling. However, some people report having pain in only one area of the body. This symptom tends to come and go, and is rarely present all the time. If you experience muscle aches or pain, it is important to talk with your health care provider before taking anything to treat the pain because some over-the-counter pain medicines are potentially harmful to the liver.

Pruritus

Pruritus is the medical word for itching. People with hepatitis C sometimes have pruritus. Often, it is limited to the palms of the hands and/or the soles of the feet. However, some people have generalized pruritus, meaning they itch all over.

Sleep Disturbances

Insomnia is difficulty sleeping, and it may be part of your experience with hepatitis C. Insomnia can occur in different forms. You may have trouble falling asleep, or you may wake up often during the night. Some people report having unusually vivid, intense, and/or frightening dreams. Such dreams can contribute to insomnia.

Spider Nevi

Spider nevi are small, red, spider shaped spots on the skin. They are usually less than ° inch around. They are most commonly seen on the face and chest, but can occur anywhere on the skin. Spider nevi are painless and do not itch.

Weakness

People with hepatitis C sometimes experience a sense of weakness. This symptom can vary from mild to severe, and tends to come and go.

Abdominal and digestive system signs and symptoms

Abdominal Pain

You may experience episodes of abdominal pain if you have hepatitis C. Pain on the right side just below the ribs is likely to be from the liver. People usually report this pain as being short, sharp, or stabbing. More constant, cramping pain closer to the middle of chest, but under the ribs, can be due to gall bladder problems that may accompany hepatitis C. You may experience pain elsewhere in the abdomen. If you experience any new pain in the abdomen, it is important for you to tell your health care provider right away so the source of the pain can be determined.

Appetite Changes and Weight Loss

People with hepatitis C frequently experience changes in their appetites. You may find you no longer want the foods you once enjoyed. Many people find they are particularly put off by fatty foods and alcohol. For some, foods that are at room temperature or cold are more appealing than hot foods. The distaste for alcohol is actually good for you because alcohol increases the damage done to the liver by HCV. People with hepatitis C should not drink any alcohol including beer, wine, wine coolers, and mixed drinks. If changes in your appetite are causing you to lose weight, you need to discuss this with your health care provider because good nutrition is particularly important for people with hepatitis C.

Bloating

Bloating is usually described by people with hepatitis C as a feeling of fullness in the abdomen. You may notice your clothes seem tight around your waist. This bloating may or may not be accompanied by weight gain.

Diarrhea and Irritable Bowel Syndrome

Diarrhea can be experienced as unusually loose stools or an increase in the frequency of bowel movements, with or without a change in the consistency of the stool. If the diarrhea is accompanied by cramping abdominal pain and persists, it is often termed irritable bowel syndrome.

Indigestion and Heartburn

Indigestion is usually experienced as an uncomfortable feeling of fullness in the stomach. It is often accompanied by queasiness and burping of a mixture of gas and stomach contents. When this occurs, you may notice a burning in your throat and/or a sour taste in your mouth. Heartburn is experienced as pain or burning in the chest under the breastbone. It, too, may be accompanied by burping of gas and stomach contents. Both indigestion and heartburn can be brought on by and last longer after a fatty meal.

Jaundice

Jaundice is a yellowish discoloration of the skin and/or the whites of the eyes. It is caused by a yellow substance in the blood called *bilirubin*. The liver normally breaks down bilirubin. If the liver is not working normally, bilirubin can build up in the blood and begin to stain the skin. If the liver starts to work more normally, jaundice will fade or go away.

Nausea

Nausea is the feeling that you may vomit. Hepatitis C may cause episodes of nausea. Although it is usually not accompanied by vomiting, it can be a very uncomfortable and debilitating symptom. If you are having nausea, talk with your health care provider because there are many ways to treat this symptom.

COGNITIVE, MOOD, AND NERVOUS SYSTEM SIGNS AND SYMPTOMS

Cognitive Changes

Your cognitive ability refers to your ability to think clearly and to concentrate. Some people with hepatitis C notice they have changes in their cognitive ability. This can take several different forms. You may find you cannot concentrate for long periods of time, or you may notice your thought processes seem slower than usual. You may have a hard time coming up with words you want to say, or you may just feel mentally tired. These cognitive changes are sometimes called 'brain fog.' Like other symptoms of hepatitis C, these cognitive changes often come and go.

Depression

Hepatitis C does not directly cause depression, but concerns about the disease and changes it may cause in your life can lead to depression. Some of the symptoms of depression include:

- sleeping more or less than usual
- eating more or less than usual
- hopelessness
- helplessness
- irritability
- lack of interest in your usual activities, and
- feelings of sadness and/or despair most of the time.

If you have one or more of these symptoms, you may have depression and should discuss what you are feeling with you health care provider. Depression can seriously interfere with your quality of life, and can make it difficult for you to do what you need to do to take care of yourself. Depression is nothing to be ashamed of, and it can be treated. If you have any of the symptoms of depression, talk to your health care provider right away.

Dizziness

Some people experience dizziness as feeling as if they are going to faint. Others experience dizziness as disorientation, or feeling as if the world is spinning around them. Both of these can be symptoms of hepatitis C. If you are experiencing dizziness, talk with your health care provider because this can be not only troublesome for you, but also dangerous.

Headaches

Headaches can be symptoms of hepatitis C. For some people, the headaches are mild, but for others, the headaches are severe. If you are having headaches, talk to your health care provider before taking any medicines for your headaches because some over-the-counter pain medicines can be harmful to your liver.

Mood Swings

Hepatitis C can sometimes cause mood swings. Some people find this symptom is worse during the winter months.

Numbness or Tingling

A significant number of people with hepatitis C have numbness or tingling in their extremities. Your extremities are those parts of your body that extend from the main part of your body, that is, your arms and legs, fingers and toes. Most people with numbness or tingling feel it in their fingers and toes, but it may extend into the arms and legs. Numbness is a decreased sense of feeling. In its most severe form, the affected areas have no sense of feeling. Tingling can sometimes be painful. People describe painful tingling as feeling like being stuck with pins. This symptom tends to come and go.

Visual Changes

There are a number of visual changes that can accompany hepatitis C infection. You may find you are not seeing as clearly as you once did. Peripheral vision, that is, the ability to see things that are at the sides of your view, can also be diminished. Some people report seeing small specks called 'floaters' moving across their view. This can occur when the eyes are open or closed. Another symptom you may experience is dryness of the eyes, or feeling as if there is something scratchy in your eyes. All of these symptoms can come and go.

Other Signs and Symptoms

Blood Sugar Abnormalities

Hepatitis C can cause blood sugar abnormalities, either high or low. High blood sugar causes symptoms such as extreme thirst, frequent urination, fatigue, and weight loss. Low blood sugar causes light-headedness or dizziness, nausea, and weakness. The symptoms of low blood sugar are worst when you have not eaten anything for several hours, and are relieved by eating or drinking something. If you are having any of the symptoms of either high or low blood sugar, tell your health care provider right away.

Chest Pain

Hepatitis C can cause chest pain. However, chest pain can also be a symptom of serious heart or lung disease. If you have chest pain, you must contact your health care provider immediately so he or she can find out the source of your pain.

Menstrual and Menopausal Changes

Women with hepatitis C may have menstrual changes such as irregular periods, spotting, or increased premenstrual symptoms. Menopausal women may experience an increase in menopausal symptoms such as hot flashes and mood swings.

Palpitations

A heart palpitation is involuntarily becoming aware of your heart beating. Palpitations occur in different forms. You may feel your heart is beating harder or faster than usual, or that it is beating irregularly. If you have palpitations, you need to tell your health care provider immediately so he or she can make sure you are not having a problem with your heart.

Sexual Changes

Some people with hepatitis C have a decreased interest in sexual activity. Decreased sexual response and lack of intensity of sexual response have also been reported. Sexual changes can be an upsetting symptom of hepatitis C. If you are experiencing sexual changes, talk with your health care provider, and your spouse or partner. There are things that you, your health care provider, and your partner can do to help you have a satisfying sex life.

SIGNS AND SYMPTOMS OF HEPATITIS C WITH CIRRHOSIS

Approximately 20-40% of people with *chronic hepatitis* C go on to develop liver cirrhosis over a period of 10-40 years. Because blood cannot flow well through a cirrhotic liver, blood backs up in the vessels leading to the liver. This back up of blood leads to an increase in pressure in those blood vessels, a condition known as *portal hypertension* . Many of the signs and symptoms of cirrhosis are related to portal hypertension.

The liver has many functions, so there are a number of things that can go wrong when the liver is not functioning normally. The liver not functioning normally causes the other signs and symptoms of hepatitis C with cirrhosis.

Ascites

Portal hypertension associated with cirrhosis can cause fluid to leak from the blood vessels leading to the liver. This fluid builds up in the abdomen and is called ascites. Ascites causes the abdomen to become *distended* or enlarged.

Bleeding Problems

The liver produces many of the substances needed for normal blood clotting. A cirrhotic liver may not produce enough of these substances for normal clotting. If you have a cirrhotic liver and begin bleeding for any reason, it may be difficult to get the bleeding stopped.

Bone Pain

Cirrhosis can lead to a deficiency in vitamin D. This can cause softening of the bones and bone pain. This pain is most often felt in the legs, hips, and spine.

Bruising

Cirrhosis can lead to a deficiency in vitamin K. This can lead to easy bruising. If you are experiencing easy bruising, tell your health care provider because this symptom can often be reversed with appropriate treatment.

Caput Medusae

Caput medusae refers to enlarged, visible veins that start at the navel and spread out and up over the abdomen. They are caused by portal hypertension.

Gastroesophageal Varices

Gastroesophageal varices are another complication of portal hypertension. These varices are enlarged, fragile veins found where the esophagus (the tube that takes food from your mouth to your stomach) meets the stomach. These veins can burst and bleed. If you have cirrhosis and begin to vomit blood, you must call an ambulance and get to an emergency room as soon as possible to get the bleeding stopped.

Glossitis

Glossitis is a sore tongue. If you have glossitis, your tongue will be redder than usual and will be sensitive to salty and sour foods, and carbonated beverages.

Hemorrhoids

Hemorrhoids are enlarged, fragile veins found around the anus (the opening through which your bowel movements pass). Hemorrhoids can be a complication of portal hypertension. If you have hemorrhoids, they may bleed occasionally. If the bleeding persists, or is frequent, be sure to discuss it with your health care provider.

Hepatic Encephalopathy

Hepatic encephalopathy is one of the most serious complications of cirrhosis. It can occur in an acute form that develops over a period of days to weeks, or it can occur in a chronic form that develops over a period of months to years. There are a number of different symptoms that can indicate hepatic encephalopathy, but all of them indicate abnormalities of the nervous system. Early symptoms include euphoria (feeling unusually happy for no apparent reason) or depression, confusion, slurred speech, or abnormal sleeping patterns. If these symptoms are not treated, they will progress to severe confusion, incoherent speech, tremors, and rigidity. It is urgent for these symptoms to be treated or you could fall into a coma. With the acute form of hepatic encephalopathy, treatment will usually reverse all of the symptoms. However, with the chronic form, some of the symptoms may not be reversible.

Melanosis

Melanosis is a gradual darkening of those areas of skin that are exposed to the sun. The skin tends to get darker over time.

Night Blindness

Cirrhosis can lead to a deficiency in vitamin A. This can lead to episodes of night blindness. If this occurs, be certain to talk about it with your health care provider because this symptom is often reversible.

Shortness of Breath

Shortness of breath can develop as a complication of portal hypertension. Some people experience this symptom only at night; others experience it during the day as well. If you are having shortness of breath, discuss it with your health care provider who can help you with this problem.

Steatorrhea

Steatorrhea is the passing of fat in your bowel movements. The presence of fat in the stool makes the stool smell particularly bad, and causes it to float in the toilet bowl. Steatorrhea is usually accompanied by an increased amount of stool and intestinal gas.

Xanthelasma

Xanthelasmas are small deposits of fat just under the surface of the skin around your eyes. They appear as small, raised, yellowish bumps on the skin.

Xanthoma

Xanthomas are small deposits of fat just under the surface of the skin over your joints and/or tendons. They appear as small, raised, yellowish nodules.

SUMMARY

The experience of living with hepatitis C is quite different from one person to another. It is also variable for each person over time. There will probably be days when you feel great. There may be other times when you feel overwhelmed by different signs or symptoms associated with hepatitis C. And there will likely be still other times when you feel somewhere in between these two states. Below are a few things you may find helpful to keep in mind about your signs and symptoms as you learn to live with hepatitis C.

- Discuss your signs and symptoms with your health care provider. There are many ways to treat the signs and symptoms associated with hepatitis C, so there is no need to suffer in silence.

- Always tell your health care providers if you start to experience a new sign or symptom. Doing this will help them in their efforts to help you feel your best.

- Keep all of your health care providers informed about what treatments, medicines, and supplements you are using to manage your hepatitis C. Sometimes, different treatments interact with one another in ways that cause side effects that you may experience as new signs or symptoms.

Do not panic if you start to experience new signs or symptoms. Although many of the signs and symptoms associated with hepatitis C can be troubling to you, they do not necessarily mean your liver disease is getting worse.

Chapter Five

LABORATORY TESTS AND PROCEDURES

Tina M. St. John, MD

INTRODUCTION

Chronic hepatitis infection is a complex disease. The course and symptoms vary from one person to another. The liver is the primary site of infection, although other cells of the *immune system* can also be infected with the virus.

The liver is one of the most important organs of the body. It performs many jobs, such as those listed below.

- making *proteins,* cholesterol, *bile, heme,* and other substances
- regulating fats in the body
- activating vitamins and drugs
- detoxifying harmful chemicals

With all of these important jobs, there are many things that can potentially go wrong if the liver is damaged. Further complicating the disease is the fact that, although the hepatitis C virus (HCV) primarily infects the liver, it can affect any organ system of the body.

One of the tools health care providers use to find out how HCV is affecting your body is laboratory testing. There are a large number of tests available to help your health care providers find out what is happening inside your body. This section describes some of the most common laboratory tests used to diagnose and/or monitor chronic hepatitis C. Your health care provider will use his or her knowledge of your disease and symptoms to decide which tests you need and when they should be done. Therefore, you should not look at this list as tests that should be done, but rather as a list of tests that may be helpful in specific situations. Also, there are other tests available that are not listed here. If your health care provider orders a test you are not familiar with, ask him or her what the test is and why it is being done.

If you are considering *interferon based therapy*, be sure to read, "What You Need to Know Regarding Therapy" in *Chapter 8: Section 2: Allopathic Medicine*, for a complete list of recommended tests before, during, and after treatment.

WHAT IS NORMAL?

Each testing laboratory has its own range of 'normal' values for each test. A laboratory's normal range means that the majority of people in good health tested by that laboratory have values within this range. Your test results will be compared to the laboratory's normal range. If you have had the same test done before, the new test result will be also be compared to previous tests so that your health care provider can look for any changes over time. It is important for you and your health care provider to know what laboratory is conducting your tests to ensure that correct comparisons are being made.

We suggest that you request copies of your laboratory test results for your own files so that you can better understand your disease process.

LIVER ENZYMES AND LIVER FUNCTION TESTS

You will probably hear your health care providers talk about *liver enzymes* and *liver function tests* (LFTs). These two broad categories of tests give your health care providers different information about what is happening in your liver.

Liver enzymes are proteins that are present inside liver cells. If liver cells are damaged, liver enzymes are released into the blood. Therefore, liver enzyme tests indicate how much damage is happening in your liver. Some examples of liver enzymes that are frequently monitored in chronic hepatitis C include *AST, ALT,* and *GGT.* Although liver enzymes indicate how much damage is being done to the liver cells, they do not tell your health care provider how much repair is taking place. Unlike many other organs, the liver has a remarkable ability to repair itself. This is important when considering liver enzymes because, although there may be ongoing damage to liver cells, it is possible that the liver is able to repair this damage.

Liver function tests give your health care providers information about how well the liver is performing its many jobs. Because the liver has so many different jobs, there are many different LFTs, each indicating how well the liver is performing a specific job. Examples of LFTs that are commonly monitored in chronic hepatitis C include *bilirubin, albumin,* and *platelet* count.

VIRAL LOAD TESTING

HCV viral load testing determines how much virus you have in your blood. Viral load is one factor your doctor takes into consideration when estimating your chance of success with interferon-based therapy. If you are already on therapy, the test is used to check if you are responding to your treatment.

There are different methods used to perform viral load testing including *PCR, b-DNA,* and *TMA.* These methods are described later in the chapter. Most laboratories buy their testing materials from companies that produce HCV testing kits. However, some large laboratories have developed their own testing materials and procedures. One example is Quest Laboratories, which has developed a very sensitive HCV viral load test called Heptimax™.

Although it is not necessary for you to understand the technical differences between these methods, you <u>do</u> need to be aware of the fact that different methods often give different test results. Sometimes these differences are quite large. Therefore, when you have HCV viral load testing, you need to be aware of what type of test was used and where the test was performed. Without this information, it is almost impossible to interpret the meaning of changes in your viral load.

In addition to the type of viral load test used, you also need to be aware of how the test result is reported. When HCV viral load tests were first developed, the results were reported as number of copies per mL (copies/mL) or equivalents per mL (equiv/mL). Recently, the World Health Organization developed a standard unit for reporting the results of HCV RNA viral load tests. The new reporting standard is International Units per mL (IU/mL). If your previous viral loads were reported as copies/mL and are now being reported in IU/mL, you may be confused about what is happening with your viral load. Below are two conversions to help you sort this out.

If PCR was used:

Take the result in IU/mL and multiply by 2.7 to get the number of copies/mL.
Example: 1,000,000 IU/mL x 2.7 = 2,700,000 copies/mL

If TMA was used:

Take the result in IU/mL and multiply by 5.2 to get the number of copies/mL.
Example: 1,000,000 IU/mL x 5.2 = 5,200,000 copies/mL

If you have questions about a change in your viral load, talk with your health care provider. He or she can explain your test results and what they mean.

SAMPLE LABORATORY REPORT

Following is a sample laboratory report. The tests on the sample report are described in the next section of this chapter.

The Testing Laboratory

100 The Road
Anytown, OH 00000

Patient: John Doe **Sex: M** **DOB: 12/01/55**

TEST	RESULT	NORMAL RANGE (see note below)
WBC	7.2	5-10 thousand/mm^3
RBC	4.8	4.70-6.10 million/ mm^3
Hemoglobin	13.6 L	14.0-18.0 g/dL
Hematocrit	41.6 L	42.0-52.0%
Platelet Count	260	140-440 thousand/ mm^3
PT	11.9	10.0-12.5 seconds (0.9-1.1 INR)
Fibrinogen	385	150-450 mg/dL
Sodium	141	140-148 mmol/L
Potassium	3.9	3.6-5.2 mmol/L
Chloride	104	100-108 mmol/L
Carbon Dioxide	24.5	21.0-32.0 mmol/L
Albumin	3.4	3.4-5.0 g/dL
Total Protein	6.2 L	6.4-8.2 g/dL
Glucose	85	70-110 mg/dL
Cholesterol, Total	216 H	<200 mg/dL
BUN	10	7-18 mg/dL
Creatinine	0.8	0.6-1.3 mg/dL
Bilirubin, Total	0.18	0.00-1.00 mg/dL
AST	42 H	15-37 IU/L
ALT	78 H	30-65 IU/L
GGT	46	5-85 IU/L
Alk Phos	74	50-136 IU/L
Ethanol	0	None detected
Ammonia	18	11-35 µmol/L
Ferritin	149	15-200 ng/mL
AFP	12	<25 ng/mL
HCV Antibodies	positive*	negative
HCV RNA	650,000*	undetectable
HCV Genotype	1b	--------
ANA	negative	negative
Cryoglobulins	negative	negative

IMPORTANT NOTE: The normal ranges in this sample laboratory report are <u>only</u> <u>examples</u> of normal ranges. Please see your own laboratory reports to find if your test values are inside or outside of your laboratory's normal range.

LABORATORY TESTS

The laboratory tests described below are in alphabetical order. For each test, you will see the name of the test, other names for the test (if applicable), what the test is, and why it is used for people with chronic hepatitis C. Note that there are other uses for many of these tests, but only their role in hepatitis C is described here.

alanine aminotransferase (ALT)

other names:

alanine transaminase

previously called glutamate pyruvate transaminase (GPT)

What?

ALT is an *enzyme* found inside liver cells. It is also found in other kinds of cells such as those of the heart and pancreas. Large amounts of ALT are found in the liver.

Why Test?

Testing the blood for ALT is one way of telling if liver cells are dying. If liver cells die, ALT is released into the blood. When liver cells die, ALT levels rise over a period of 7-12 days, and then slowly return to normal. If liver cells continue to die, the ALT level will stay elevated. The level of ALT tells your health care provider how much ongoing damage is happening in your liver. However, an elevated ALT level does not necessarily mean your liver disease is getting worse because this test cannot determine how much repair is occurring and how many new liver cells are being produced.

albumin

What?

Albumin is the most abundant protein in the blood. It is made in the liver.

Why Test?

In advanced cirrhosis, the liver begins to fail at its many jobs. Since albumin is made in the liver, when the liver begins to fail, it may not make enough albumin. Measuring albumin is one way of telling how well a *cirrhotic* liver is doing at making proteins.

alcohol

What?

Alcohol is the intoxicating substance in beer, wine, and hard liquor. It may also be found in over-the-counter medications such as cough syrups, and in certain mouth washes and other products.

Why Test?

Alcohol is toxic to the liver. If you have hepatitis C, you should not consume **any** alcohol. Research has shown that even small amounts of alcohol will make the damage done to your liver by the hepatitis C virus much worse. Your blood alcohol should always be zero.

alpha-fetoprotein

What?

Alpha-fetoprotein is a protein normally found in only trace amounts in the body.

Why Test?

People with chronic hepatitis C are at higher risk for developing *liver cancer* than are people without the virus. Alpha-fetoprotein is a tumor marker for liver cancer, meaning it may indicate the presence of a cancerous liver tumor when it is found in abnormally high amounts. Elevated alpha-fetoprotein does not always mean someone has liver cancer, but it is often used to screen for the disease in people with HCV.

alkaline phosphatase (ALP or alk phos)

What?

ALP is an enzyme found in nearly every tissue in the body. The highest concentrations of ALP are found in the liver, bones, intestines, kidneys, and the placentas of pregnant women. In normal adult men and normal, non-pregnant adult women, most of the alkaline phosphatase in the blood comes from the liver and the bones.

Why Test?

Testing the blood for ALP is one way to know if the bile ducts of the liver are working normally. When liver cells die, scarring takes place. If there is a significant amount of scarring, the bile ducts can become partially blocked, and bile flow through the liver is slowed. This condition is called *cholestasis*. When there is cholestasis, the liver starts to make more ALP. Some of this ALP is released into the blood. ALP is also elevated if there is blockage of bile flow outside the liver. A common cause of this type of blockage is gallstones.

alkaline phosphatase isoenzymes (ALP isoenzymes)

What?

ALP from different tissues is chemically different. The test for ALP isoenzymes measures the different forms of ALP.

Why Test?

If ALP is elevated in the blood, it is important to know what tissue(s) it came from. The test for ALP isoenzymes measures how much ALP is from the liver, and how much is from other tissues. Elevated ALP from the liver indicates that the flow of bile is blocked either inside or outside the liver.

aminopyrine clearance test

What?

Aminopyrine is a chemical used to determine how well the liver is metabolizing and detoxifying substances.

Why Test?

Two of the liver's many important jobs are to metabolize drugs and detoxify foreign chemicals. The aminopyrine clearance test is used to determine how well the liver is performing these jobs. A single test does not give very much information, but comparing a series of tests done over time can show if liver function is decreasing.

ammonia

What?

Ammonia is a chemical normally found in very low levels in the blood. It comes from the normal breakdown of proteins in the body.

Why Test?

One potential complication of cirrhosis and portal hypertension is a condition called *hepatic encephalopathy.* See *Chapter 4: Signs and Symptoms That May Be Associated with Hepatitis C* for an explanation of hepatic encephalopathy. Ammonia levels are high in hepatic encephalopathy and testing for ammonia can help make the diagnosis.

anti-HCV antibodies

other names:

HCV antibodies

What?

After being exposed to the hepatitis C virus, the body develops several different types of *antibodies* to the virus. The anti-HCV test detects these antibodies.

Why Test?

Testing for HCV antibodies will tell you if you have been exposed to HCV. There are several different tests available to detect HCV antibodies. Depending on which test is used, there are differences in how soon hepatitis C antibodies can be detected in the blood after exposure to the virus. If this screening test is positive, a second test called a confirmatory test may be performed so you and your health care provider will know for sure whether you have been exposed to HCV. The anti-HCV antibody test cannot tell whether or not you have the hepatitis C virus in your body, only that you have been exposed to the virus.

anti-liver-kidney microsomal antibodies (anti-LKM)

What?

Anti-liver-kidney microsomal antibodies are a type of autoantibody. Normally, the body makes antibodies only against foreign substances such as bacteria and viruses. Autoantibodies are abnormal antibodies that act against your own cells.

Why Test?

More than half of all people with chronic hepatitis C have one or more autoantibodies in their blood. This is important to know because these autoantibodies can cause additional symptoms and disease.

anti-nuclear antibodies (ANA)

What?

Anti-nuclear antibodies are a type of autoantibody. Normally, the body makes antibodies against foreign substances such as bacteria and viruses. Autoantibodies are abnormal antibodies that act against your own cells.

Why Test?

More than half of all people with chronic hepatitis C have one or more autoantibodies in their blood. This is important to know because these autoantibodies can cause additional symptoms and disease.

anti-smooth muscle antibodies (anti-SMA)

What?

Anti-smooth muscle antibodies are a type of autoantibody. Normally, the body makes antibodies only against foreign substances such as bacteria and viruses. Autoantibodies are abnormal antibodies that act against your own cells.

Why Test?

More than half of all people with chronic hepatitis C have one or more autoantibodies in their blood. This is important to know because these autoantibodies can cause additional symptoms and disease.

aspartate aminotransferase (AST)

other names:

aspartate transaminase

previously called glutamate oxaloacetate transaminase (GOT)

What?

AST is an enzyme found inside liver cells. It is also found in other kinds of cells such as those of the heart and muscles. The largest amounts of AST are found in the heart and liver.

Why Test?

Testing the blood for AST is one way of telling if liver cells are dying. When liver cells die, AST is released into the blood. The level of AST rises over a period of 7-12 days, then slowly returns to normal. If liver cells continue to die, the AST level will stay elevated. The level of AST tells your health care provider how much ongoing damage is happening in your liver. However, an elevated AST does not necessarily mean your liver disease is getting worse because this test cannot determine how much repair is occurring and how many new liver cells are being produced.

bicarbonate (HCO3)

other names:

total carbon dioxide

What?

Bicarbonate is a charged particle called an *electrolyte*. It is one of four major electrolytes in the body.

Why Test?

Electrolytes perform many important jobs in the body. Two of the most important jobs are keeping the amount of water in your body regulated, and keeping your blood pH normal. Some people with hepatitis C hold more water in their bodies than they need. This can cause abnormal bicarbonate levels. This is more likely in people with cirrhosis than in those without cirrhosis.

bilirubin, conjugated

other names:

direct bilirubin

What?

Bilirubin is a yellow chemical that comes from the normal breakdown of red blood cells. Bilirubin is normally processed in the liver into other substances that can be eliminated from the body. There are two forms of bilirubin in the body, conjugated (direct) bilirubin and unconjugated (indirect) bilirubin. Conjugated bilirubin is bilirubin that is attached to another chemical called glucuronic acid in a process called conjugation. Conjugation takes place inside liver cells. Conjugated bilirubin is excreted in the bile. Normally, conjugated bilirubin makes up less than 10% of the total bilirubin.

Why Test?

If the total bilirubin in the blood is high, it is important to know how much of it is conjugated because this tells your health care provider what process in the liver is not working normally. High amounts of conjugated bilirubin mean the bile flow is blocked either inside or outside the liver. Problems inside the liver such as hepatitis, *fibrosis*, and cirrhosis can cause increased conjugated bilirubin. Problems outside the liver such as gallstones can also cause increased conjugated bilirubin. A high level of conjugated bilirubin in the blood can also be detected in the urine.

bilirubin, total

What?

Bilirubin is a yellow chemical that comes from the normal breakdown of red blood cells. Bilirubin is normally processed in the liver into other substances that can be eliminated from the body.

Why test?

Testing the blood for bilirubin in one measure of how well the liver is working. When the liver cells are not working normally, bilirubin can build up in the body. If bilirubin levels get very high, the skin and/or the whites of the eyes will become yellow, a condition called *jaundice*. However, bilirubin levels can be elevated without jaundice.

bilirubin, unconjugated

other names:

indirect bilirubin

What?

Bilirubin is a yellow chemical that comes from the normal breakdown of red blood cells. Bilirubin is normally processed in the liver into other substances that can be eliminated from the body. There are two types of bilirubin in the body, conjugated (direct) bilirubin and unconjugated (indirect) bilirubin. Conjugated bilirubin is bilirubin that is attached to another chemical called glucuronic acid in a process called conjugation. Conjugation takes place inside liver cells. Conjugated bilirubin is excreted in the bile. Unconjugated bilirubin has not undergone this conjugation process. Normally, unconjugated bilirubin makes up over 90% of the total bilirubin.

Why Test?

If the total bilirubin in the blood is high, it is important to know how much of it is unconjugated because this tells your health care provider what process in the liver is not working normally. In hepatitis, fibrosis, and cirrhosis, high amounts of unconjugated bilirubin means the liver cells are not conjugating bilirubin normally, causing it to build up in the blood.

blood urea nitrogen (BUN)

What?

BUN is a chemical produced by the liver in the process of breaking down proteins.

Why Test?

BUN is most commonly measured to check how well someone's kidneys are working. BUN is normally eliminated from the body in the urine. If the kidneys are not working normally, the BUN will increase. Some people with advanced liver cirrhosis and *liver failure* develop a condition called hepatorenal syndrome. With this syndrome, the kidneys begin to fail because the liver is failing. BUN is one test used to check for hepatorenal syndrome in people with cirrhosis and liver failure.

If there is no kidney failure, the BUN is often lower than normal in people with cirrhosis and liver failure. This is because the failing liver does not metabolize proteins normally, and as a result, lower than normal amounts of BUN are produced. Because of this, the BUN is one test that can be used to see how well the liver is performing one of its many jobs in people with cirrhosis and liver failure, but no kidney failure.

branched DNA test for HCV (b-DNA)

What?

The branched DNA (b-DNA) test for HCV is a test to check for the presence of the virus in the blood.

Why Test?

The b-DNA test is used to measure the amount of detectable HCV in the blood. This is called the *viral load*. Viral load tests are used to check a person's response to treatment.

In order for a b-DNA test to be positive, there has to be a certain amount of virus in the blood. For this reason, a negative b-DNA test is reported as 'undetectable,' not zero. A negative b-DNA test does not mean there is no HCV in the blood, only that there is no detectable virus. The b-DNA test for HCV is not as sensitive as the HCV PCR test, another test used to check viral load. This means that the b-DNA test cannot detect as low a viral load as the HCV PCR test.

It is important to note that viral loads in hepatitis C naturally fluctuate, and a high viral load does not necessarily mean more symptoms. Because of the normal fluctuation of viral loads in hepatitis C, not all changes in viral load are significant. If you have a viral load test, talk about the results with your health care provider. He or she will be able to tell you whether the change is significant.

calcium

What?

Calcium is an electrolyte. It is needed for many important functions of the body, including bone formation and muscle contractions.

Why Test?

People with cirrhosis can have lower than normal vitamin D levels because it is not being absorbed normally in the intestines. When the level of vitamin D is too low, the amount of calcium in the blood also drops. Many different symptoms can occur if your calcium is too low.

If cirrhosis has led to development of hepatorenal syndrome in which both the kidneys and the liver fail, the blood calcium can actually become elevated, which can cause other problems.

chloride (Cl)

What?

Chloride is a charged particle called an electrolyte. It is one of the four major electrolytes in the body.

Why Test?

Electrolytes perform many important jobs in the body. Two of the most important jobs are keeping the amount of water in your body regulated and keeping your blood pH normal. Some people with hepatitis C hold more water in their bodies than they need. This can cause abnormal chloride levels. This is more likely in people with cirrhosis than in those without cirrhosis.

cholesterol

What?

Cholesterol is a *lipid* or fat that is both absorbed from the food we eat and manufactured by the liver. Normally, most of the circulating blood cholesterol comes from the liver, not from what we eat.

Why Test?

The liver is responsible for both production and breakdown of cholesterol. The liver breaks down cholesterol and excretes it into the bile. If there is any blockage of bile flow either inside or outside the liver, the amount of cholesterol in the blood increases. The more obstructed the flow of the bile, the higher the amount of cholesterol in the blood. Cirrhosis can block bile flow in the liver, and gall stones can block bile flow outside of the liver. Both of these situations can occur with chronic hepatitis C infection.

complete blood count (CBC)

What?

A CBC is a group of tests indicating the concentration and characteristics of blood cells circulating in the blood. A CBC typically includes the following tests: RBC count, WBC count, hemoglobin, hematocrit, and platelet count. Other tests may also be included.

Why Test?

See individual tests for an explanation of the role of each test in chronic hepatitis C.

coproporphyrin

What?

Coproporphyrin is a substance that is produced in the liver and bone marrow during the process of making a chemical called heme. Heme is the chemical that binds oxygen to red blood cells.

Why Test?

Since the liver is one of two sites for heme production, liver cell damage can interfere with the production of heme. If heme production is abnormal, the substances used to make heme begin to build up in the blood. Coproporphyrin is used to determine how well the liver is performing its job of making heme.

creatinine

What?

Creatinine is a waste product of muscle cell *metabolism*. Creatinine is excreted by the kidneys in the urine.

Why Test?

Creatinine is most commonly measured to check how well someone's kidneys are working. If the kidneys are not working normally, the blood creatinine will increase. Some people with advanced liver cirrhosis and liver failure develop a condition called hepatorenal syndrome. With this syndrome, the kidneys begin to fail because the liver is failing. Creatinine is one test used to check for hepatorenal syndrome in people with cirrhosis and liver failure.

cryoglobulins

What?

Cryoglobulins are *immunoglobulins* that are joined together.

Why Test?

Some people with hepatitis C develop cryoglobulins in their blood, a condition called *cryoglobulinemia*. It is important to know if someone has cryoglobulinemia because it can cause kidney damage.

ferritin

What?

Ferritin is a protein found in the cells of the liver, spleen, and intestine. It binds iron.

Why Test?

Ferritin is measured to see if there is an overload of iron in the body. High amounts of ferritin in the blood means there is too much iron in the body. This is important because iron overload is often seen with chronic hepatitis C. This condition must be treated because too much iron will add to the amount of damage being done to the liver by the hepatitis C virus.

fibrinogen

What?

Fibrinogen is a protein produced by the liver. It is an important part of the body's ability to form blood clots in response to bleeding.

Why Test?

A cirrhotic, failing liver may be unable to produce normal amounts of fibrinogen. Measuring the amount of fibrinogen is one way of telling how severely the liver is failing. Testing the amount of fibrinogen in the blood is also important because, if the level gets very low, a person may not be able to form a blood clot if he or she begins to bleed for any reason.

gamma-glutamyl transferase (GGT)

other names:

glutamyl peptide

What?

GGT is an enzyme found in all cells of the body except muscle cells.

Why Test?

GGT is elevated in all forms of liver disease. It is highest when bile flow is blocked either inside or outside the liver.

genotyping

What?

There are different strains of the hepatitis C virus. A *genotyping* test tells what strain of the virus a person has.

Why Test?

At present, this test is used primarily for research purposes and to determine potential response to *interferon-based therapy*. There are currently over 90 known strains of HCV. Researchers have discovered that certain strains are more likely to respond to treatment than others are. Future studies will hopefully discover why this occurs. This may allow researchers to come up with more effective treatments.

glucose

What?

Glucose is another name for blood sugar.

Why Test?

People with chronic hepatitis C can have blood sugar abnormalities, either too high or too low. A glucose test is done to see if your blood sugar level is abnormal.

glutathione

What?

Glutathione is an amino acid found throughout the body.

Why Test?

Glutathione protects cells from a type of injury called *oxidative stress*. Scientists believe that oxidative stress is one of the key ways HCV damages liver cells. This damage is done by agents called free radicals. Glutathione prevents free radicals from causing damage to cells. Measuring the amount of glutathione in the blood is one way your health care providers can tell how capable your liver is of preventing and/or repairing liver damage.

HCV polymerase chain reaction (HCV PCR)

What?

HCV PCR is a test to check for the presence of HCV in the blood.

Why Test?

There are two different types of HCV PCR tests. The first type of test is a qualitative test. A qualitative HCV PCR test does not measure the amount of virus in the blood, but rather determines if there is detectable virus in the blood. The second type of test is called a quantitative test. It is used to measure the amount of detectable HCV in the blood. This amount of detectable virus is called the viral load. Viral load tests are used to check a person's response to treatment.

In order for a PCR test to be positive, there has to be a certain amount of virus in the blood. For this reason, a negative PCR test is reported as 'undetectable,' not zero. A negative PCR test does not mean there is no HCV in the blood, only that there is no detectable virus.

It is important to note that viral loads in hepatitis C naturally fluctuate, and a high viral load does not necessarily mean more symptoms. Because of the normal fluctuation of viral loads in hepatitis C, not all changes in viral load are significant. If you have a viral load test, talk about the results with your health care provider. He or she will be able to tell you whether the change is significant.

HCV transcription mediation amplification (HCV TMA)

What?

HCV TMA is a new test used to measure the amount of detectable HCV in the blood.

Why Test?

The TMA test for HCV is used to measure the amount of detectable HCV in the blood. This amount of detectable virus is called the viral load. Viral load tests are used to check a person's response to treatment.

In order for a TMA test to be positive, there has to be a certain amount of virus in the blood. For this reason, a negative TMA test is reported as 'undetectable,' not zero. A negative TMA test does not mean there is no HCV in the blood, only that there is no detectable virus.

It is important to note that viral loads in hepatitis C naturally fluctuate, and a high viral load does not necessarily mean more symptoms. Because of the normal fluctuation of viral loads in hepatitis C, not all changes in viral load are significant. If you have a viral load test, talk about the results with your health care provider. He or she will be able to tell you whether the change is significant.

HCV TMA may eventually replace the PCR test because early results with this test show that it may be more sensitive than the PCR test, meaning it can detect lower concentrations of the virus than the PCR test.

hematocrit (HCT)

What?

A hematocrit test measures what percentage of the blood are red blood cells.

Why Test?

Liver disease can lead to a shortage of red blood cells, a condition called *anemia*. The hematocrit is used to test for anemia.

hemoglobin (HGB)

What?

Hemoglobin is the *protein* inside red blood cells that carries oxygen.

Why Test?

Liver disease can lead to a shortage of hemoglobin. The hemoglobin test is used to check if there is enough hemoglobin in the blood.

immunoglobulins (Igs)

What?

Immunoglobulins are a group of proteins that act as antibodies in the body.

Why Test?

When the Igs are tested in the laboratory, the different proteins of the group are separated and each is measured. Different patterns show how much of each type of protein is present, and may point to different types of problems in the liver. For example, one pattern will show damage is being done to liver cells, while a different pattern will show that cirrhosis has developed.

iron (Fe)

What?

Iron is a metal found in red blood cells. It helps red blood cells carry oxygen to all the cells of the body.

Why Test?

The liver is one of the main places in the body where iron is stored. When liver cells are damaged, iron is released into the blood. Therefore, the amount of iron in the blood is one way to check how much damage is being done to the liver cells by HCV. If the body becomes overloaded with iron, this will add to the damage being done to the liver by HCV.

liver biopsy

What?

A liver biopsy is a surgical procedure to remove two or three tiny pieces of the liver using a long needle that is inserted into the liver through the skin of the abdomen. The samples are stained and looked at under a microscope.

Why Test?

A liver biopsy is the only way to be certain what is happening in the liver as a result of hepatitis C infection. The three main things that will be looked for are inflammation (the presence of inflammatory cells in the liver), fibrosis (scar tissue that forms when liver cells are destroyed by the virus), and cirrhosis (wide-spread damage to the liver resulting in abnormal liver structure and function).

5'-nucleotidase (5'NT)

other names:

5'-ribonucleotide phosphohydrolase (NTP)

What?

5'NT is an enzyme found in many tissues throughout the body, including the liver.

Why Test?

5'NT is increased from 2-6 times the normal amount when the bile flow is blocked either inside or outside the liver. Hepatitis, fibrosis, and cirrhosis can block bile flow inside the liver. Gall stones can block bile flow outside the liver.

partial thromboplastin time (PTT)

other names:

activated partial thromboplastin time (APTT)

What?

A partial thromboplastin time is a test to see how quickly the blood is able to form a clot.

Why Test?

The liver produces many of the proteins needed for the blood to clot. People with cirrhosis and liver failure may not be able to produce normal amounts of these proteins. The PTT is one indicator of the liver's ability to make proteins. It is also important to know if someone cannot form blood clots normally because he or she may not be able to stop bleeding should bleeding begin for any reason.

platelet count

What?

Platelets are small pieces of cells circulating in the blood. Platelets help the blood clot.

Why Test?

Liver disease can cause a shortage of platelets. The platelet count is used to test for such a shortage.

porphyrins

What?

Porphyrins are a group of substances produced in the liver and bone marrow during the process of making a chemical called heme. Heme is the chemical that binds oxygen to red blood cells.

Why?

Since the liver is one of two sites for heme production, liver cell damage can interfere with the production of heme. If heme production is abnormal, the substances used to make heme begin to build up in the blood. Testing for porphyrins is done to check how well the liver is performing its job of making heme.

potassium (K)

What?

Potassium is a charged particle called an electrolyte. It is one of the four major electrolytes in the body.

Why Test?

Electrolytes perform many important jobs in the body. Two of the most important jobs are keeping the amount of water in your body regulated and keeping your blood pH normal. Some people with hepatitis C hold more water in their bodies than they need. This can cause abnormal potassium levels. This is more likely in people with cirrhosis than in those without cirrhosis.

prothrombin time (PT)

What?

Prothrombin time (PT) is a test to see how quickly the blood is able to form a clot.

Why Test?

The liver produces many of the proteins needed for the blood to clot. People with cirrhosis and liver failure may not be able to produce normal amounts of these proteins. The PT is one indicator of the liver's ability to make proteins. It is also important to know if someone is not able to form blood clots normally because he or she may not be able to stop bleeding should bleeding begin for any reason.

red blood cell count (RBC)

What?

Red blood cells carry oxygen from the air we breathe to all of the organs and tissues of the body.

Why Test?

Liver disease can lead to a shortage of red blood cells, a condition called anemia. The red blood cell count is used to test for anemia.

rheumatoid factor (RF)

What?

Rheumatoid factor is a type of autoantibody. Normally, the body makes antibodies against foreign substances such as bacteria and viruses. Autoantibodies are abnormal antibodies that act against your own cells.

Why Test?

More than half of all people with chronic hepatitis C have one or more autoantibodies in their blood. This is important to know because these autoantibodies can cause additional symptoms and disease.

sodium

What?

Sodium is a charged particle called an electrolyte. It is one of four major electrolytes in the body.

Why Test?

Electrolytes perform many important jobs in the body. Two of the most important jobs are keeping the amount of water in your body regulated, and keeping your blood pH normal. Some people with hepatitis C hold more water in their bodies than they need. This can cause abnormal sodium levels. This is more likely in people with cirrhosis than in those without cirrhosis.

thyroid stimulating hormone (TSH)

other names:

thyrotropin

What?

Thyroid stimulating hormone (TSH) is produced by the *pituitary gland*. It acts on the thyroid gland to cause it to produce the two thyroid *hormones*.

Why Test?

Some people with hepatitis C develop thyroid problems because of autoantibodies. Measuring the TSH along with the levels of the thyroid hormones in the blood tells your health care provider if the thyroid gland is working normally.

thyroxine (T4)

What?

Thyroxine is one of two hormones produced by the thyroid gland.

Why Test?

Some people with hepatitis C develop thyroid problems because of autoantibodies. Measuring the thyroxine in the blood is one way to test whether the thyroid gland is working normally.

total iron binding capacity (TIBC)

What?

The total iron binding capacity (TIBC) is a measurement of how much iron the blood is able to capture.

Why Test?

TIBC is one of the tests used to see if there is too much iron in the body. The more iron there is in the body, the lower the TIBC. An abnormally low TIBC means there is too much iron in the body. This is important because iron overload is often seen with chronic hepatitis C. This condition must be treated because too much iron will add to the amount of damage being done to the liver by HCV.

triiodothyronine (T3)

What?

Triiodothyronine is one of two hormones produced by the thyroid gland.

Why Test?

Some people with hepatitis C develop thyroid problems because of autoantibodies. Measuring the triiodothyronine in the blood is one way to test whether the thyroid gland is working normally.

total protein (TP)

What?

Total protein is a measurement of all proteins in the blood.

Why Test?

The liver produces many of the proteins found in the blood. Measuring the total protein in the blood is one way of testing how well the liver is performing its job producing proteins.

transthyretin

other names:

prealbumin

What?

Transthyretin is a small protein made by the liver. It is used to make the larger protein called albumin.

Why Test?

Transthyretin is a sensitive indicator of how well the liver is able to produce proteins. The lower the transthyretin level in the blood, the poorer the liver is performing its job of making proteins.

vitamin A

other names:

retinol, retinoic acid

What?

Vitamin A is a fat-soluble vitamin.

Why Test?

Absorption of vitamin A from the intestines requires bile. If bile is not being made and secreted in normal amounts, the body isn't able to absorb as much vitamin A as it needs. In extreme cases, this can result in night blindness, dry skin, brittle hair, and brittle nails.

vitamin D

other names:

ergocalciferol

cholecalciferol

What?

Vitamin D is a fat-soluble vitamin.

Why Test?

Absorption of vitamin D from the intestines requires bile. If bile is not being made and secreted in normal amounts, the body isn't able to absorb as much vitamin D as it needs. Further, liver cells convert absorbed vitamin D into its active form. In cirrhosis and liver failure, the liver may not be performing this job normally. In extreme cases, vitamin D deficiency can result in softening of the bones and bone pain.

vitamin E

other names:

alpha-tocopherol

What?

Vitamin E is a fat-soluble vitamin.

Why Test?

Absorption of vitamin E from the intestines requires bile. If bile is not being made and secreted in normal amounts, the body isn't able to absorb as much vitamin E as it needs. In extreme cases, vitamin E deficiency can cause a shortage of red blood cells and muscle loss.

vitamin K

other names:

phylloquinone

antihemorrhagic factor

What?

Vitamin K is a fat-soluble vitamin.

Why Test?

Absorption of vitamin K from the intestines requires bile. If bile is not being made and secreted in normal amounts, the body isn't able to absorb as much vitamin K as it needs. Vitamin K is required for the production of proteins needed for blood clotting. Vitamin K deficiency can lead to easy bruising and bleeding problems.

white blood cell count

other names:

WBC count

What?

White blood cells protect your body against infections. They are part of the body's immune system. There are several different kinds of white blood cells including neutrophils, lymphocytes, and macrophages.

Why Test?

An elevated white blood cell count often accompanies acute infection. Changes in your white blood cell count can indicate a change in your hepatitis C disease status.

SUMMARY

Laboratory tests and procedures give a great deal of useful information to your health care providers. They can provide information about how well your liver is doing its many jobs, and about how much damage HCV is doing to your liver. In deciding what tests you need, your health care provider will consider several things. They will consider such things as:

- How have you been feeling?
- Are you having any new signs or symptoms?
- What treatments or medicines are you taking?
- Where are you in your treatment plan?

Since the answers to these questions are different for each person, and may be different from one clinic visit to the next, there is no one group of laboratory tests that are considered standard for people living with hepatitis C.

If you have questions about why you need a certain test or what the results mean, ask one of your health care providers. Understanding your laboratory tests can help you understand how your body is responding to your HCV and to the management plan you have chosen.

Chapter Six

PROMOTING LIVER HEALTH
Lorren Sandt

INTRODUCTION

The human body is amazingly resilient. It can recover from devastating trauma and disease. It can continue to function with missing or malfunctioning limbs or even some organs. However, the human body cannot survive for more than 24 hours without a liver. The liver is an incredibly complex organ involved in more than 500 body functions. It is responsible for such things as detoxifying drugs and alcohol, making vital substances such as blood *proteins*, and processing nearly every class of nutrient.

Many things we do or are exposed to in life can increase the work our livers must do to keep us healthy and alive. Alcohol, environmental pollutants, food preservatives and additives, drugs, and other *toxic* substances can pose challenges to the liver's ability to function effectively. *Hepatitis C* infection makes these challenges even more difficult for the liver.

One way to help your liver perform its best despite being infected with the hepatitis C virus (HCV) is to reduce other challenges to the liver. This chapter discusses some ways you can accomplish this in your own life.

A POSITIVE ATTITUDE

How do you meet the demands of a disease like hepatitis C and also live a full life? Having a positive, healing attitude helps many people meet this challenge head-on.

Negative feelings can drain your body of the energy necessary for healing. Without qualities like endurance, integrity, honor, and self-esteem, healing the physical body is a difficult task. It has been said, "If you *believe* you can, you probably can. If you *believe* you won't, you most assuredly won't. Belief is the ignition switch that gets you off the launching pad."[1]

For many people with a life-changing illness, a positive attitude is not just a cliché, it is what gets them through the day. Consider positive thinking as the process of creating thoughts that produce and focus energy that, in turn, bring about a positive outcome. Positive thinking is a powerful tool to which we all have access, but which few of us put into full use.

One research study of cancer patients who had a spontaneous *remission* found only one factor common to each person they examined. Everyone in the study had changed his or her attitude prior to remission and, in some way, had found hope. Each had become more positive in his or her approach to the disease.[2] Acceptance of reality is the first step toward taking responsibility for and control of one's life. Each of our lives is influenced by a number of outside factors, many of which we cannot control. Your attitude, however, reflects the ways in which you respond to what is happening to you. And your attitude is completely within your control. How you adapt to situations and the actions you take can impact your health and may influence your chance for recovery.

Some believe that every thought you have produces a reaction in each cell in your body, from the top of your head to the tips of your toes. They believe the body is constantly reacting to thoughts, whether those thoughts are based on real situations or your imagination. According to this belief, your body becomes an obedient servant of your mind, reacting with the emotional intensity that you associate with your thoughts. Pleasant thoughts produce pleasant feelings, and unpleasant thoughts produce unpleasant feelings.

How do you begin to practice having a positive attitude? Every time your life is not going according to plan or presents you with a challenge, try thinking of it as an opportunity. Challenges and disappointments can be opportunities to try new approaches, to amass more know-how, and to exercise your brain power.

There is still so much we do not know about the human body and how it works. We are only beginning to discover the powerful interactions between our minds and bodies. When you consider the miracle of the human body, it is not at all hard to believe that it is capable of contributing to its own healing.

LIFESTYLE CHANGES AND PERSONAL HABITS

Changing your lifestyle and personal habits to reduce the effects of *chronic hepatitis* C may be one of the hardest things you do in your life. Try to remember that you are not alone in facing these difficult tasks. Ask for help if you need it. It is much easier to address problems you may experience if you have support and proper medical care.

Sleep

Our society tends to focus on health issues . We spend billions of dollars on *nutritional supplements* and pills. We try to keep ourselves physically fit and mentally stable. We exercise and strive for more quality time with our families. But we often overlook the most fundamental aspect of good health – sleep. Many professionals consider sleep to be the most fundamental practice associated with good health. Sleep enhances immune function, and immune system activity enhances sleep.[3]

Getting enough sleep in our fast-paced world is not always easy. We all experience situations that can keep us up around the clock, if we allow that to happen. While adequate sleep is crucial for everyone, it is particularly vital for those of us living with a chronic disease such as hepatitis C.

Ambitious schedules are not the only enemy of sleep. Anxiety and/or *depression* are experienced by many people with chronic hepatitis C. These problems are often associated with sleeping difficulties. Lack of sleep often then intensifies anxious and/or depressed feelings creating a vicious cycle. It is important to get the help you need to end this cycle, and to ensure yourself a healthy amount of sleep.

It has been suggested that adults need nine or ten hours of sleep each night.[4] However, the amount of sleep a person needs varies from one person to another. One way to determine how much sleep you need is to keep an activity diary for a month. Keep track daily of the quantity and quality of your sleep, your daytime activities, and your mood. By looking at the patterns in your diary, it will become clear what amount sleep is best for you.

A person's measurable intelligence, his or her intelligence quotient (IQ), drops with each hour of sleep lost. The more sleep deprived you are, the lower your IQ is.[4] Since many people living with hepatitis C experience what is commonly referred to as 'brain fog,' getting enough sleep appears to be especially important for reducing this symptom.

Exercise

Many health care professionals and people in the general public do not realize the importance of exercise in maintaining good health. People who exercise regularly not only feel better, but also often respond more positively to medical treatment.[5]

Exercise boosts the immune system. As an added bonus, it gives us self-esteem and self-confidence by providing a sense of accomplishment and a feeling of independence.

Exercise causes the *pituitary* gland to release substances called *endorphins*. Endorphins remain in the body for hours and have a number of effects. They improve mood, relieve pain, increase red blood cell production, and reduce the amount of cortisol in the blood. Increased red blood cell production provides better *oxygenation* to the body tissues. Better oxygenation helps us feel more energetic and allows our brains to function better. Cortisol is a hormone linked to stress and depression. Reduced levels of cortisol may lead to reduced stress and better mood.

For someone living with hepatitis C, the key to exercise is moderation. Moderate exercise performed regularly boosts the immune system and increases resistance to disease. However, extreme exercise such as running a marathon causes an immediate suppression of the immune system. Extreme forms of exercise may be particularly harmful if you have cirrhosis.

HCV increases your risk of *osteoporosis*, a weakening of the bones. To counter this risk, some experts advise people with liver disease to incorporate weight bearing exercises into their exercise routine because weight bearing strengthens bones. Weight training also reduces the amount of fat in your liver.[5] In advanced liver disease, the body may use its own muscle tissue as a source of energy. Moderate exercise may help counter and/or reduce the impact of this muscle destruction. By building strong bones and muscles, you can build up a reserve to help fight off some of the physical complications of liver disease.

It is important to drink plenty of water after any type of exercise to prevent dehydration. Many people who exercise like to have a massage after their workout. If you have a massage after exercising, it is especially important to drink plenty of water to flush out the toxins that are released into the blood by the massage.

Review your exercise program with your health care provider to make sure your routine is healthy for you. It is also important to be aware of what your body tells you. There may be days, or even weeks or months, during which you may not be able to engage in your normal exercise routine. When you are not feeling up to your normal exercise, you may want to consider other forms of body work such as massage, qi gong, tai chi, or yoga. See *Chapter 11: Mind:Body Medicine and Spiritual Healing* for more information on these forms of body work.

Exercise and Weight Management

Exercise can be an effective tool for managing your weight. Maintaining or achieving your ideal body weight has several benefits for someone infected with HCV. Recently, researchers in

Australia reported that weight loss improved the *fibrosis, ALT, insulin* and *triglyceride* status in people with HCV.[6] Although this was a small study, the results suggested some significant benefits. The *grade* of *steatosis* (fat in the liver) decreased in all seven patients, and the fibrosis score was reduced in three of the seven patients. See *Chapter 7: Nutrition and Hepatitis C* for more ideas on how to achieve and/or maintain your ideal weight.

Sexual Activity

When they are first diagnosed with hepatitis C, many people become fearful about continuing their sex life. What is normal is different for everyone, but according to a recent study by researchers at Wilkes University, sexual activity can benefit your immune system.[7] The arousal, desire, excitement, and physical release of sexual activity enhance the ability of the immune system to ward off illness.

Many people find that thinking of themselves as sexual beings, regardless of whether or not they participate in sexual activity, helps them develop a greater ability to enjoy life. The feeling we have when we are sexually aware is sufficient to alleviate a variety of physical and emotional ills. Being or feeling sexual can be good for your self-esteem. It can help fight off depression. As a form of physical exercise, sexual activity helps trigger endorphin release creating a more positive attitude. Sexual activity allows you to relax and, at least for a time, to forget about some of your troubles. Your sexuality can go a long way toward enhancing the healing process and creating an environment for a better functioning immune system.

Sexual Transmission of HCV

The most recent statistics gathered by the Centers for Disease Control and Prevention (CDC) suggest that HCV may be a sexually transmittable disease. However, CDC has not changed its recommendations for longterm *monogamous* relationships. In summary, CDC states that people with HCV who have one longterm sexual partner do not need to change their sexual practices.

People with HCV who are not in monogamous relationships are cautioned to practice safe sex. This means using latex condoms correctly and consistently with every sexual encounter. This practice will prevent the transmission of HCV to others, and will keep you from being exposed to other HCV *genotypes*. It will also help you avoid other sexually transmitted diseases such as HIV, *hepatitis B*, and gonorrhea. If it is appropriate to your situation, talk to your health care provider about whether you should avoid certain sexual practices such as rough sex, 'high risk' sexual activities, and sex while menstruating.[8]

Stress

Stress does not cause disease directly, but it can contribute to disease. Stress can suppress your immune system, which may cause you to be more vulnerable to disease. Hepatitis C can be a frightening diagnosis. Your stress may be compounded by the fact that you may never know how, when, or where the infection occurred since most people are not diagnosed until well after the initial infection. Stress-reduction techniques such as warm baths, yoga, meditation, visualization, and/or keeping a journal can help soothe your soul and thereby strengthen your immune system.

Asking questions and trying to understand as much as you can about hepatitis C can go a long way toward reducing your stress level. Without knowledge, you run the risk of having your decisions controlled by fear and misinformation. Regardless of how well-informed you are, there will be times when fear and stress will dominate your thought processes. These feelings make it difficult for you to concentrate on the important issues you need to in order to make informed decisions about your health and, ultimately, your life. It is in those times of fear and stress when it most important to realize you are not alone.

Many people turn to friends, loved ones, and advisors during times of stress. If you do not already have a trusted support network of friends, advisors, and mentors, you may want to consider developing such a network. If you choose to pursue this option, seek out people with whom you can openly share your experiences and feelings. Look for people with whom you can speak freely, and from whom you can gain information and insight. You may also want to consider pursuing individual counseling with a mental health professional or clergy member. These people can further help you adjust to the new realities of your life with hepatitis C. Your physical, mental, and emotional health can all benefit when you share your voice with others, exchange ideas and concepts, and engage in thought-provoking discussions. You can gain much useful information from others who are facing similar circumstances. However, try to keep in mind that each person's experiences are different.

Stressful situations may cause people to seek an escape from their troubles. This can lead some people to take drugs or turn to alcohol. This is very dangerous for people with hepatitis C. Be very cautious about taking **any** drug (legal or not). Drugs have the potential to seriously complicate the situation for a person with HCV. Similarly, people with HCV should not drink **any** alcohol because alcohol is known to increase the liver damage done by chronic HCV infection.

If you are feeling overwhelmed by your situation, we strongly urge you to ask for help. You are not alone! Many people can help you make your situation more manageable and tolerable.

Prescription Medicines and Over-the-Counter Drugs

Some prescription medicines and over-the-counter drugs can have toxic effects on the liver. Many over-the-counter compounds contain *acetaminophen* (also known as APAP and by the brand name Tylenol®). If acetaminophen is taken in quantities over the recommended or prescribed amount, it can cause liver failure even in people with a healthy liver. If you are considering taking acetaminophen, discuss it with your health care provider first to determine if it is safe for you. This same advice holds true for any medicinal product you are considering taking. Always ask your health care provider before you begin taking a new product to make sure it is not toxic to the liver.

The Physician's Desk Reference (PDR) is available at most local libraries. It provides information about prescription drugs. However, the PDR is written for health care professionals and contains very technical language that can be quite difficult to understand. There are several books written for people with hepatitis C that contain excellent lists of prescription drugs about which people with hepatitis C need to be aware. Two examples are, *The Hepatitis C Handbook* and *The Hepatitis C Help Book: A Groundbreaking Treatment Program Combining Western and Eastern Medicine for Maximum Wellness and Healing*. See *Appendix VII, HCV/HIV Coinfection* for a list of some prescription and over-the-counter medicines that can be harmful to the liver.

Street Drugs and Other Recreational Drugs

People with hepatitis C need to be very cautious about taking drugs of any kind. Nearly all drugs are metabolized by the liver. Some drugs are *hepatotoxic* meaning they have the potential to directly damage the liver. Many other drugs suppress the immune system even if they are not directly hepatotoxic. For example, marijuana is not hepatotoxic, but it is *immunosuppressive* and *carcinogenic*. The immunosuppression makes the body more susceptible to infections. Carcinogens induce chemical changes in the body that can eventually lead to cancer. People with hepatitis C already have an increased risk for *hepatocellular carcinoma* (liver cancer). Using a drug that is carcinogenic adds to this risk.

The liver damage caused by HCV can prevent the liver from effectively *metabolizing* and processing drugs. This may cause the effects of drugs to be intensified, increasing the possibility of an overdose.

Even if you already have HCV, you can still be infected with other *quasispecies* of the virus. This can make it more difficult to treat your hepatitis C. If you are an intravenous drug user, do not share any equipment, and take every precaution possible to keep a sterile environment to avoid transmitting HCV to someone else. One microscopic drop of blood containing HCV can change another person's life forever.

Tobacco

We know the far-reaching dangers of tobacco use including lung cancer, head and neck cancer, mouth cancer, emphysema, chronic bronchitis, and other conditions. Tobacco contains much more than nicotine, the addictive substance that hooks people. Tobacco contains many naturally occurring chemical carcinogens. During the manufacturing process, many other chemicals are added to all forms of tobacco including cigarettes, cigars, pipe tobacco, and chewing tobacco. Many of these chemical additives are also known carcinogens. Hepatitis C infection and smoking are each known risk factors for liver cancer. Therefore, combining these two risk factors increases your risk for liver cancer. Keeping your body free of tobacco is one important way to help preserve the health of your liver.

Toxic Chemicals

Every chemical we are exposed to has the potential to stress the liver. Repeated exposure to the following known toxic chemicals should definitely be avoided: benzene, carbon monoxide, carbon tetrachloride, chlorine, dioxin, dry cleaning fluids, exhaust fumes, fluoride, fluorine, organophosphorous pesticides, paints, petroleum-based chemicals (such as gasoline), radioactive substances, and solvents.[9]

Vaccinations

People with HCV who are not already infected with *hepatitis A* or *B* should be vaccinated against these viruses. This will prevent the potentially serious complications that can occur if two types of hepatitis viruses infect the liver simultaneously.

SUMMARY

Regular exercise, adequate sleep, and a positive attitude can help promote the health of your liver. Avoiding addictive substances and environmental toxins will also help keep your liver healthy. Behaviors that enhance your immune system should be practiced every chance you get. Anything you can do to promote the health of your liver will help you live a longer, healthier life with hepatitis C.

For more tips on promoting liver health, see *Chapter 11: Mind/Body Medicine and Spiritual Healing*.

Chapter Seven

NUTRITION AND HEPATITIS C

Lark Lands

INTRODUCTION

Nutrients provide the building blocks for the body's physical structure—its cells, tissues, and organs. This includes that all-important organ, the liver. A wide variety of nutrients are also needed to support the body's immune response to infection. While both of these roles are important for anyone, they are particularly crucial for someone living with *hepatitis C.*

The ongoing presence of the hepatitis C virus (HCV) means the *immune system* is always responding to it. Since an active immune system requires energy, there must be a steady intake of nutrients to provide that energy.

The immune system must be able to create a constant flow of immune cells and chemicals to fight the virus. Those cells and chemicals, fundamental components of the body's immune response to HCV, are created from nutrients. This means a steady supply of nutrients are necessary for viral control.

Any damage to the body done by HCV, in the liver or elsewhere, must be repaired. This also requires a constant intake of the nutrient building blocks needed to make new cells.

Finally, having proper amounts of nutrients may actually help prevent liver damage. There is also evidence that certain nutrients may help prevent *liver cancer*, a major risk for those living with *chronic hepatitis* C.[1]

There are two sources for the nutrients that meet all these needs: the foods we eat and drink, and micronutrient supplements including vitamins, minerals, and amino and fatty acids. It is important to know that supplements cannot substitute for a healthy diet. Gulping down handfuls of pills will not make up for eating a bad diet. On the other hand, even the best diet may not provide the amount of certain nutrients needed to protect and repair the liver in someone living with hepatitis C.

Only a steady intake of nutritious foods can provide the needed nutrients we are aware of, as well as the many nutrients we have not yet identified. Research continues to show us that newly discovered nutrients play critical roles in the body's immune function and in maintaining overall health. It is safe to say there are probably many nutrients yet to be discovered. You cannot depend on supplements to provide your basic nutrition needs because manufacturers cannot put into a tablet or capsule ingredients that have not yet been discovered. To ensure good health, it is critical to take in all the nutrients Mother Nature designed, not just the ones we have studied. In addition, whole foods contain countless components that help nutrients work better in the body.

Many studies have shown certain vitamins, minerals, *amino acids,* and fatty acids help improve the health of people living with hepatitis C. Although higher than normal levels of certain nutrients may be needed for liver protection and repair, only a healthy diet can provide the nutrient base that is absolutely necessary for good health. See *Chapter 13: Naturopathic Medicine* and *Chapter 14: Nutritional Supplementation* for more information on supplements.

HEALTHY EATING: A PYRAMID OF GOOD FOOD

The first step toward ensuring you are getting all the nutrients you need is to make the most of what you eat. This means eating a wide variety of whole foods every day, along with plenty of water and other healthy liquids your body needs to function at its best. The most nutritious food is usually that which is closest to its natural state. Too much processing, refining, and overcooking can chip away at any food's nutrients.

Eating the following types of nutritious food every day will help build good health into every cell of your body.

- fresh or lightly cooked vegetables and fruits
- raw or lightly toasted nuts and seeds
- whole grains such as brown rice and barley
- whole-wheat breads, pastas, cereals, and crackers
- mixed grain/nut/seed/bean combinations, eggs, poultry, fish, and lean meat for good quality protein

Many people find the mathematical formulas that give standard diet directions using 'percentages of this' and 'grams of that' are difficult to follow. Therefore, many experts recommend a simpler approach for designing your meals: the food pyramid. Picture a pyramid with layers made up of food groups. Just like any pyramid, the base is the largest and each level above that decreases in size. The idea is to eat from the bottom up, with the largest amount of your food coming from the base layer, the second largest amount from the second level up and so on.

Food Guide Pyramid
A Guide to Daily Food Choices

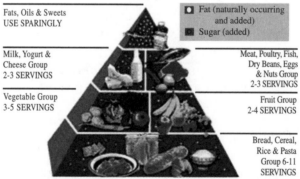

The food pyramid is reprinted courtesy of the U.S. Department of Agriculture and the U.S. Department of Health and Human Services

The pyramid base is the bread, cereal, rice, and pasta group. This group contains primarily complex *carbohydrates* that provide a substantial portion of the energy you need every day. It is recommended that you eat 6-11 servings from this group each day. Some examples of an average serving from this group would be one slice of bread, one-half of a bagel or English muffin, one cup of most flaky cereals, six crackers, two corn tortillas, one-half cup of cooked pasta, or three squares of graham crackers.

The next level up is split in half. One side is the vegetable group, and the other side is the fruit group. It is recommended that you eat 3-5 servings of vegetables and 2-4 servings of fruit each day. Eating the recommended amounts of fruits and vegetables will help you get all the nutrients and fiber needed for healthy body functions, especially immune function. One serving of vegetables is approximately one cup of raw vegetables or one-half cup of cooked vegetables. One serving of fruit is approximately one-half cup of fresh, chopped, or canned fruit.

The third level is the protein level, and it is also split. One side is the meat, poultry, fish, dry beans, eggs, and nuts/seeds group. The other side is the milk, yogurt, and cheese group. Most people need to eat at least 2-3 servings per day from each of these groups in order to get an adequate amount of protein.

The top level of the pyramid is the fats, oils, and sweets group. It is recommended that you eat the least from this group. Although a moderate amount of good fats is healthy, keeping the overall fat content of the diet low is important. Researchers have shown that high fat intake is tied to an increased risk of progression to *cirrhosis* in those with chronic hepatitis C.[2] Although an occasional sweet treat can be fun, most sweets contain few nutrients and often substitute for more healthy foods you might otherwise be eating. Limiting your intake of sweets is a good way to improve your chances for a total daily intake of nutrients that is supportive of your good health.

Another important and easy way to increase your daily nutrient intake is to go for variety and color. Each food is rich in certain nutrients, but not in others. Choosing a wide variety of foods at each pyramid level will help ensure intake of all the nutrients nature can provide. You run the risk of limiting your nutrient intake if you tend to eat the same foods over and over. Emphasizing color when you select a wide variety of foods is additional nutritional insurance. Think of it as, 'the rainbow theory of shopping.' When you are in the bread, pasta, cereals, and cracker aisles, choose brown, whole-grain varieties instead of white. White varieties contain processed grains, and processing tends to remove many of the natural nutrients of the grain. When you are in the produce section, pick up a variety of colors: red, purple, green, orange, yellow, blue, etc. Any time you see natural color, you are seeing nutrients. The more your shopping basket looks like a rainbow of color, the better your diet will be.

Adjusting the Food Pyramid to Your Individual Needs

The food pyramid is a simple way to look at your overall diet. Its guidelines provide a basic approach to eating. However, some of the recommendations might need to be modified based on your individual needs.

One possible modification is adjusting the number of servings from the food groups that will be required to meet your calorie or energy needs. Both your *metabolism*, the rate at which your body uses energy, and your lifestyle can significantly affect your calorie requirements. These individual characteristics make it difficult to come up with generic recommendations on how many calories someone needs each day. You may have a high rate of metabolism and an energy-demanding job such as construction work or an intensive daily exercise schedule, which increase your calorie needs. On the other hand, you may have been born with a very low rate of metabolism and have a sedentary desk job or a lifestyle that does not include much exercise, which lessen your calorie needs. However, regardless of these individual variables, the total intake of food that you need daily is somewhat increased by chronic hepatitis C. Your immune system has an ongoing response to the virus and this response is constantly burning up calories.

Dietary adjustments may also be needed in those people with a significant level of liver damage from the virus. Since adequate protein is generally so important, it is easy to jump to the conclusion that more is better. However, in the presence of serious liver disease, too much protein can actually be dangerous. A damaged liver cannot process protein as well as a healthy liver. Too much protein can result in protein overload that may lead to *encephalopathy*, a brain condition that causes mental confusion, and, in advanced stages, coma. If you have significant liver damage, it is very important for you to discuss your dietary needs with your health care provider to ensure that your nutritional needs are met without placing undue stress on your liver.

Another dietary change that may be very important for some people is salt reduction. *Ascites* is a complication of cirrhosis that results in an abnormal accumulation of fluid in the abdomen. Too much salt in the diet can significantly worsen ascites.

People who are coinfected with HCV and *human immunodeficiency virus* (HIV), may have additional problems that require dietary changes. For example, many people living with HIV suffer from lactose intolerance, an inability to properly digest the milk sugar lactose. This results in gas and/or diarrhea when dairy products are eaten. People with lactose intolerance often need to reduce or eliminate milk and milk products (cheese, yogurt, ice cream, etc.) from their diet. A reduced ability to absorb fats, called *malabsorption*, is also common in HIV disease. This can be another cause of gas and/or diarrhea. Therefore, people living with both viruses may need to keep the fat content of their diets even lower than those who have HCV alone. Finally, some of the drug regimens taken by many coinfected people require additional dietary adjustments.

For all these reasons, it is very important to discuss the details of your personal situation with your health care provider, and ask for advice about dietary adjustments that may be needed. You and your health care provider will need to consider your health history, laboratory results, the state of your liver, and any other conditions such as diabetes or heart disease that may require dietary adjustments. For those who are coinfected, you will also want to discuss all aspects of your HIV disease. Your health care provider may want you to make an appointment with a nutritionist or dietitian who specializes in hepatitis C. A qualified nutrition counselor can help you create an individualized dietary program. Just make sure your counselor is truly knowledgeable about the nutritional needs of people living with HCV.

All that can be offered to you in this manual is a generalized look at what we know about nutrition for those living with hepatitis C. Consider the information in this manual to be a base of knowledge that absolutely must be modified by your health care provider based on all aspects of your current health status. A diet that has been adjusted to precisely meet your current health status and individual needs is ideal.

With this in mind, we will now go back to the food pyramid and provide some specific suggestions on healthy choices for each of the food layers.

The Bottom of the Pyramid: Carbohydrates

Carbohydrates are the main source of your body's energy and should be the largest part of your diet. Carbohydrates are classified according to their structure as either simple or complex. Simple carbohydrates are found in sweet foods and sweeteners such as fruit, fruit juice, sugar, and honey. Complex carbohydrates are found in potatoes, root vegetables such as carrots, beans, peas, winter squashes, and grains such as wheat, rice, corn, and oats. Most of the carbohydrates you eat should be the complex variety, although a reasonable amount of simple carbohydrates, mostly from fruit, is acceptable.

Whole grains (those that are largely unrefined) provide vitamins, trace minerals, and fiber, all of which are important to the immune system and your overall health. One of the best ways to increase your nutrient intake is to substitute whole grains for the white foods that are common in our society. For example, use brown rice instead of white. Eat whole grain bread instead of white bread. Be sure to read the label and make sure your bread is all or mostly whole grain, such as whole wheat or whole rye. If the label says, "enriched flour," "white flour," or "wheat flour," be aware that this really means nutrient-poor white flour. Use whole grain pasta instead of white flour spaghetti, macaroni, or noodles. Eat whole-grain rye, wheat, or rice crackers instead of white flour saltines. Again, do not be tricked by the name on the box; read the label carefully. Whole grain flaked cereals and whole grain hot cereals such as oatmeal have more nutrients than the usual cold breakfast cereals.

Beans of all varieties are also excellent sources of complex carbohydrates and low-fat protein. Do not think of beans as a boring side dish. Make up a spicy bean dip, add them to a pasta dish, or sprinkle a tasty variety on your salad. And do not forget about corn and winter squashes. They are loaded with nutrients and can be a tasty source of complex carbohydrates from breakfast (whole corn grits) to dinner (baked spaghetti squash used in place of pasta in your favorite Italian dish).

Pyramid Level 2: Fruits and Vegetables

Fruits and vegetables are nature's most abundant source of most vitamins and minerals. In addition, they provide a great deal of fiber that is important for your health. Including a variety of vegetables and fruits in your diet every day is one of the most important things you can do for good health. Most experts recommend eating 5-9 servings of fruits and vegetables every day, but many people do not even come close to that amount. That makes fruits and vegetables an important area to emphasize for improving nutrient intake.

Fresh fruits and vegetables, lightly steamed or sautéed vegetables, and fresh-squeezed fruit and vegetable juices (made with a juicer that retains pulp) are the most nutrient-rich choices in this group because there has been little or no processing to degrade the nutrients. These fruit and vegetable options contain all of the vitamins and minerals nature intended. Cooking at high temperatures destroys *enzymes* and some nutrients. Therefore, including fresh or lightly cooked fruits and vegetables in your daily diet can be a particularly potent source of nutrients.

Whether raw, steamed, sautéed, or cooked into soups or sauces, the greater the variety of vegetables you eat, the better your chances are for getting all the important nutrients you need. Thus, do not eat the same vegetables day after day. Choose from the entire produce section and include several helpings each day. Your choices are many and include such things as carrots, zucchini, yellow summer squash, broccoli, cauliflower, red and green cabbage, green beans, peas, snow peas, kale, mustard and collard greens, spinach, red, yellow and green peppers, celery, Brussels sprouts, red and green lettuce, and so on. If you cook these with onions, garlic, ginger, peppers, and tomatoes, you will add the healing nutrients of these ingredients to your body's health store, too.

Several helpings of fruit each day are also important for your diet. Take advantage of the wide variety of fruits available in modern supermarkets. Choices include apples, bananas, oranges, grapefruits, tangerines, red and green grapes, peaches, plums, apricots, melons, pineapples, papayas, mangoes and so on,. It is important to eat fresh fruit rather than just drinking fruit juice since juice often does not contain the fiber and pulp that provide many of the fruit's most important nutrients. Do not forget that fruit is the best and most healthy dessert you can eat. Fruit is also a far healthier snack food than the common sugar-loaded variety.

Increasing your fruit and vegetable intake to reach the recommended 5-9 servings daily can seem impossible to some people, but it may not be as difficult as you think. For one thing, the amounts of these foods that make up a serving are rather small. One serving of fruit equals one-half cup of fresh chopped fruit. To reach the recommended 2-4 servings of fruit, just think in terms of trying to have 1-2 cups of fruit each day. One serving of vegetables equals one cup of raw vegetables or one-half cup of cooked vegetables. Therefore, to get your 3-5 servings of vegetables, think in terms of a mixture of raw and cooked vegetables that equals about one quart per day. Eating the recommended amount of fruits and vegetables is not very difficult if you concentrate your food choices appropriately. Have a piece of fresh or stewed fruit as a dessert and for some of your between-meal snacks. Eat a couple of servings of vegetables with your main meal of the day, and include at least one or two other vegetable servings at another meal or as a snack. In the morning, sauté a mixture of vegetables such as onions, spinach, mushrooms, tomatoes, and potatoes and stir them into an omelet for a nutrient-loaded breakfast. Add a variety of vegetables to rice, barley, couscous, or any other grains you are cooking. Bake some carrots or winter squash along with your baked potato.

Vegetables cooked into soup count as a serving or two, depending on how many vegetables you put into the soup and how much of it you eat. Making up a big pot of hearty vegetable soup can help provide vegetables for a number of meals. You can eat the soup over several days or freeze individual portions to use when other vegetable preparation feels too difficult. If you add beans, chicken, or fish to your soup, you will also be getting lots of protein. For days when eating seems like a difficult chore, getting good nutrition can be made easier by pureeing or blending soup in a blender or food processor so that it becomes an easily drinkable, liquid meal.

If you can purchase organic fruits and vegetables, you will limit your exposure to the pesticides that are used when growing non-organic produce. If you cannot purchase organic fruits and vegetables due to budgetary constraints or lack of availability, be sure to carefully wash your produce with a mild soap and water solution for two minutes.

Pyramid Level 3: Protein

The third level of the pyramid consists of proteins, without which your body cannot survive. Recall one side of this level is the meat, poultry, fish, dry beans, eggs, and nuts/seeds group. The other side is the milk, yogurt, and cheese group. Eating 2-3 servings from each half of this pyramid level generally provides the protein needed each day.

You need protein to build and maintain cells, keep muscles and organs healthy, produce enzymes and *hormones*, make the *hemoglobin* that carries oxygen to your cells, and maintain your immune system. When your protein intake is too low to maintain your protein stores, the immune system cannot function normally. A loss of immune function created by protein deficiency can cause a lowered resistance to infections, improper wound healing, and a lessened ability to control viruses including HCV. Too little protein can also result in weight loss, *fatigue*, and a decreased ability to respond to drug therapy.

Proteins are made of building blocks called amino acids. When making protein choices, it is important to remember that we require all of the amino acids necessary for the body to build the proteins it needs. The eight so-called essential amino acids are those the body cannot make on its own. They must be obtained from your diet. The so-called nonessential amino acids are those your body can manufacture for itself, provided it has the necessary materials. To manufacture non-essential amino acids, the body uses other amino acids, vitamins, minerals, and enzymes. If any of these are in short supply, even the nonessential amino acids may become deficient.

Complete proteins contain all of the essential amino acids. Complete proteins are found in animal foods such as eggs, dairy products, meats, fish, and poultry. Essential amino acids can also be obtained through complementary proteins created by combining grains, nuts, seeds, and legumes such as beans, peas, and nuts. However, building tissue from complementary proteins requires more energy than building it from complete proteins. Therefore, if you have already experienced muscle loss and/or your appetite is low, it may be better for you to concentrate on eating animal foods that contain complete proteins.

On the other hand, plant foods are generally less expensive than animal foods. If cost is a concern, remember that including some combination of beans, peanut butter, peas, rice, corn, nuts, seeds, and other grains and legumes in your daily diet will give your body the protein it needs. Small amounts of animal proteins added to a mostly plant-based diet can ensure that such combinations work without increasing the cost too much. Always remember that eggs top the list for high quality, inexpensive protein.

Some good, concentrated sources of protein are listed below.

- eggs
- poultry - skinless to lower the fat content
- fish - preferably deep-water, cold-ocean varieties since these are less likely to contain the liver-stressing toxins that fish from polluted waters may have
- complementary proteins found in mixed grain/nut/seed/bean combinations
- lean meat

Unless lactose intolerance is a problem, cheese and other dairy products can add to your protein intake. Adding things like alfalfa sprouts, chickpeas or other beans, or sesame seeds to your salad, or having beans as part of your meal can increase your protein intake substantially. Snacking on sunflower seeds will do the same. Just be careful not to overdo on seeds or nuts as they also contain substantial amounts of fat. With a reasonable combination of such protein foods in your three daily meals and occasional snacks, you should easily be able to eat the amount of protein you need.

Remember, this is a case where more is *not* necessarily better. A health care provider who knows the details of your health and liver status should prescribe the exact amount of protein you need to eat each day.

The Top of the Pyramid: Less is More

The top and smallest part of the food pyramid includes fats, oils, and sweets. Some fat is necessary for good health, but fat intake should be limited in people living with hepatitis C. Fats should come from healthy sources which means focusing on natural fats. The best fat choice is monounsaturated fat such as that found in extra-virgin, cold-processed olive oil or canola oil.

It is very important to eliminate partially hydrogenated fats from your diet. Hydrogenation is a process that uses heat and chemicals to change the structure of fatty acids in vegetable oils so that the oils are solid at room temperature. For example, hydrogenation is how liquid corn oil is converted into solid margarine. You will see partially hydrogenated fats referred to as *trans* fats. During hydrogenation, the normal chemical *cis* bond found in the fat is changed to a trans bond. Do not worry, you do not need to study organic chemistry to understand this. Just know that trans fatty acids may contribute to blocking some of the body's normal chemical processes, including those related to fat metabolism. Researchers who have studied this believe that artificially created trans fats have many negative health effects. A group of Harvard researchers stated, "Federal regulations should require manufacturers to include trans fatty acid content in food labels and should aim to greatly reduce or eliminate the use of partially hydrogenated vegetable fats."[3]

Partially hydrogenated fats are found in countless foods. These include margarine, shortening, most standard breads, crackers, cookies and other baked goods, many condiments such as mayonnaise, most commercial salad dressings, and some processed meats and snack foods such as potato chips, corn chips, ice cream, and French fries. It is crucial to read labels carefully in order to eliminate these unhealthy fats from your diet. If the words "partially hydrogenated" appear anywhere on the label, do not eat that food. Seek out brands of foods that have eliminated these bad fats in favor of healthy, natural ones. Luckily, many whole-food companies manufacture fat-healthy foods of all kinds. When eating out, be aware that most fast-food establishments use partially hydrogenated oils in their cooking processes. If you just have to have burgers and fries, you are better off making them at home from healthy ingredients. Even in better restaurants, it is a good idea to ask what kinds of fats they use in cooking and what is in the bread they put in front of you.

In general, try to make sure that you are consuming fats that nature made. Green, cold-processed olive oil not only makes great salad dressing, it is also a wonderful spread on bread. You can even use it for sautéing garlic, onions, or vegetables, as long as you keep the temperature fairly low since it has a low smoke point. Nut and seed butters are another source of healthy and tasty fat, whether they are spread on bread or used in salad dressing. If you really want a more traditional fat for cooking or spreading on your toast, plain old-fashioned sweet cream butter is definitely preferable to a partially hydrogenated margarine. Just be careful not to eat too much of any of these foods since your overall fat level needs to be moderately low to help reduce your chance of disease progression to *cirrhosis*.

When looking at possible ways to reduce fat, remember that much of it is hidden. Most meats (other than very lean varieties) and dairy products (other than those made from skim milk) are loaded with fat. Bacon, sausage, hot dogs, luncheon meats, and other similar products are very high in fat content. Almost all snack foods are also loaded with fat. This includes most chips, peanuts, nuts, many types of crackers, cookies, granola bars, candy bars, and many others. The fats found in salad dressings, peanut butter or other nut butters, and many sauces can add huge amounts of fat calories to your diet. Fried foods of all kinds (such as hamburgers, French fries, fried chicken, fried fish, fried or deep-fried vegetables) are often incredibly high in fat. Finally, the addition of fatty products such as butter, vegetable oils, mayonnaise, whipping cream, and sour cream can dramatically increase the fat content of any dish.

Relatively simple dietary and food preparation changes can significantly reduce the fat content of your diet. Some useful tips are noted in the following list. Any one of these can go a long way in increasing both the appetite-stimulating smell and flavor of foods while at the same time reducing the fat in your diet.

- Bake, broil, or grill your meats, poultry, and fish instead of frying.
- Use skim milk and skim milk cheeses and yogurt instead of whole milk and whole milk products.
- Avoid high-fat bread products like croissants, doughnuts, muffins, and most cornbread. Use whole-wheat pita bread or low-fat whole grain breads instead. If you are making

your own baked goods or sauces, use unsweetened condensed skim milk in place of cream.

- Avoid high-fat sauces, gravies, and butter. Substitute herbs and other seasonings to improve the flavor of foods.
- Unfortunately, removing the fat from dishes often seems to remove a lot of the flavor to which we are accustomed. Try using salsas, roasted garlic or shallots, flavored vinegars, chicken broth, and various hot sauces to spice up low-fat dishes.
- Thicken sauces or soups with pureed white beans, instant mashed potatoes, or corn-starch and skim milk instead of heavy cream.
- Make mashed potatoes using fat-free chicken broth instead of butter and milk.
- Avoid fried potatoes or other vegetables, substituting steamed or baked versions.
- Sauté foods like onions, garlic, mushrooms and so on using water or poultry broth instead of butter or oil. Alternatively, just 'sweat' such foods by placing the chopped onions or garlic in a frying pan. Use moderate heat just until they begin to brown around the edges, then pour in stock or vinegar to deglaze the pan.
- Prepare your own popcorn using grated skim-milk cheese and various seasonings instead of butter as the topping.
- Use toasted sesame oil or other strongly flavored oils when you just **have** to have a little fat for flavor.

One caution in this discussion of fat is that you should not carry fat avoidance to an extreme. You want a whole-foods diet that includes moderate amounts of good fats. You do not want a diet with no fat at all. In our concern to educate people about the need to lower dietary fat content, it is sometimes forgotten that fat is necessary at appropriate levels and in appropriate forms. Essential fatty acids are just that, essential. Both the omega-3 and omega-6 fatty acids are very important for human health.

When fat intake drops so low that the levels of essential fatty acids in the body are compromised, many negative health consequences can result. These consequences include skin problems, *neurological* problems, energy problems, and suppressed *immunity*. Fat provides the body's storehouse of energy. Fat in the diet is required for the absorption of the fat-soluble vitamins A, D, E, and K. In your attempt to decrease your intake of unhealthy fats, be sure you do not eliminate the good ones in the process. Moderate amounts of healthy fats are essential for a nutritious diet. Too much or too little fat are **both** unhealthy.

A healthy diet involves limiting the amount of concentrated sweets you eat. Many people consume too many nutrient-poor snack foods and desserts that are often loaded with excessive sugar and fat. Then they are not hungry for all the nutrient-rich foods on the lower levels of the food pyramid. The end result is a diet loaded with empty calories that do not promote good health. Try to make both sweets and fatty foods occasional treats instead of a major part of your diet.

HEALTHY LIQUIDS

Drinking plenty of healthy liquids is just as important as eating nutritious foods. Water is a dietary essential. Your diet must include plenty of water. The old adage about drinking eight large glasses of water per day (approximately two quarts) is actually a good beginning. However, because your size affects how much water you need, a better and simpler rule is to divide your body weight in pounds in half, and then drink at least that number of ounces of water every day. For example, if you weigh 140 pounds, divide that in half and drink at least 70 ounces of water (almost nine cups) each day. Many people drink far too little water thinking they can substitute other water-based beverages like soft drinks, coffee, or tea. However, these drinks are not a substitute for pure water.

You need to drink plenty of fresh, pure water every day because without sufficient water, the body simply cannot function properly. Anytime you are running a fever, have diarrhea, are suffering from nausea and vomiting, or have daytime or nighttime sweats, you run the risk of *dehydration*. Dehydration describes the state your body is in when it does not have enough water. Under these circumstances, you should put drinking plenty of fluids at the top of your list of priorities.

It is especially important for those who are coinfected with HIV to remember that the water you drink must be free of all disease-causing organisms. You can ensure the safety of your water by boiling it or using a water purifier that is designed to kill or filter out bacteria, protozoa, and other disease-causing organisms. The risk of water-borne infections is too high to ignore this.

Many people find herbal teas to be an enjoyable addition to their list of healthy liquids. Make sure you consult with your pharmacist or health care provider to make sure the herbs you are drinking have no potential for liver *toxicity* and will not interact with any of your medications. Fresh fruit and vegetable juices are also healthy liquids. Remember, many of the nutrients in vegetables and fruits are in the pulp. If you are preparing fresh juice, it is best to use a juicer that retains the pulp so you get the most nutrient value from your juice

Bottled fruit juices are another source of good liquids and are widely available. Be sure to pick the varieties with no added sugar. There are also canned or bottled juice spritzers that are sweet, cold, and carbonated. They have no added sugar, but taste great and are just as fizzy as carbonated soft drinks. These spritzers are good alternatives to soft drinks and other high calorie drinks such as many so-called sports drinks.

Soups, already mentioned as a good source of protein and vegetables, can also contribute to your fluid intake. Warm liquids such as soups, herbal teas, and roasted-grain coffee substitutes are not only nutritious, but are also less demanding on the body than icy cold drinks. Anything that is drunk icy cold requires some of your body's energy to warm it up. Drinking large quantities of very cold beverages can actually drain away calories your body needs.

DIET DANGERS

There can be hidden dangers lurking in certain foods and liquids. Both alcohol and salt (especially if ingested in excess) are bad for people with hepatitis C. The facts are simple.

Alcohol is highly toxic to the liver and can cause serious disease and/or death, even in those with no active viral infection. In people with HCV, alcohol intake has been linked to increased risk of cirrhosis, a more advanced degree of liver *fibrosis*, and a higher death rate. If you are considering *interferon-based therapy*, you should know that alcohol consumption has been associated with a decreased response to the drug.[4, 5]

Another hidden dietary danger is the large amount of salt (sodium) contained in the typical American diet. High salt intake is not healthy for anyone, but for those with cirrhosis, it can be particularly dangerous since it can lead to or exaggerate ascites. Anyone with ascites must be on a salt-restricted diet. It is estimated that every 1,000 mg of sodium consumed can result in the accumulation of approximately 1 cup (200 mL) of ascitic fluid. The more the salt content of the diet can be reduced, the better the chances of avoiding this excessive fluid accumulation. For people with advanced disease, liver experts recommend limiting sodium intake to no more than 500-1,000 mg daily.[6] This level of salt restriction requires careful shopping and scrupulous attention to food labels. Most fast foods and snack foods (especially chips, pretzels, and crackers) are dangerously loaded with sodium and must be avoided if you are on a salt-restricted diet. Even foods that might otherwise be considered healthy can be dangerously loaded with salt. For example, one cup of chicken noodle soup may contain an amazing 1,108 mg of sodium.

The only way to cut salt intake is to look at the sodium content of all the foods you are eating. Use food labels on prepared foods and a chart that shows sodium levels for other food ingredients to determine your total daily intake of sodium. One easy way to cut sodium intake is to avoid prepared foods. As many people with high blood pressure are placed on low sodium diets, there are many cookbooks and dietary plans available to help you avoid salt. People with hepatitis C who have not developed ascites usually do not need severe sodium cutbacks, but moderating your salt intake is likely to be beneficial.

Another possible dietary danger is eating too many iron-containing foods. This is a particular concern for those who have had a *liver biopsy* showing an abnormal accumulation of iron. Iron is stored in the liver and is used by the body for many different processes such as producing red blood cells. Iron is also a very important component of the enzymes involved in energy production and the manufacture of DNA, the building block of life. Therefore, the human body requires some amount of iron. However, because of its ability to act as a source of substances called *free radicals*, iron can cause liver damage in people with hepatitis C. This damage can lead to inflammation and scarring. See *Chapter 13: Naturopathic Medicine* and *Chapter 14: Nutritional Supplementation* for discussions of free radical damage.

Studies have shown that iron appears to be much more likely to contribute to liver damage in people who have hepatitis C than in those who do not. A study in India with *hepatitis B* and C patients showed that a low-iron diet significantly lowered blood iron and *ALT* (a liver enzyme), especially in those who started with high iron levels.[7] Many iron-rich foods are also high in protein. Although it is not a good idea to sacrifice protein for the sake of a low-iron diet, it is fairly simple to avoid foods that contain very high amounts of iron or are fortified with iron while still getting enough protein.

In general, dietary iron is poorly absorbed. The iron from meats is better absorbed (10-20%) than the iron from plants (2-5%). If you already have a high iron level in your liver, it may be advisable to decrease your animal protein intake as a way to lower your intake of iron. You can substitute plant proteins for the animal proteins. Be aware that many processed foods are fortified with iron and can significantly increase your iron intake. Unless your physician has recommended iron supplements because of iron-deficiency *anemia*, it is best to avoid iron supplements. While the exact role of iron in hepatitis C is still under study, eliminating excess iron from your diet appears to be a good idea.

As a final cautionary note, people with hepatitis C should avoid raw fish and shellfish. These foods can be contaminated with the hepatitis A virus. The chance of contracting *hepatitis A* from raw fish or shellfish is not worth the risk for people already infected with HCV, as the complications can be severe.

THE BOTTOM LINE

A summary of dietary guidelines for people living with hepatitis C is rather simple. Try to avoid junk food and fast food. Avoid other nutrient-poor foods that are made with white flour or white sugar, deep-fried in chemically altered oils, overcooked, or loaded with chemicals.

Create your meals from whole foods, using a wide variety of properly prepared fruits and vegetables, whole grains, and high-quality protein. Include plenty of healthy liquids.

Put care and thought into what you put into your body so that every mouthful adds nutrients and increases your capacity to heal. If you have created each cell in your body from healthy foods and liquids, then there is no question that you will have dramatically increased your body's ability to resist the assault of any disease, including hepatitis C.

Chapter Eight

WESTERN (ALLOPATHIC) MEDICINE
Section 1
OVERVIEW OF ALLOPATHIC
TREATMENT FOR HEPATITIS C
Douglas LaBrecque, MD

INTRODUCTION

If you are like most people reading this manual, you get all or most of your health care from medical doctors (MDs) or doctors of osteopathy (DOs). MDs practice allopathic medicine, the most common form of health care in the United States and the western world. Allopathic medicine is more commonly called western medicine. When selecting your own approach to maintaining health and treating disease, it is important to understand the basic concepts and philosophy that underlie the western medical approach to treating *hepatitis C*.

THE PRINCIPLES OF WESTERN TREATMENTS FOR HEPATITIS C

Three basic concepts guide the western medical approach to the treatment of hepatitis C.

- to understand and eliminate the cause of the disease (the virus)
- to treat the disease with medicines that have been shown to be effective against the virus in controlled, scientific studies and have been approved by the Food and Drug Administration (FDA)
- to improve the health and sense of well-being of those with hepatitis C by relieving their *symptoms*, even if the virus is resistant to therapy

Understanding and Eliminating the Cause of Disease

Allopathic medicine is based on an understanding of the causes of disease and eliminating those causes. The hepatitis C virus (HCV) is understood to be the cause of *chronic hepatitis* C and the symptoms it causes. Many studies have shown that eliminating HCV from the body prevents the disease from progressing further.[1-8] Both short and longterm improvements in liver health and quality of life are associated with having undetectable levels of HCV in the blood.[1, 9-11] An undetectable level of virus is also associated with decreasing the rate of progression to *liver failure* and/or *liver cancer*.[12-18] At least 95% of people in whom the virus has been eliminated continue to have undetectable virus, normal liver tests, and improved health 5-15 years after treatment.[19, 20] The primary goal in attempting to improve the health and sense of well-being of those with hepatitis C is elimination of the virus.

Treating the Disease with Effective, FDA Approved Medicines

Western physicians make decisions about which treatment will be most helpful for their hepatitis C patients based on controlled, scientific studies. This approach is known as evidence-based medicine, and the studies are commonly called *clinical trials*. In controlled, clinical trials, a new drug or treatment is compared to a *placebo* (an inactive pill or treatment) or the best currently available therapy. These trials are conducted to avoid the possibility of misinterpreting a patient's improvement as resulting from a particular treatment when it was actually due to the natural course of the disease, spontaneous improvement, or pure coincidence. Most western doctors have had the experience of a new drug or therapy producing almost miraculous results in one person, only to find it to be a total disappointment in many other people. While it is possible that the treatment was the cause of the improvement in these cases, it is more likely that the improvement would have occurred without any therapy. The apparent benefit was a coincidence of timing, that is, the treatment was started just before the person was about to improve on his or her own. Even if the treatment did improve the health of one person, without scientific studies, we have no way to separate those people who might benefit from the treatment from the many others who will not benefit or may even be harmed by the treatment.

Regardless of who recommends them, we strongly advise our patients to be wary of therapies for which fantastic claims are made if there is no scientific evidence to support the claims. If such treatments were clinically effective, many health care providers would gladly recommend them. There is a saying in western medicine that states, "The degree of enthusiasm for a treatment is inversely proportional to the degree to which it has been studied." In other words, once new treatments have been studied in a controlled, scientific way, many initially exciting new approaches prove to be ineffective or no better than safer, less expensive therapies.

The Placebo Effect

The placebo effect of mind over matter is well documented. A person who strongly believes that a particular treatment will make him or her feel better often does feel better, even if an inactive placebo is used.[21, 22] Because of the placebo effect, western doctors insist on specifically measurable results and carefully controlled trials when evaluating a new therapy. In these trials, neither the trial participants nor their doctors know who is taking placebo and who is taking active drug. This is done to eliminate even unintentional bias on the part of the trial participants or the health care providers.

Natural versus Manufactured Drugs

Western doctors consider any compound that is ingested to improve health or fight disease to be a drug. The distinction between so-called natural compounds and those that are manufactured is often an artificial one. Many manufactured drugs are derived from natural sources by taking extracts from plants, living organisms, or other naturally occurring materials. Other manufactured drugs are exact copies of naturally occurring compounds. For example, the drug alpha interferon, the basis of all current western therapies for HCV, is a copy of the alpha interferon the human body manufactures to combat viruses. The flu-like side effects of *interferon therapy* are not surprising when you realize that the same symptoms occur when the body releases its own interferons to combat a viral infection.

Any manufactured drug can have uncomfortable, even dangerous, side effects. The same holds true for natural drugs; most of our best-known poisons are found in nature. Western doctors consider it wise to regard anything we take into our bodies as potentially dangerous. They look for evidence-based proof not only that a drug is effective, but also that it has been adequately studied to be certain that it is not harmful. The FDA requires documentation of both safety and usefulness for each newly approved drug. However, the FDA does not evaluate or regulate natural additives, herbal therapies, or dietary supplements. Therefore, you must read the advertisements for such products carefully. The phrase, "meets all FDA guidelines" does **not** mean a substance is FDA approved. In fact, the FDA has no guidelines for the use of natural additives, herbal therapies, or dietary supplements. Do not be fooled by slick advertising, whether it is for an FDA approved treatment, an herbal remedy, or any other product.

GOALS OF WESTERN TREATMENT FOR HEPATITIS C

The goal of western treatment for people infected with HCV is to eliminate the virus so that:

- progression of the disease to *cirrhosis*, liver failure, and/or liver cancer (*hepatocellular carcinoma*) can be prevented,
- symptoms can be relieved,
- *signs* and symptoms of hepatitis C infection can be reduced or prevented, and
- quality of life can be improved.

Defining Response to Therapy

Chronic hepatitis C is considered to be responding to therapy if:

- your *ALT* levels are below 30 IU/mL,
- your *viral load* is undetectable using the most sensitive PCR test, and
- there is no progression of *inflammation* and/or *fibrosis* on *liver biopsy*.

Interferon-based therapy is not always successful in ridding the body of HCV. However, several studies have shown that these therapies can still benefit most patients by slowing disease progression, reducing the risk of liver cancer, and reducing liver cell *necrosis*, inflammation, and fibrosis.[5, 19, 23-26] Virtually none of the severe, life-threatening complications of hepatitis C occur until a person develops cirrhosis. Therefore, preventing progression to cirrhosis is critical, even if the virus cannot be eliminated. Interferon has been shown to decrease the activation of stellate cells (the cells that produce fibrosis or scarring in the liver) in laboratory experiments[27, 28] and in human studies.[29] This effect occurs even when interferon fails to decrease the amount of circulating virus. Interferon also reduces liver cell death (necrosis) and inflammation.

SUMMARY

The two basic tenants of western medicine regarding the treatment of hepatitis C are to understand the disease and to eliminate its cause. Our goal in treating people with hepatitis C is to eliminate the virus in order to stop disease progression, relieve the symptoms associated with the disease, prevent the spread of the infection outside the liver, and improve quality of life.

With recent advances in the treatment of chronic hepatitis C, many people are candidates for treatment. If you have elevated ALT levels, other conditions related to your HCV infection, a detectable viral load, and/or chronic inflammation on liver biopsy, you might be a candidate for therapy. Statistically, at least 95% of people in whom the virus has been eliminated using western drug therapies continue to have undetectable virus levels 5-15 years after treatment has ended.

WESTERN (ALLOPATHIC) MEDICINE
Section 2
TREATMENT OPTIONS FOR THOSE
WHO HAVE NOT HAD PRIOR TREATMENT
Douglas LaBrecque, MD

INTRODUCTION

It has only been possible to diagnose *hepatitis C* since 1990. However, great progress has been made in the treatment of hepatitis C in this short period. Currently, all western therapy for hepatitis C is based on the use of alpha *interferons*. However, alpha interferons alone (*monotherapy*) have provided only limited success. The allopathic standard of care as of this writing (December 2002) is combination therapy with *pegylated interferon* plus *ribavirin*. *Hepatologists* generally agree that it is no longer advisable to treat people with hepatitis C with interferon alone <u>unless</u> the use of ribavirin is *contraindicated*.

TREATMENT OPTIONS

The term used in western medicine for people who have never been treated for hepatitis C is treatment naïve. Generally, therapy is considered when a person's *liver enzymes* have been elevated for more than six months. At that point, he or she is considered to have *chronic hepatitis* C.

When a western doctor determines a person is a candidate for treatment, he or she has five major goals in mind:
1. to eliminate the virus from the person's body,
2. to return the person's liver function to normal (as shown by liver-specific blood tests),
3. to prevent further damage to the person's liver (shown by improvement or stabilization on the *liver biopsy*),
4. to improve the person's overall health and sense of well-being, and
5. to produce a maintained response to therapy (a *durable* or *sustained response*) for the rest of the person's life.

Interferon Monotherapy

Interferon alpha-2b (Intron AÒ) injections (three times a week for six months) was the first therapy approved by the Food and Drug Administration (FDA) for chronic hepatitis C. The results of that therapy were somewhat disappointing.[1,2] Approximately 30-40% of those who received this treatment experienced a normalization of their liver enzymes and undetectable levels of the hepatitis C virus (HCV) while on treatment. However, half of these people who experienced a response while on treatment relapsed during the six month follow-up period after therapy ended. As a result, the overall durable response rate was less than 20%. Less than 10% of people with pre-existing *cirrhosis* and/or HCV *genotype* 1 had durable responses.[3-5] The results were similar with two other types of interferon, alpha-2a (Roferon A®)[6-10] and consensus interferon alpha (Infergen®).[11, 12] It was quickly discovered that 12 months of treatment rather than six approximately doubled the durable response rate to 20-25%.[13-18] It also became clear that those with genotypes 2 and 3 had a much higher durable response rate than those with genotype 1. Those with cirrhosis showed the poorest response.

Anecdotal Story of Successful Interferon Therapy

A 36-year-old female with a history of alcohol and intravenous (IV) drug abuse was found to have hepatitis C while undergoing drug rehabilitation. She had one tattoo, but had not received any blood transfusions. Her *ALT* level was 2-3 times above normal. Her liver biopsy showed mild activity with mild-to-moderate *fibrosis* and marked fatty infiltration. She had HCV genotype 3a. She was *asymptomatic*, and her physical exam was unremarkable. At the time of evaluation, she had been drug and alcohol free for 20 months. She was treated with 3 million units of interferon alpha-2b three times per week for 48 weeks. Her ALT returned to normal, and her *HCV RNA* fell from 28,000,000 to 500 within four weeks. HCV RNA was undetectable at 12 weeks. Two years after completing therapy, the patient continues to have undetectable virus, normal liver enzyme levels, and is in good health. A liver biopsy taken six months after completing therapy showed clear improvement with no *inflammation* or fibrosis. The patient experienced mild *fatigue* and mild hair loss during therapy. Both side effects disappeared after therapy was completed.

This patient's experience demonstrates the rapid clearance of even very high levels of HCV that is seen in people who have a durable response to therapy. It also demonstrates the relationship between having the virus become undetectable, maintaining a sustained response, and improved liver health.

Combination Therapy with Ribavirin

A big breakthrough in western treatment of hepatitis C was the addition of ribavirin to interferon therapy. Ribavirin is an oral drug taken daily along with three injections per week of interferon. This *combination therapy* was initially given for one year, and was the standard western treatment until the introduction of the pegylated interferons.[12-21] Combination therapy with interferon plus ribavirin produces an overall durable response rate of approximately 40%. Among those with genotypes 2 or 3, the durable response rate is 60-70%, and therapy is generally reduced to only six months. Those with genotype 1 have a more modest 30% durable response rate.[22-25]

Anecdotal Story of Success with Combination Therapy

RT was first noted to have elevated liver enzymes in 1990 at the age of 36. He had briefly used IV drugs 18 years previously. He drank two beers per day. He had no history of blood transfusions, and was *monogamous* and heterosexual. A liver biopsy showed mild activity and minimal fibrosis. He had no symptoms. Despite discontinuing alcohol, his ALT level remained 3-4 times the normal level. A repeat biopsy 18 months later revealed liver disease progression with moderate-to-severe activity.

RT was treated with 3 million units of interferon alpha-2b three times a week for six months. His ALT levels quickly dropped to normal. However, he relapsed within one month of stopping the interferon in July 1993. A follow-up biopsy in March 1994 showed only mild activity. However, because his ALT remained 3-4 times above normal, he enrolled in a *clinical trial* in which he was treated with repeated 6-month courses of

3 million units of interferon alpha-2b three times a week. Between June 1994 and January 1998, he underwent six courses of therapy. During each treatment course, his enzyme levels dropped to normal, but his viral *HCV PCR* test generally remained positive. His ALT always went back up within one month of stopping interferon. In addition, a follow-up liver biopsy in 1996 showed significant disease progression with moderate-to-severe fibrosis.

In December 1998, RT began treatment with 3 million units of interferon alpha-2b three times a week plus 600 mg of ribavirin twice each day. Again, his enzyme levels promptly dropped to normal, and on the combination *protocol*, his virus also became undetectable. Therapy was stopped after six months in July 1999. When last seen, more than 3 years after the completion of combination therapy, RT's liver enzyme levels remained normal and the virus continued to be undetectable.

RT's experience demonstrates the importance of using *viral clearance* rather than normalization of *enzyme* levels to determine success with any given therapy. He also demonstrates the important advantage of adding ribavirin to interferon therapy. Interestingly, RT proved to have HCV genotype 3a, a subtype of the virus that is generally more responsive to therapy than genotype 1, and that usually requires only six months of treatment. RT's follow-up liver biopsy at the end of therapy showed marked improvement with a decrease in both activity and fibrosis. This demonstrates the *histologic* improvement seen in patients after successful therapy.

Pegylated Interferons

The hepatitis C virus replicates very rapidly, doubling in number every 2-3 hours. Standard interferon is cleared from the body very quickly, within 6-7 hours. When standard interferon is given three times a week, there are long periods when there is no interferon circulating in the blood. This gives the virus time to recover from the effects of the interferon. Studies have shown larger or more frequent doses of standard interferons produce more side effects with no significant improvement in durable response rates. The development of pegylated interferons came about from an effort to solve these problems and to keep interferon continuously circulating in the blood.[26, 27] It was hoped that a longer-acting form of interferon would provide a great improvement in the success rate with treatment, and this has proven to be the case. It was already known that the attachment of polyethylene glycol (a long-chain sugar molecule known as 'peg') to a protein such as interferon slows its absorption, and decreases its breakdown and clearance from the body. Based on this knowledge, pegylated interferons were developed and have been recently tested.[28-35]

Studies completed to date indicate that treatment with pegylated interferon provides a constant level of interferon in the blood when given only once a week. This makes it more convenient (one injection each week rather than three) and produces a continuous interferon level to combat the virus. Without continuous, consistent levels of interferon in the body, the virus has time to replicate when the interferon levels are low. Landmark studies have shown that approximately 80% of people with genotypes 2 and 3 who receive pegylated interferon plus ribavirin achieve a durable response. Just under 50% of people with genotype 1 achieve a durable response with this treatment protocol.[32, 36] Side effects are similar to those seen with standard combination therapy.[31, 32, 36, 37] Studies also suggest that pegylated interferons may be better tolerated than standard interferon therapy.[32, 36, 38-41] Pegylated interferon plus ribavirin is now the allopathic standard of care for chronic hepatitis C as approved by the FDA and the recent National Institutes of Health Consensus Development Conference Management of Hepatitis C: 2002.[42]

Recent data presented at the meeting of the American Association for the Study of Liver Diseases in November 2002 (available at the time of publication only in abstract form) indicate that aggressive treatment with the combination of ribavirin and consensus interferon (interferon alfacon-1, Infergen®) may be effective in historically difficult to treat patients such as those with a high viral titer (>2,000,000 copies), genotype 1 infection, those with cirrhosis, and/or non-responders to standard combination therapy.[43-45] Full details of these small studies have not yet been published and combination therapy with consensus interferon has not as of yet been approved by the FDA.

SPECIAL SITUATIONS

Treatment of Acute HCV Infection

The initial hepatitis C infection, called *acute hepatitis* C, generally goes undetected because the *symptoms* are usually mild and are often mistaken for the flu. We do not know the actual rate of *spontaneous clearance* of HCV in people with acute infection. However, small studies in the past have shown that treating individuals who have acute hepatitis C with interferon alone can produce response rates of 39-64%. A more recent study in Germany found 43 out of 44 patients with acute hepatitis C who were treated with interferon monotherapy had undetectable levels of HCV RNA and normal ALT levels both at the end of therapy and at follow-up.[46] Expected spontaneous clearance without therapy is 15-20%. It should be recognized that these studies included only small numbers of patients and were uncontrolled. The role of interferon plus ribavirin in people with acute hepatitis C is unknown. Clinical trials will need to be conducted to see if it combination therapy is a valuable therapeutic option to reduce the frequency of chronic hepatitis C.

Treatment of HCV Infected Individuals with Normal Liver Enzymes

It is not known if there is any benefit to be gained from treating people with acute or chronic HCV infection who have normal liver enzyme levels. Many of these individuals appear to clear the virus following treatment in a way similar to those who have elevated liver enzymes. Some studies have shown an actual rise in enzyme levels during treatment in a few patients who had normal enzymes prior to therapy.[47] Other studies have shown a much better response rate in patients who have at least a three-fold elevation of ALT levels prior to treatment.[28]

Clinical trials need to be conducted to look at the natural course of hepatitis C disease when ALT levels remain normal, and to see if combination therapy or alternative therapeutic approaches are helpful in this situation. It is hoped that a more standardized approach will be developed for defining what normal liver enzyme levels are. This should include correction for body weight or body mass, and gender. Often, the upper limit of what is considered a normal ALT level in women is lower than the upper limit of normal in men.

Treatment of Chronic Hepatitis C in Patients with Cirrhosis

A study that evaluated the effectiveness of interferon monotherapy in people with cirrhosis found ALT levels returned to normal in 27% of people with cirrhosis, but only 5-10% of these patients maintained an undetectable viral load for more than six months after the trial ended.[13] Small studies in which interferon plus ribavirin were used found undetectable virus in 20% of those with cirrhosis following treatment. These data support the belief that some people with cirrhosis are able to eliminate the virus, and possibly have fewer complications of liver disease. [22-24, 48]

A more recent study of pegylated interferon monotherapy showed similar response rates in people with and without cirrhosis. Thirty percent of those in the study with cirrhosis achieved a durable response, suggesting this newer therapy might provide a better outlook for people with cirrhosis.[29] This notion was confirmed in two studies using combined pegylated interferon plus ribavirin. In these studies, 43% and 44% of patients with cirrhosis achieved a durable response. While these response rates are lower than the durable response rates seen in patients without cirrhosis, they represent a great improvement. These study data indicate that even patients who are already cirrhotic may benefit from state of the art *interferon-based therapy*.[32, 36]

Potential Therapy-Related Complications

If you have cirrhosis and are undergoing treatment, you are at risk during therapy for serious bacterial infections and other liver disease complications that may occur because your liver is not functioning properly. You are also more liable to have low *neutrophil, platelet*, or *hemoglobin* levels than someone without cirrhosis. Neutrophils are a type of white blood cell, and a low level makes you more susceptible to bacterial infections. A low platelet count makes it more difficult for your blood to clot normally, and may cause you to bleed and/or bruise easily. A low hemoglobin level can make you feel more fatigued than normal.

If you have cirrhosis and are undergoing treatment, it is very important that you tell your health care provider about any problems you experience. Your health care provider should check your blood counts frequently to identify potential complications early.

Treatment Options for Patients with HCV-Related Diseases Outside the Liver

HCV has been associated with a wide variety of diseases outside the liver, including *cryoglobulinemia, lichen planus*, and *porphyria cutanea tarda*.[49, 50] All of these cause disfiguring skin problems. Cryoglobulinemia can also cause kidney, nerve, blood vessel, and other tissue damage that may be life threatening.

If you have an *immune complex disease* that is the result of your HCV infection, you may still be a candidate for therapy with interferon alone, which may decrease or control the disease by reducing or clearing the HCV virus. This is true even if you have little evidence of liver disease. There are few data available on the effects of standard or pegylated interferon plus ribavirin on long-term control of *extrahepatic* HCV-related diseases. However, since combination therapy is more effective than monotherapy in clearing HCV, it is also likely to be more effective in the control of extrahepatic disease.

Options for People Coinfected with Hepatitis B Virus or Human Immunodeficiency Virus

Hepatitis B Virus

Coinfection with HCV and the *hepatitis B* virus (HBV) increases your risk of developing cirrhosis and other liver complications compared to infection with either virus alone. If you are coinfected with HBV and HCV, your health care provider may consider interferon therapy including the higher doses used to treat patients who are infected only with HBV.

Human Immunodeficiency Virus

People who are infected with both HCV and the *human immunodeficiency virus* (HIV) often have poor treatment outcomes such as end-stage liver disease, although this is <u>not</u> always the case. Those coinfected with HIV and HCV have been reported to have higher HCV viral loads and more rapidly progressive liver disease compared to people infected with HCV alone.[51-53] A number of studies have shown that HCV/HIV coinfected people have a lower antibody response rate to the HCV infection than do people infected with only HCV.

A similar rate of response to interferon has been shown for patients coinfected with HIV and HCV compared to patients infected with HCV only, provided the *CD4* cell count is greater than 500. No response to interferon has been observed when the CD4 cell count was less than 180. A low CD4 count (less than 200), high alcohol consumption (more than 1.75 ounces per day), and older age at the time of HCV infection are associated with an increased rate of progression to liver fibrosis.[52]

If you are coinfected with HIV and HCV, you could be a candidate for interferon-based combination therapy if aggressive liver disease is found on liver biopsy and you have a significantly long life expectancy (based on your CD4 cell counts, history of opportunistic infections, and HIV viral load). The use of anti-HCV drugs may cause more frequent treatment complications among people who are coinfected.

The treatment of HCV/HIV coinfected people remains an area of active investigation, and firm recommendations cannot yet be made. You should discuss your options with a hepatologist or infectious diseases specialist. Regardless of whatever treatments you decide upon, you should definitely eliminate all alcohol intake.

RESPONSE TO THERAPY

Western medicine's key measurement of successful treatment of hepatitis C is undetectable virus in the blood. Among those for whom therapy is successful, this usually occurs very early during the treatment course. If therapy fails to produce an undetectable or very low viral load test after 12 weeks of treatment, it is very unlikely that the therapy will be successful.[32, 36] Most doctors will discontinue therapy if viral levels are not undetectable by 12 weeks, though some will continue therapy for another 12 weeks if the viral load has dropped by at least two logs, that is, by a factor of 100 (for example from 1,000,000 to 10,000). It is a rare and unusual occurrence for a doctor to continue therapy for an additional 12 weeks if there is no viral response to treatment within the first 12 weeks.

If a durable response is to occur, the virus should be undetectable after 24 weeks of therapy. It is important to recognize that measurements of viral levels are not very precise and will vary greatly from one laboratory to another. Therefore, you should make sure the same laboratory always performs your viral tests. Also, be aware that small changes in viral load are not significant. Recall that viral levels must fall at least 100-fold to be considered significant. For example, even a seemingly large drop from 800,000 to 200,000 would not be considered significant, and would not be an indication of successful therapy.

Undetectable viral load at completion of therapy is currently the determinant of a successful response to treatment. A durable or sustained response to treatment is declared if the virus remains undetectable six months after you have completed therapy. A relapse is defined as having an undetectable viral load during treatment, but the return of a detectable viral load after treatment ends. If your viral load becomes detectable after treatment, there are usually no symptoms but ALT levels usually begin to rise. A relapse usually occurs within 4-24 weeks after completing therapy. Developing a detectable viral load more than 12-24 weeks after completing treatment is rare and occurs in less than 5% of those treated. [15, 63] Relapse beyond two years after completing therapy is exceedingly rare. Retreatment for people who have a relapse is discussed in *Section 3: Options for Those Whose Treatment Failed to Clear the Hepatitis C Virus* of this chapter.

The best measure of treatment success is improvement on liver biopsy. However, a follow-up liver biopsy after successful therapy is rarely performed outside of research studies. This is because a liver biopsy is an invasive procedure with potential complications such as bleeding and infection. It is also much more costly and time-consuming to do than simple blood tests for liver enzyme levels and viral load. If the virus is undetectable and ALT levels have returned to normal, it is assumed that the biopsy will show improvement based on a large amount of information obtained from carefully controlled research studies. In addition to improved liver histology, there is some evidence that antiviral therapy may reduce the risk of developing *hepatocellular carcinoma* (*liver cancer*). [53-59]

SIDE EFFECTS FROM THERAPY AND THEIR MANAGEMENT

Most therapies produce one or more uncomfortable side effects in at least a small percentage of individuals. There are side effects from treatment with both interferon alone (monotherapy) and combination therapy. Many of these potential side effects can be managed. However, side effects are unpredictable and quite variable. Some side effects can be severe enough that your doctor will either reduce the dose of the drug you are taking or discontinue therapy altogether. Combination therapy is more likely to lead to reductions in dosage or discontinuation of therapy than treatment with interferon monotherapy.

Side Effects of Interferon

The currently available interferons all have similar side effects. The most common side effects are flu-like symptoms. Other potential side effects include thyroid abnormalities, injection site reactions, *bone marrow suppression*, and hair loss. The most serious side effects of interferons are depression, and the worsening of existing depression or other psychiatric disorders. With the exception of *hypothyroidism*, virtually of all of these side effects will go away after treatment has ended. Following are brief discussions of these potential side effects of interferon therapy.

Flu-Like Symptoms

Up to 66% of people taking interferon experience flu-like symptoms including fever, chills, fatigue, *myalgia* (muscle pains), *arthralgia* (joint pains), and weight loss. These symptoms usually lessen after the first two or three treatments. Taking acetaminophen or a *nonsteroidal analgesic* such as ibuprofen or naproxen 30-60 minutes prior to treatment can further reduce these symptoms. However, you should discuss using these or any medicines with your doctor before taking them.

Most patients prefer taking their interferon in the late afternoon or early evening, so that the worst side effects occur while they are asleep. However, this must be individualized as some patients do better when they get their injections early in the morning. The timing of injections appears to be less critical with long-acting, once-a-week pegylated interferons. People also find that drinking at least eight eight-ounce glasses of a non-caffeinated or decaffeinated beverages per day markedly reduces their flu-like symptoms. Those who have tried this approach swear by the value of increasing their intake of fluids. A good rule of thumb to determine how much water you should be drinking each day is to divide your weight in pounds in half, and drink that many ounces of fluid per day. For example, a 120 pound female should drink at least 60 ounces of fluid, preferably water, per day. Good indicators that you are drinking enough fluids are clear to very pale yellow urine, and having to get up at least once during the night to urinate.

Bone-Marrow Suppression

Mild bone marrow suppression, especially leukopenia (low white cell count) and thrombocytopenia (low platelet count) are frequently seen. This can be easily monitored and managed.

Thyroid Abnormalities

Hypothyroidism among people taking interferon is usually due to stimulation of an unsuspected autoimmune *thyroid* disorder. This side effect of treatment can occur in 3-5% of patients. Hypothyroidism is managed with thyroid hormone replacement therapy. Patients may require continued thyroid hormone replacement after treatment has ended.

Injection Site Reactions

The development of redness and warmth with or without itchiness at the injection site is a common side effect of interferon treatment. This often does not occur until 24-48 hours after the injection. This is a common local reaction and does not lead to complications. However, it is important to rotate injection sites in order to avoid injecting the same spot over and over again. This is particularly true with the pegylated interferons, which are absorbed more slowly and may stay in the skin for a prolonged period. Injection sites can take 2-3 weeks to clear. It is important not to get an interferon injection in an area that is still red from a prior injection. Repeated injections into the same area can lead to severe skin reactions including deep skin ulcers that take many weeks or months to heal.

Hair Loss

Limited hair loss occurs in about 20% of patients taking interferon.

Depression and Psychiatric Disorders

Interferon can worsen existing depression and other psychiatric disorders, and can lead to new depression among people who have not previously suffered from this condition. Studies show that about one-third of those on interferon therapy suffer from depression. However, suicidal thoughts or attempts occur in less than 1% of those taking interferon. It is very important to tell your health care provider before you consider treatment if you have had any psychiatric counseling or have been dealing with depression. If you have ever attempted or even seriously considered suicide, you must tell your doctor. You should not be treated with interferon if you have recently struggled with thoughts of or have attempted suicide because interferon could cause you to reconsider suicide. Once you and your health care provider are confident that you have successfully dealt with any issues of suicide, you may consider therapy. Discontinuation of therapy is most frequently due to depression and emotional disturbances attributed to interferon. However, depression and suicidal thoughts can usually be managed with counseling and/or antidepressant medications.

Anecdotal Story of Success with Interferon Therapy Despite Psychiatric Complications

A 44-year-old female was found to have elevated liver enzymes when she donated blood in 1990. A liver biopsy showed mild activity and no fibrosis. She tested positive for hepatitis C in 1992. Enzyme levels remained 1-2 times normal until 1998 when they were noted to be 4-6 times above normal. The patient had abused alcohol and used multiple oral and IV drugs until 1994. She was asymptomatic, and her physical exam was unremarkable. She had a history of depression while actively using drugs, but no suicide attempts. A liver biopsy showed moderate activity and moderate fibrosis. She had genotype 1b virus.

The patient was treated with pegylated interferon 2b plus ribavirin for 48 weeks. Enzyme levels dropped to normal within four weeks. Fever, decreased appetite, "weird dreams," and increased moodiness complicated the patient's therapy during the first few weeks. These symptoms resolved except for worsening mood swings. Three months into therapy, the patient was referred for psychiatric help due to decreased ability to concentrate, insomnia, excessive crying, anxiety, feelings of loss of control, and hopelessness. She was diagnosed with a mood disturbance related to interferon and started taking Xanax® and Effexor.® Because of intolerance to Effexor®, she was switched to Prozac® with occasional Xanax®. Xanax® was changed to Klonopin® to manage residual anxiety. This was later switched to Ativan® due to over-sedation with the Klonopin®. The patients was also started on intensive psychotherapy to address her personal problems. She remained on Prozac® and a variety of antianxiety drugs throughout therapy with no more active depression. She has continued with psychotherapy since completing her hepatitis C treatment

The patient remains virus free with normal liver enzymes for more than one year after completing therapy. Follow-up liver biopsy showed a definite decrease in activity and fibrosis.

This patient's experience demonstrates the importance of close follow-up for early recognition of the development of psychological problems. It also shows that the majority of such problems can be successfully overcome and therapy completed successfully with the cooperation of a psychiatrist experienced in the management of interferon-related depression. This patient's experience stresses the concept that there is no simple 'one drug fits all' approach to interferon-related psychiatric problems. Patient therapy must be individualized.

Side Effects of Ribavirin

Ribavirin can lead to side effects such as cough, *dyspnea* (difficulty breathing), insomnia, *pruritus* (itching), rash, and reduced appetite (anorexia). These side effects are generally mild and usually do not require discontinuation of therapy or dose modification. Most side effects go away over several weeks to months after stopping therapy.

Ribavirin is also associated with two serious side effects, *hemolytic anemia* and birth defects, which are discussed below.

Hemolytic Anemia

The most serious side effect of ribavirin is hemolytic anemia, which occurs in approximately 10% of patients. The severity of this type of *anemia* depends on the amount of ribavirin you are taking. Hemolytic anemia means your red blood cells are breaking down. Red blood cells are necessary to carry oxygen from your lungs to all the tissues of the body. Without sufficient oxygen, your cells cannot function well. With anemia, you will feel increasingly tired as the number of red blood cells decreases. To test for hemolytic anemia while taking ribavirin, your blood will be tested frequently during the first few months of therapy. Your hemoglobin should be checked at least at 2, 4, 8, and 12 weeks after starting therapy. After 12 weeks, it should be checked every 4-8 weeks. This is especially important if you have coronary artery disease, or have suffered a stroke or *transient ischemic attacks* (TIAs) in the past.

Hemoglobin in most patients receiving ribavirin decreases by 2-3 grams/dL in the first 4-8 weeks of therapy. Adding interferon does not make this side effect worse. If your hemoglobin value falls below 10 grams/dL, your health care provider will probably reduce your dose of ribavirin. Hemolytic anemia is the most common cause for reducing the dose of ribavirin, however it rarely causes therapy to be stopped. Hemoglobin levels usually increase within 4-8 weeks of completing therapy.

If you already have severe anemia, active coronary artery disease, peripheral vascular disease, or if you cannot tolerate anemia for any other reason, you are not a suitable candidate for combination therapy. Your health care provider may suggest you consider treatment with pegylated interferon monotherapy or may advise no treatment. Erythropoietin, the hormone the body produces to stimulate production of red blood cells, may be given to increase your production of red blood cells and reduce your anemia to an acceptable level to allow you to complete therapy.[60-62]

Anecdotal Story of Pegylated Interferon and Use of Erythropoietin to Manage Anemia Due to Ribavirin

A 49-year-old nurse was diagnosed with hepatitis C in 1993, two years after an accidental needle stick from a known hepatitis C patient. She also had a remote history of IV drug use in 1969. She was asymptomatic and had a normal physical exam. A liver biopsy revealed minimal nonspecific changes with no fibrosis. She had genotype 2b virus. The patient's ALT remained elevated two-fold or less above normal over the next six years. A repeat liver biopsy in 1999 showed the development of mild activity and moderate fibrosis.

The patient was treated with pegylated interferon a-2b plus ribavirin, but suffered a 5.4 gram drop in hemoglobin to a level of 8.7 grams/dL. She had severe fatigue and was unable to carry out her normal work. Ribavirin was initially stopped, allowing her hemoglobin to rise back to 10.4 grams/dL. Ribavirin was then restarted at half dose, but her hemoglobin again fell to 8.7 grams/dL. Erythropoietin therapy was added to stimulate red blood cell production. This allowed the patient to continue ribavirin therapy and to return to work with a hemoglobin of 11.0-12.1 grams/dL. Three years after completion of therapy, the patient has undetectable virus and her liver enzymes remain normal.

This patient's experience demonstrates the value of working through side effects to complete therapy if early tests show viral clearance indicating that therapy is likely to be successful.

Birth Defects

Another major concern with ribavirin is its ability to harm a developing baby. If you are a woman of child-bearing age and have not had a hysterectomy, you should have a pregnancy test prior to starting therapy, and periodically thereafter. Reliable birth control is essential during therapy as ribavirin will cause birth defects. Neither the male nor the female in a partnership can take ribavirin if the female is pregnant or could become pregnant. Ribavirin cannot be given to pregnant women, or to men or women who cannot comply with the requirement for adequate contraception for the duration of treatment and six months following discontinuation of treatment. If you are planning to have children, it is important that you discuss this with your health care provider.

MAKING THERAPY WORK

As discussed elsewhere in this manual, the most important risk factors contributing to rapid progression of hepatitis C are being over 40 years of age, being male, and drinking alcohol. Of course, you cannot change your age or sex. Therefore, the single most important thing you can do to slow progression of your hepatitis C is to eliminate all alcohol from your diet (hard liquor, beer, and wine), and avoid all products that may contain alcohol such as certain over-the-counter cough remedies, mouth washes, and other products. Remember that even so-called nonalcoholic beer contains some alcohol.

Your liver is damaged by infection with the hepatitis C virus. It has to both fight the virus and repair itself. As discussed in other chapters in this manual, a well-balanced diet will give your liver the building blocks and energy it needs to repair itself. Adequate exercise and sleep will also help the repair process and improve your immune function. Finally, a positive attitude is critical. A positive attitude helps your body fight disease and repair damage. It also makes it easier to tolerate the side effects of both the disease and its treatment.

Alternative approaches to managing the symptoms of hepatitis C and the side effects associated with interferon and ribavirin treatment are discussed elsewhere in this manual. It is critical to make sure your allopathic doctor is aware of everything you are taking so that he or she can integrate all of your medicines including both prescription drugs and over-the-counter medicines. This includes all supplements such as your daily vitamins, aspirin, cough and cold remedies, Chinese and Ayurvedic herbs, and any other nutritional supplements. In other words, you should tell your doctor about anything you ingest, put on your skin, inject, or in any other way introduce into your body. Your doctor must have the full picture in order to best advise you on your care and evaluate the results of your treatment.

The 80-80-80 Mantra

Taking combination interferon plus ribavirin therapy is not easy. It requires serious commitments from both you and your health care provider. Recent studies have shown that if you do not take at least 80% of the prescribed interferon and ribavirin doses at least 80% of the time, your chances of long-term success are dramatically reduced. Studies showed that achieving this 80-80-80 goal increased overall durable response rates to 60% among those who participated. Careful attention on the part of you and your health care provider to prevent and treat side effects, anticipate complications, and support each other in this treatment regimen will produce a high likelihood of success. Failure to make every effort to achieve at least the 80-80-80 goal described above is likely to be a fruitless exercise, wasting your effort and causing discomfort. While this goal may sound like a formidable task, remember that you are only committing to a 12-week trial. At the end of that period, it should be clear if therapy is not working and should be stopped. However, if therapy appears to be successful at 12 weeks, every effort should be made to complete the full course of treatment. In one study, 75% of patients who had an early virologic response (at 12 weeks) and completed more than 80% of their therapy achieved a sustained virologic response. Only 12% of those who discontinued therapy achieved a sustained response. Among patients who were forced for one reason or another to decrease their therapy to less than 80% but completed the full 48 weeks of treatment, 67% had durable response.[36]

REASONS FOR USING THE ALLOPATHIC APPROACH AND WHO MIGHT BENEFIT

Hepatitis C is often a silent disease in the early years of infection, but eventually progresses to liver cirrhosis, liver failure, and/or liver cancer in 20-30% of those infected. Now that successful therapy is available, these serious consequences can be avoided in over 50% of patients. Most of those infected will remain asymptomatic until the disease is quite advanced. However during this time, infected people can pass HCV on to others.

You are urged to consider combination therapy if you are in one or more of the following circumstances.

- If you have HCV genotype 2 or 3, combination therapy should be considered because the durable response rate is greater than 70-80% after 24 weeks of therapy with pegylated interferon plus ribavirin.

- If your liver biopsy shows stage 2-3 fibrosis and/or grade 2-4 necrosis/inflammation, you should consider therapy regardless of your genotype. Without treatment, you will inevitably progress to cirrhosis. Almost all serious complications and deaths due to hepatitis C are related to the development of cirrhosis.

- If you have active disease, stage 4 fibrosis (cirrhosis), and your liver disease is compensated, you should consider combination therapy because if your disease cannot be stabilized, the next step is liver transplantation.

REASONS FOR NOT USING THE ALLOPATHIC APPROACH

You may wish to wait to begin therapy if you are asymptomatic, have minimal disease on liver biopsy (stage 0-1, grade 0-1), and have no manifestations of hepatitis C outside the liver. This is particularly true if you have had the disease for over 20 years, are over 60 years of age, and/or have HCV genotype 1 or 6 (the most difficult genotypes to treat). However, even if you decide not to have treatment at this time, you will still require regular follow-up and a repeat liver biopsy in 3-5 years to look for evidence of progression.

You cannot safely take interferon if you have had a severe psychiatric condition, a history of suicide attempt(s) or suicidal thoughts, continued alcohol and/or drug abuse, severe heart disease, very low neutrophil or platelet counts, organ transplantation (except liver), and/or uncontrolled seizures. If you have *decompensated* cirrhosis, you should be promptly referred to a transplant center to be evaluated for liver transplantation. You may be put on carefully monitored therapy in an attempt to reduce HCV viral load prior to transplant.

Other conditions such as uncontrolled diabetes and hypertension, moderately decreased neutrophils (less than 1000/mm^3) or platelets (less than 75,000/ mm^3), uncontrolled autoimmune disease, psoriasis, and rheumatoid arthritis may make treatment with interferon unsafe. Your doctor will determine if it is safe for you to take interferon if you have any of these conditions.

Pregnant women and women of child-bearing age who do not use a reliable form of birth control cannot take ribavirin because of the risk of birth defects. Because ribavirin is cleared from the blood by the kidneys, patients on hemodialysis or with end-stage renal failure cannot take ribavirin. Severe anemia (hemoglobin less than 11gm/dL), *hemoglobinopathies*, or other conditions in which anemia can be dangerous may also make it unsafe to take ribavirin.

WHAT YOU NEED TO KNOW REGARDING THERAPY

There are a number of things you and your doctor need to know about your situation before you decide to begin therapy and at various stages of treatment once it has begun. Most of this information can only be gained through testing.

Before Starting Therapy

Before therapy begins, you will need to have the following tests, and discuss these aspects of your medical history.

- viral genotype
- viral load
- liver biopsy grade (inflammation/necrosis) and stage (fibrosis)
- hemoglobin level
- white blood cell count with neutrophil count
- platelet count
- cryoglobulin level
- thyroid stimulating hormone (TSH) level to check thyroid status
- electrocardiogram (EKG) if you are over 50 years of age
- presence or absence of other liver diseases (for example, hepatitis B, alcoholic liver disease, etc.), autoimmune diseases, heart or kidney disease, seizure disorder, diabetes, and/or severe lung disease
- presence or history of any psychiatric disorder, especially depression or suicidal thoughts; psychiatric consultation may be required if one of these is present
- pregnancy or ability to become pregnant and the use of appropriate means to prevent pregnancy

During Therapy

During therapy, the following tests need to be done.

- *complete blood count* (CBC) and differential cell count (neutrophils) at 2, 4, 8, and 12 weeks, and then every 4 to 8 weeks until therapy is completed

- ALT levels are usually checked at the same time points as your CBC

- TSH at 12, 24, and 48 weeks

- a standardized test for depression (for example, Beck's Inventory or the Hospital Anxiety Index) as well as a clinical evaluation for depression at the time of each visit to screen for the development of psychological problems

You must eliminate <u>all</u> alcohol and strive to take more than 80% of your prescribed interferon and ribavirin doses more than 80% of the time in order to have the best chance of achieving a durable response.

After Therapy

If your viral load is negative at the end of treatment, the following tests need be done after therapy is completed.

- ALT at 4, 12, 24, and 48 weeks
- viral level at 12, 24, and 48 weeks, or at any time your ALT becomes elevated
- yearly tests after these time points

If your viral load is not negative at the end of treatment, see *Section 3: Options for Those Whose Initial Treatment Failed to Clear the Hepatitis C Virus.*

SUMMARY

With recent advances in the treatment of chronic hepatitis C, many people are candidates for treatment. You may be a candidate for therapy if you have elevated ALT levels, other conditions related to your HCV infection, a detectable viral load, and/or chronic inflammation or fibrosis on liver biopsy. Currently, the best initial therapy is pegylated interferon plus ribavirin. This combination has resulted in a sustained response in 54-56% of patients studied in clinical trials. If you are not a candidate for combination therapy, you may be a candidate for pegylated interferon monotherapy.

Therapy for hepatitis C is rapidly changing with the primary goals of eliminating the virus, improving quality of life, and alleviating the effects of HCV infection on organs other than the liver. The recommendations for therapy will probably change every few years, and it is hoped that new approaches will provide effective therapy for the majority of people infected with hepatitis C.

WESTERN (ALLOPATHIC) MEDICINE

Section 3

**TREATMENT OPTIONS FOR THOSE
WHOSE INITIAL TREATMENT FAILED TO CLEAR
THE HEPATITIS C VIRUS**

Gregory T. Everson, MD

INTRODUCTION

Up to 56% of people who are treated with *interferon-based therapy* have sustained clearance of the hepatitis C virus (HCV) from their bodies.[1] Sustained clearance or sustained response means the virus can no longer be detected in your body even after treatment has stopped. Studies show that the lowest rates of sustained response are seen when *interferon* is given alone for a short period of time. Only 5-15% of people clear virus with this treatment given for six months.[2] The highest sustained response rates occur in people who are treated with a combination of pegylated interferon plus *ribavirin* for 12 months. The reported *sustained response* rate is 54-56% for this treatment protocol.[1, 3] The impressive increases in response rates have provided considerable hope to those seeking treatment for *hepatitis C* and those of us who treat them. However, it is still true that about half of the people treated with the maximum amount of our best current therapy still will not clear HCV.

This chapter covers a number of topics that are relevant if your initial treatment with interferon-based therapy failed to clear HCV. These topics include:

- What are the goals of retreatment?
- Who should consider retreatment?
- Should I be retreated with pegylated interferon plus ribavirin?
- What is the evidence that retreatment clears virus?
- What is the evidence that treatment slows disease progression?
- What is the evidence that treatment reduces the risk of *liver cancer*?
- Should I be screened for liver cancer? If so, what tests should be done?

WHAT ARE THE GOALS OF RETREATMENT?

There are three main reasons to consider retreatment:

- To clear the virus from your body, or if the virus cannot be eliminated,
- To slow disease progression, and
- To reduce the risk of liver cancer (as known as *hepatoma, hepatocellular carcinoma, and HCC*).

The goals of retreatment vary from person to person. Table 1 summarizes the issues doctors take into account when recommending retreatment to people with hepatitis C. Each of these issues is important. We must determine which therapy gives a particular patient the best chance to clear the virus. We must also determine if there are supportive care measures we need to take to slow the rate of injury to the liver. These measures could include reducing the amount of iron in the body, *antioxidant* therapy, and/or long-term treatment with low-dose, pegylated interferon.

Table 1: Management Issues in Retreatment of Non-responders to Previous Interferon-Based Therapy

- Attempt to eradicate HCV with pegylated interferon plus ribavirin
- Prevent disease progression
  - antioxidants (vitamin E, silymarin, vitamin C, SAMe, and others)
  - iron unloading in patients with increased iron in the liver
  - maintenance interferon
  - anti-fibrotic agents
  - others
- Detect liver cancer in patients with *fibrosis* and/or *cirrhosis*
  - *alpha-fetoprotein* every six months
  - radiologic imaging such as *ultrasound*
- Monitor for liver *decompensation* (with biochemical tests) and the need for referral to a liver transplant center

Clearing the Virus

Viral clearance is the elimination of HCV from the blood and the liver. The most common test used to measure viral load is the polymerase chain reaction (*PCR*) assay. Sustained viral clearance means HCV *RNA* is undetectable in the blood for six months or more after completing a course of *antiviral* therapy. Clearance of HCV from the blood is usually accompanied by clearance of virus from the liver. This is known as a virologic cure. A virologic cure is assumed to occur when a person maintains a sustained response for at least six months following completion of therapy. A small percentage of people (less than 5%) who have a sustained response may *relapse*, meaning the virus becomes detectable again. This sometimes occurs a year or more after therapy has ended.[4]

Certain characteristics predict the likelihood of clearing HCV with retreatment using pegylated interferon plus ribavirin.

- Relative effectiveness of prior treatment: Patients who received the least effective initial therapy are most likely to respond.
- Features of the infected person: Young individuals, women, and people without cirrhosis are more likely to respond than others are.
- Viral status: Patients with non-1 *genotype* and relatively low levels of virus are more likely to respond than others are.

Slowing Disease Progression

If viral clearance cannot be achieved, the secondary goals of treatment are to reduce the extent of liver damage, slow disease progression, and reduce the risk of complications.

A *non-responder* is at risk for disease progression and should be monitored for signs of *liver failure*. If you are a non-responder, any clinical sign of liver function deterioration should prompt your health care provider to refer you to a treatment center experienced in liver transplantation for evaluation.

Clinical information, laboratory tests, and/or *liver biopsy* results define the progression of liver disease. See *Chapter 4: Signs and Symptoms That May Be Associated With Hepatitis C* and *Chapter 5: Laboratory Tests and Procedures* for further explanation of the following criteria that point toward disease progression.

Clinical criteria:

- ankle *edema*
- *ascites*
- *encephalopathy*
- gastrointestinal bleeding from *varices*
- skin manifestations (spider telangiectasia, palmar erythema)
- varices

Blood tests:

- increased *bilirubin*
- increased *prothrombin time*
- reduced *albumin*
- reduced *platelet* and/or *neutrophil* counts

Liver biopsy findings:

- increased fibrosis
- development of cirrhosis

Despite increased awareness of the potentially serious consequences of hepatitis C, many people ignore early warning signs and only see their health care provider when they already have late-stage disease. Unfortunately, it is more difficult to treat people with late-stage disease using interferon-based therapy. Many of these patients will progress to liver failure and may ultimately need a liver transplant.

Reducing the Risk of Liver Cancer

The third goal of retreatment is to reduce or eliminate the risk of developing liver cancer. Among people with chronic hepatitis C, the risk of liver cancer is mainly limited to those with cirrhosis.[5] Screening tests for liver cancer often include twice yearly blood tests for alpha-fetoprotein and ultrasound imaging of the liver. Despite aggressive screening efforts, at least one-third of liver cancers are not detected in the early stages of the disease. Later stage tumors may not be curable with surgery, and cannot be cured with a liver transplant.

Current studies suggest but have not proven that interferon may reduce the risk of developing liver cancer.[6] It has also been suggested that interferon may slow the growth of liver cancer. This would allow more time to find the cancer at a potentially curable stage. Detection of slow growing cancers at an early stage of disease can allow effective and possibly curative therapies such as liver transplant. The new procedure *living donor liver transplantation* may be of particular benefit for people with liver cancer since it can be performed relatively quickly once the cancer has been diagnosed.[7]

WHO SHOULD CONSIDER RETREATMENT?

You may want to consider retreatment with interferon-based therapy if:

- the initial therapy you received failed to clear the virus (non-response), or
- the initial therapy cleared the virus, but the virus recurred after treatment was stopped (relapse).

Non-response

Non-response is the inability of the treatment to clear HCV both during and after a course of antiviral therapy.

There are five main reasons that a person's treatment may have failed, making him or her a non-responder.

- The type of hepatitis C infection was resistant to interferon-based treatment.
- The therapy used was inferior to best current therapy.
- The person did not comply with the prescribed treatment regimen.
- Treatment doses had to be reduced because of low levels of white cells, red cells, and/ or platelets.
- The length of treatment was reduced due to side effects and/or poor quality of life.

Relapse

Relapse is not the same as non-response. In people who relapse, the virus is undetectable during treatment, but becomes detectable again after treatment ends. Relapse is a common occurrence with interferon *monotherapy* (interferon used as single agent therapy). It is less common with the combination of interferon plus ribavirin, especially when pegylated interferon is used.

SHOULD I BE RETREATED WITH PEGYLATED INTERFERON PLUS RIBAVIRIN?

You and your doctor have a number of options if your prior treatment was interferon monotherapy and you are considering retreatment. These include:

- interferon alfa-2b plus ribavirin combination therapy,
- pegylated interferon monotherapy, or
- pegylated interferon plus ribavirin combination therapy.

There are fewer available treatment options if your initial treatment was combination therapy using interferon alfa-2b plus ribavirin. The only western treatment options for retreatment would be the combination of pegylated interferon plus ribavirin, or enrollment in a *clinical trial* involving a new, novel treatment.

The retreatment regimen with the greatest chance of clearing the virus is the combination of pegylated interferon plus ribavirin. Although there are no published trials involving retreatment of non-responders with pegylated interferon plus ribavirin, the estimated chance of response to this retreatment can be projected from the results of existing trials of previously untreated patients.[8] The estimated chances for virologic cure in non-responders after retreatment with pegylated interferon plus ribavirin are 52% for people who were previously treated with six months of interferon monotherapy, and 18-27% for people who were previously treated with 12 months of combination therapy using interferon alfa-2b plus ribavirin (see Table 2 on the following page).

Table 2: Estimated Rates of Sustained Response After Retreatment with Pegylated Interferon Plus Ribavirin

Prior Antiviral Therapy	Predicted Sustained Response (%)	
	After Retreatment with Pegylated Interferon Plus Ribavirin	
	All Patients	Patients with Genotype 1
Interferon, thrice weekly, 6 months	52%	41%
Interferon, thrice weekly, 12 months	48%	38%
Rebetron®, 6 months	35%	31%
Rebetron®, 12 months	18-27%	8-19%
Pegasys® monotherapy, 12 months	27-36%	19-34%
Peg-intron® monotherapy, 12 months	40%	33%

From <u>Living with Hepatitis C: A Survivor's Guide. 3ʳᵈ Edition.</u> Everson GT, Weinberg H. Hatherleigh Press, Inc., NY, NY. Copyright 2001**8**

This table depicts the expected rates of response to retreatment of non-responders with 48 weeks of pegylated interferon plus ribavirin. The spectrum of non-responders includes those who failed to clear HCV after short-term or long-term treatment with either interferon monotherapy or Rebetron, or those who failed 12 months of monotherapy with pegylated interferon. The derivation of the data in this table is described in Chapter 9 of reference 8.

Please note that the sustained response rates reported in this table were derived from existing literature describing the treatment of naïve patients. The response rates for non-responders listed in the table have not yet been verified by controlled clinical trials.

Your doctor may not recommend pegylated interferon plus ribavirin for clinical reasons. In this situation, options include retreatment with either interferon alfa-2b plus ribavirin or pegylated interferon monotherapy. The chance for a virologic cure with these regimens is less than that for pegylated interferon plus ribavirin. Pegylated interferon monotherapy might be preferred over interferon plus ribavirin for patients with *renal* failure, cardiac conditions, *anemia*, or for women of childbearing age.

WHAT IS THE EVIDENCE THAT RETREATMENT CAN CLEAR THE VIRUS?

The probability that retreatment will clear HCV is affected by the type of prior treatment, your personal characteristics, and viral characteristics.

For example, there is a good chance retreatment will provide virologic cure in a person without cirrhosis who did not respond to six months of interferon monotherapy, and who has less than a million copies of genotype 2b per milliliter of blood. This is true whether the person is re-treated with a combination of interferon alfa-2b plus ribavirin or pegylated interferon plus ribavirin.

In contrast, retreatment is only likely to clear virus in 8-19% of people with cirrhosis whose initial treatment was interferon alfa-2b plus ribavirin, and who have high levels of genotype 1b HCV. Virus levels greater that 2 million copies of virus per milliliter of blood are considered high. The treatment goals for a person in this situation are to slow disease progression and reduce the risk of liver cancer.

In my opinion, there is adequate evidence that retreatment of non-responders with more effective regimens can provide virologic cure for a significant proportion of patients. The best evidence comes from the retreatment of non-responders to monotherapy who were successfully retreated with the combination of interferon alfa-2b plus ribavirin.

A recent report examined multiple studies from many parts of the world in which non-responders to interferon monotherapy were retreated with six months of interferon plus ribavirin combination therapy.[9] This analysis found that 13.2% of non-responders who received this shortened course of treatment cleared HCV. Rates of viral clearance varied considerably among the studies ranging from 0-40%. In one large study from a single center, 30.6% of patients who received 6-12 months of retreatment with combination therapy achieved viral clearance.[10]

My own experience retreating people who did not respond to monotherapy has been encouraging. At our center, we recruited 96 patients into a prospective study involving 48 weeks of retreatment with interferon-alfa2b plus ribavirin. The study involved 67 men and 29 women. They ranged in age from 30 to 64. Forty-three percent had contracted HCV through intravenous drug use. Sixty-eight percent had HCV genotype 1, one of the most difficult genotypes to treat. Sixteen percent of the patients in this study had already developed cirrhosis. About 30% of those enrolled in the study had sustained viral clearance.[11]

WHAT IS THE EVIDENCE THAT TREATMENT SLOWS DISEASE PROGRESSION?

Patients treated with interferon monotherapy may potentially gain secondary clinical benefits even if the treatment fails to provide sustained virologic clearance. Potential benefits include reducing liver *inflammation* and the rate of fibrosis, slowing the rate of progression to cirrhosis, and reducing the rate of liver decompensation.

Data from existing clinical trials suggest that interferon therapy reduces liver damage. Eighty percent of people who clear virus show significant improvement on post-treatment liver biopsy. The major improvement is reduced liver injury and inflammation, but the amount of fibrosis may also decrease. Importantly, 40% of those who do **not** clear virus also show improved liver *histology* after treatment. Once again, the biggest improvement is reduced inflammation. Because inflammation stimulates fibrosis, it has been suggested that long-term interferon therapy may slow fibrosis and progression to cirrhosis.

One published trial evaluated the effectiveness of long-term interferon therapy in preventing progressive fibrosis in patients who had not responded to therapy.[12] Patients had a pre-treatment liver biopsy, and a second biopsy following a six-month course of interferon therapy. Those patients whose liver biopsies showed improvement were randomly assigned to stop interferon therapy or to continue on interferon treatment for a two year follow-up period. Those who continued interferon therapy had a reduction in liver inflammation and a decline in liver fibrosis. Those who did not continue therapy had an increase in liver inflammation and fibrosis.

The National Institutes of Health is currently conducting a multi-center clinical trial (HALT C) to determine if maintenance therapy with pegylated interferon alfa-2a blocks the progression of disease in patients with chronic hepatitis C. See *Appendix III: Western (Allopathic) Medicine* for additional information on the HALT C trial.

WHAT IS THE EVIDENCE THAT TREATMENT REDUCES THE RISK OF LIVER CANCER?

Several studies suggest that prior treatment with interferon reduces the risk of developing liver cancer. Data indicate that interferon therapy has anti-inflammatory, anti-fibrotic, and *anti-proliferative* effects. [13] These effects may slow disease progression and prevent liver cancer. The HALT C trial will examine the ability of maintenance therapy with low dose pegylated interferon alfa-2a to prevent liver cancer.

A study involving patients with cirrhosis showed that only 4% of those who were previously treated with interferon developed liver cancer, while 38% of those who were not treated with interferon went on to develop liver cancer.[14] The patients in this study were followed for an average of 4.4 years after treatment. There were two surprising aspects of this study. The first was that the reduction in cancer risk was achieved with a limited, six-month course of interferon therapy. The second was that the beneficial effect occurred in both those who cleared the virus and in those who did not.

A review article reported the results of three studies addressing the effect of interferon therapy on the development of liver cancer in hepatitis C patients with cirrhosis.[6] These three studies involved a total of 272 patients who received no treatment, 371 patients who received but did not respond to interferon treatment, and 60 patients who had a sustained response to interferon treatment. The incidence of liver cancer was 15% among those who received no treatment, 4% among those who did not respond to treatment, and 0% among those who had a sustained response. The greatest reduction in the incidence of liver cancer was among those who had sustained viral clearance. However, even those who did not respond to interferon therapy had a reduced risk of liver cancer.

The studies cited above appear to support the use of interferon therapy to prevent liver cancer in cirrhotic patients. However, analysis of these and other data suggest that clinical differences in the patients at the time of their entry into the trials and **not** interferon therapy may have been the reason for the reduced incidence of liver cancer. Additional analyses suggest that progression from cirrhosis to liver cancer may be related to such factors as HCV genotype 1b, male gender, and age greater than 60 years. This supports the unproven theory that the characteristics of the person (the host) infected with the virus and variations in the virus itself may be more important in the development of liver cancer than treatment with antiviral therapy. This conclusion was also reached in a study that reviewed the cases of 163 hepatitis C patients with cirrhosis. In these patients, the apparent reduction in the incidence of liver cancer was associated with less advanced disease among the participants.[15]

It is important to conduct properly controlled trials to determine if antiviral therapy can slow the progression of fibrosis to cirrhosis, and reduce the risk of cancer. These trials must involve large populations of hepatitis C patients who have significant fibrosis or cirrhosis, and are willing to be treated with antiviral therapy for an extended period of time. We hope the HALT C trial will allow us to determine the role of antiviral therapy in preventing of liver cancer and slowing disease progression.

SHOULD I BE SCREENED FOR LIVER CANCER?

IF SO, WHAT TESTS SHOULD BE DONE?

Because chronic hepatitis C increases your risk for liver cancer, screening is recommended for people with advanced fibrosis or cirrhosis. However, there are no screening guidelines with which everyone agrees. Liver cancer can be effectively treated if detected early. For this reason, I recommend that people with bridging fibrosis or cirrhosis have *ultrasonography* of the liver and an alpha-fetoprotein blood test every six months. A persistent, progressive rise in alpha-fetoprotein levels or the development of a new liver mass indicates the need for additional tests. These tests might include special radiologic studies of the tumor or a biopsy of the mass. If liver cancer is diagnosed, it can be treated with surgery, liver transplantation, and/or other nonsurgical approaches.

CASE HISTORIES OF RETREATMENT

Non-responder to Monotherapy

The following is a case study of a man who came to me after his initial treatment with interferon monotherapy failed to clear the virus.

> After interferon monotherapy taken three times per week for six months failed to clear HCV, this 35-year-old man consulted me for retreatment. At week 24 of his prior therapy, his *ALT* was 88 IU/L and his HCV RNA was 88,000 vEq/mL (vEq = viral equivalents). At six months following treatment, his ALT was 145 IU/L and his HCV RNA was 1,180,000 vEq/mL. His only complaints were *fatigue* and poor concentrating ability. He indicated he had no symptoms of severe liver disease such as gastrointestinal bleeding, fluid retention, or altered mental state. His physical exam was unremarkable.

> His laboratory results were: platelet count 155,000, ALT 196 IU/L, HCV RNA 1,800,000 copies/mL, and HCV genotype 2b. His most recent liver biopsy showed *grade* II inflammation and *stage* II fibrosis.

> This individual's clinical course is typical of a non-responder to monotherapy. He was treated for six months with a standard dose of interferon monotherapy, but remained HCV positive. His ALT was abnormal both during and after initial treatment. When he came to me for consultation, he had minor symptoms, an elevated ALT level, and a positive HCV RNA. His liver biopsy revealed mild-to-moderate inflammation and some increase in fibrosis, but no cirrhosis. Because he had genotype 2b HCV, he had more than a 50% chance of responding to combination antiviral treatment.

> I retreated this patient with combination therapy. His response to treatment is shown in Figure 1. His retreatment cleared HCV, and he remains free of the virus two years following retreatment.

Figure 1:

Response to IFN-alfa2b, 5 MU tiw (three times per week)
plus Ribavirin 1.2 g/day

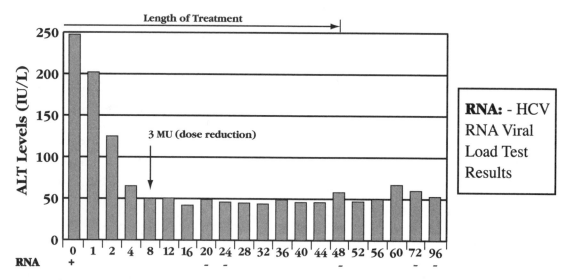

Non-responder to Combination Therapy

The following is a case study of a woman who sought consultation with me after her initial treatment with combination therapy failed. Retreatment also failed to clear the virus.

This 45-year-old woman with chronic HCV failed to respond to combination therapy. At week 48 of her initial therapy, her ALT was 68 IU/L and her HCV RNA was 182,000,000 vEq/mL. At six months following initial treatment, her ALT was 115 IU/L and her HCV RNA was 5,180,000 vEq/mL. She complained only of fatigue and poor concentrating ability.

Her laboratory results were: platelet count 115,000, ALT 226 IU/L, HCV RNA 4,800,000 copies/mL, and genotype 1b. A liver biopsy revealed grade II inflammation and stage IV fibrosis (cirrhosis).

She complained of only minor symptoms, however examination showed evidence of early liver decompensation: spider telangiectasia, an enlarged spleen, low platelets, and low albumin. Because she had genotype 1b with a viral load of almost 5 million vEq/mL, retreatment was not likely to clear the virus. Many doctors would not recommend retreatment. Because viral clearance was unlikely, the goals of therapy for this person were shifted to limiting the rate of disease progression and reducing the risk of liver cancer.

She was enrolled in the HALT C trial. The level of HCV RNA did not decline with pegylated interferon alfa-2a, but blood ALT levels declined. The patient is currently on long-term maintenance with pegylated interferon alfa-2a in the HALT C trial to try to slow progression of liver disease and reduce the risk of liver cancer.

OPTIONS FOR THOSE WHO ARE NOT CANDIDATES FOR RETREATMENT OR WHO CHOOSE NOT TO BE RETREATED

Despite many advances in antiviral treatment for HCV, some people decide against retreatment with currently available combination therapies. They may choose different therapies, or decide not to have any therapy.

Alternatives to interferon-based treatment protocols include:

- Western clinical trials
    - protease, *helicase*, or *polymerase* inhibitors
    - interferon plus ribavirin-like drugs or IMPDH inhibitors such as *mycophenolate mofetil*
- *Complementary and alternative medicine therapies (CAM)*, or
- No treatment.

Factors such as religious beliefs, lifestyle, lack of financial resources or insurance coverage, and/or health conditions that might make undergoing existing interferon-based treatment difficult can affect the decision each person makes.

Clinical Trials

If you are being treated at a major teaching hospital and/or by a hepatitis C specialist, you may have access to any of a number of clinical trials. Some of these trials will study new formulations of standard interferon and other antiviral agents. Others will be looking at completely new drugs or new approaches to the treatment of hepatitis C. Talk with your doctor about which of these trials might be available and appropriate for you. The Internet is a good source of information about clinical trials. Check the *Resource Directory* at the back of this manual for Internet addresses.

Many new drugs are under development and preliminary evaluation of them may have a therapeutic role in the management of those who do not respond to conventional, interferon-based therapy. These options may include thymosin alpha-1, histamine analogues, oligonucleotides, *amantadine* and its *analogues*, inhibitors of IMPDH, and protease inhibitors. To date, none of these agents has been completely evaluated, nor have they been shown to slow disease progression or reduce the risk of liver cancer.

Complementary and Alternative Medicine

If your treatment with western medicine failed to clear the virus and there is little hope that retreatment will be successful, you may choose a CAM treatment approach. Treatment strategies for most CAM approaches are generally focused on reducing the amount and rate of liver damage caused by the virus and slowing the progression of liver fibrosis.

CAM approaches include antioxidant therapy, Chinese herbal remedies, and Ayurvedic practices, among others. The rationale, goals, and objectives of these treatment approaches are described in other chapters of this manual.

Because of the lack of controlled clinical trials for many of the CAM approaches, there is no concrete evidence of their effectiveness in clearing HCV, slowing disease progression, or reducing the risk of liver cancer.

No Treatment

You may decide against retreatment with any of the above options. This is a personal decision, but it must be made after you have carefully weighed the information concerning the natural progression of hepatitis C and the various treatment options. The reasons why people choose not to be treated vary. Often, these decisions are related to cost, inconvenience, and the severity of side effects of the treatments.

There are major health issues that are important for you to understand even if you elect not to be retreated. You need to understand the natural history of hepatitis C and the long-term consequences of infection. You need to know how the virus affects other parts of the body in addition to the liver. This is particularly crucial if you have advanced fibrosis or cirrhosis. If you have advanced fibrosis or cirrhosis, you are at risk for liver deterioration, liver failure, and the development of liver cancer. You may eventually need a liver transplant. Your doctor or health care provider will need to regularly examine you for signs of clinical deterioration and may order tests to screen for the development of liver cancer.

SUMMARY

This chapter addresses several important clinical issues for an increasingly large population of patients with chronic hepatitis C: those in whom treatment failed to clear HCV. You have been provided with information to help you determine if you should consider retreatment with pegylated interferon plus ribavirin. You have also learned about some of the issues surrounding maintenance interferon.

The goals of retreatment are to clear virus, slow disease progression, and reduce the risk of liver cancer. This chapter identifies criteria for selection of patients for retreatment and provides definitions for response. Studies are summarized that provide information on expected response rates should you elect to undergo retreatment with interferon-based therapy.

Results from past and current clinical trials suggest retreatment can clear virus in a subset of non-responders. They also show that viral clearance is especially dependent upon viral genotype. Even if you fail to clear virus, there is evidence that suggests you may still benefit from retreatment by slowing disease progression and reducing your risk for liver cancer. Definitive clinical trials such as HALT C are currently underway to attempt to prove whether these impressions from smaller trials are accurate. Regardless of whether you decide on retreatment, if you have advanced fibrosis or cirrhosis you must have regular clinical follow-up to monitor for liver decompensation, liver failure, and the development of liver cancer.

WESTERN (ALLOPATHIC) MEDICINE
Section 4
THE FUTURE OF ALLOPATHIC TREATMENT
FOR HEPATITIS C
Robert G. Gish, MD

INTRODUCTION

Despite ongoing advances in treatment options for *chronic hepatitis* C infection, more effective and safer treatments are clearly still needed. About one-half of people infected with the hepatitis C virus (HCV) worldwide will not have a long-term response to our best current western therapy, nor to any of the western therapies on the immediate horizon.

Hopefully, we will soon find out exactly how HCV infects human cells. This will tell us more about the receptor sites that allow HCV to enter cells, and the processes in liver cells that allow HCV to thrive. We also need to learn more about the virus itself. We need to know more about its protein make-up. We need to gain a better understanding of how the *immune system* responds to the virus. Finally, we need a better understanding of disease progression. What causes *hepatitis C* to progress in some people but not in others? All of this information will lead to the development of new *antiviral* agents. These new therapies may be used as single agents. However, it is more likely that new therapies will be used in combination with current agents such as *interferon* or interferon plus *ribavirin*.

This section discusses some of western medicinescurrently being studied as potential treatments for hepatitis C. Though some of the concepts are technical and may be challenging to understand, try not to let that keep you from seeing what the future might hold for hepatitis C treatment. Many of the medical and technical terms are defined in the *Glossary*. These definitions should make it easier for you to understand the concepts in this section.

PEGYLATED INTERFERON

Scientists have recently learned how to attach molecules called polyethylene glycol (peg) to different sites on the interferon molecule. The result is *pegylated interferon* or peginterferon. Pegylated interferon molecules are not cleared by the kidneys as quickly as molecules of standard alpha 2a and 2b interferon. They remain active in the body for a much longer period.[1, 2] In theory, long-acting pegylated interferons deliver a more constant interferon dose than standard interferons. Because the drug is not rapidly cleared from the body, pegylated interferon can be given once a week. The effects of weekly pegylated interferon on the immune system and the virus are an enhanced version of the effects produced by standard interferon taken three times a week, once or twice each day.

The Food and Drug Administration (FDA) approved Peg-Intron® (pegylated interferon alfa 2b) as single agent therapy for treatment of chronic hepatitis C in January 2001. It was approved for use in combination with ribavirin (*Rebetol*®) in August 2001. Pegasys® (pegylated interferon alfa 2a) was approved by the FDA for use as monotherapy in October 2002. It is expected to be evaluated for use in combination with ribavirin in late 2002 or early 2003. The sustained response rates with these two interferons in combination with ribavirin are approximately 55%. Differences between the two treatment combinations are subtle and will only be defined if there is a large head-to-head *clinical trial*. Emerging data show that overall response rates with pegylated interferon plus ribavirin may be in the 60% range, and nearly 50% in patients with HCV *genotype* 1 virus. These numbers would apply to those patients who take more than 80% of the prescribed medicines for the full time interval specified by their genotype or *viral load*.

A *phase II trial* involving previously untreated hepatitis C patients without *cirrhosis* suggested that 180 micrograms of pegylated interferon alpha 2a is the optimal dose. The results showed a 36% sustained response rate with pegylated interferon compared to a 5% sustained response rate with interferon alpha 2a. A larger *phase III trial* involving 1,219 patients compared pegylated interferon alpha 2b with standard alpha 2b. The sustained response was 24% with pegylated interferon alpha 2b compared to 12% with interferon alpha 2b.[3, 4, 5]

Only two trials have evaluated pegylated interferon in patients with cirrhosis and compensated liver disease. One of the trials enrolled only patients with cirrhosis. This study found a 29% sustained response rate with pegylated interferon alpha 2a compared to a 6% response rate with interferon alpha 2a. In the other international, multi-center trial, 28% of the patients had cirrhosis. This group of patients had an overall sustained response rate of 39% for pegylated interferon alpha 2a compared to a 19% sustained response rate for interferon alpha 2a.[6]

Early studies indicate there may be a difference in the sustained response rates between pegylated interferon alpha 2a and pegylated interferon alpha 2b. However, the data from these studies have not been analyzed by HCV genotype and viral load, which could influence study results. Further, these are not head-to-head studies. Therefore, no conclusion can be made about the differences in overall effectiveness between these two forms of pegylated interferon. Only a detailed analysis of these trials will tell us if there is a difference between the two currently available pegylated interferons.

We do not yet know how effective either type of pegylated interferon will be when given with ribavirin in the general public. See *Section 3* of this chapter for the clinical trial results on this therapy. Pegylated therapies are currently being investigated. Ongoing studies will tell us if these agents have an equal or better side effect profile than other therapies. They will also tell us how the addition of ribavirin will affect the side effect profile of pegylated interferon.

THERAPIES THAT MODULATE THE IMMUNE RESPONSE

Vaccines

Vaccine research has historically centered on trying to prevent infection. Recently, vaccine research has taken a new direction. The trend has been toward developing vaccines capable of protecting people from chronic infection, or modifying the course of a chronic infection. There are preliminary data suggesting an HCV vaccine used in chimpanzees can stimulate them to make *antibodies* and inflammatory *CD4+ T-cell* (immune cell) responses. The vaccine is made of recombinant envelope proteins, proteins on the outside of the virus. The antibody and T-cell response prevented chronic infection in the majority of the animals in this very small study.[7] Recent advances in recombinant protein technology, novel adjuvants, and *DNA*-based vaccines will play a major role in providing new techniques for the development of HCV vaccines.

Despite these data, there are several reasons it will probably take many years to develop an HCV vaccine.

- In the past, the virus was found only in humans and chimpanzees. The recent discovery at the University of Alberta, Canada of a mouse model that supports HCV replication should help dramatically advance drug development and vaccine research.[8]
- The virus is highly susceptible to *mutation*, making it difficult for antibodies to provide long-term protective *immunity*.
- The virus can avoid being detected by the human immune system.
- The body's neutralizing antibodies (specific CD4 and *CD8* T-cells) are not efficiently produced.
- The virus can easily become resistant to treatments. These resistant viruses are spread to others.
- The virus replicates poorly in cell cultures in the laboratory.

MOLECULAR APPROACHES TO THE DEVELOPMENT OF NEW THERAPIES

Although there are many variations of HCV, one part is the same in all variants. This part is called the 5' untranslated region, or 5'UTR.[9] Scientists have learned how to add molecules called *antisense molecules* to this region of the virus. These additions can prevent the virus from replicating, thereby making it unable to cause disease. Early clinical trials have recently begun to evaluate the safety of this new approach in humans. The development of one antisense product has been slowed after finding liver *enzyme* elevations greater than 1,000 IU/mL in patients who were treated for a short time.

Another approach uses a normal cell enzyme called a *ribozyme*. Ribozymes are special *RNA* molecules that can be modified to attach to and break other RNA molecules. Researchers are working on ribozymes that can disrupt HCV RNA sequences (specific pieces of RNA) that are required for the virus to replicate. If the virus cannot replicate, it cannot cause disease. Recently, synthetic ribozymes have been developed to specifically target and break up the 5'UTR portion of the HCV RNA. These synthetic anti-HCV ribozymes have been tested in cell cultures and in animals. Unfortunately, there have been serious side effects in the animals tested and development has been halted for the time being.

PRODUCTS DERIVED FROM THYMUS EXTRACTS

Thymosin fraction 5 and thymosin a-1 are *cytokines* derived from the *thymus gland*. Cytokines are *proteins* produced by many cell types in the body. Cytokines produce specific reactions. The thymus gland is important in the immune system's ability to fight infections. These thymus-derived proteins appear to be able to change a person's response to HCV infection.[10] They may be able to prevent a chronic infection, or slow or halt disease progression.

Thymosin a-1 is an immune-stimulating protein. It has been found in less than normal amounts in the blood of patients chronically infected with the *hepatitis B* virus (HBV).[11] Initial studies in animals and humans infected with HBV suggest that thymosin a-1 and thymosin factor 5 increase the rate of clearance of HBV *DNA* (the genetic material of the virus). Tests in animals and in people in these studies show a change from positive to negative for the hepatitis B surface *antigen* (*HBsAg*) which is one marker for the presence of the HBV.[12, 13, 14] However, another study showed no difference between thymosin a-1 and a *placebo* (an inactive substance). Therefore, the results from these various studies are mixed. The same response can probably be expected in studies on HCV. Thymosin a-1 has been approved in more than 20 countries for the treatment of patients with viral hepatitis infections. A large study of thymosin in combination with Pegasys® (without ribavirin) is now in progress in the U.S.

Cytokines such as interleukin-10 (an anti-fibrotic agent), interleukin-2, and interleukin-12 have not shown any significant antiviral or antifibrosis activity.

MODULATING HCV ACTIVITY WITH IMMUNE GLOBULIN

There is evidence that up to 15% of those who become infected with HCV clear the virus through some naturally occurring immune process. HCV has the ability to rapidly change its genetic structure. This helps the virus survive by allowing it to escape detection and recognition by both *B cells* (immune cells that produce antibodies called globulins) and *T cells* (other cells that are directly involved in the body's immune response). Civicir, an antibody preparation targeted specifically to HCV, is now in clinical trials for HCV-infected patients after liver transplantation.

TARGETING FUNCTIONAL SITES IN THE HCV GENOME

The HCV *genome* (the genetic material of the virus) has been studied extensively over the last nine years.[15, 16, 17, 18] From these studies, we have been able to identify various HCV proteins involved in different steps of viral replication including *translation* and packaging. Each of these proteins is a potential target for antiviral therapy. As they are produced, drug developers will test them for activity against HCV.

The first step in the development of new treatments for HCV is identifying antiviral compounds that can be taken by mouth. This will allow them to reach the liver in an active state so that the cells in the liver can take them up. Of course, these products must inhibit viral replication and be safe for the users. As we have found with HIV treatment, the best HCV treatment will probably involve using multiple drugs. If antiviral drugs can be used with cytokines such as interferon, they could dramatically decrease the level of viral replication, mutation, and diversity. The hope is that this kind of drug combination would result in cure. It is likely that doctors will one day be using a cocktail of antiviral therapies (a group of drugs taken in combination) to treat the millions of people worldwide who are HCV-infected.

One enzyme, the HCV RNA-dependent RNA *polymerase*, is responsible for the replication of the entire HCV genome.[18] It may be possible to develop drugs that target this enzyme and prevent the replication of the virus. These drugs would need to very closely resemble the enzyme in order to act at the enzyme's active site. X-ray crystallographic data have identified the three-dimensional structure of the HCV *RNA* polymerase. This discovery will allow drug design to move forward.[19] By blocking the replication of the complete viral genome, mutation rates may also be decreased. If mutation is limited, the escape of mutant viruses from detection by the immune system may occur less often. In addition, the production of special enzymes called *proteinases* that are required to produce smaller viral proteins should be decreased. The result would be a fall in the production of complete viral particles.

Other areas within the HCV genome are also likely targets for drug development. These are the *helicase* enzyme, the internal ribosomal entry site (IRES), and the interferon sensitivity-determining region (ISDR). Each of these areas is being studied carefully by drug developers as possible antiviral targets. Despite the promise of these proteinase, helicase, and RNA-dependent RNA polymerase inhibitors, development of these agents has been slowed by the lack of suitable cell culture or animal models to use for testing these new agents. It has been difficult for drug developers to test the many thousands of possible compounds that must be developed before one is found that is effective and safe. Hopefully, the recent development of a mouse model will speed up this process, but for now, that remains to be seen.

Alpha glucosidase inhibitors and similar medications have an apparent ability to inhibit viral packaging (the way the various parts of the virus are put together). This ability makes them candidates for treating and suppressing HCV replication. This approach may greatly reduce the ability of HCV to develop resistance to treatment.[20] New ribavirin-like products such as VX497, Levovirin®, and Viramidine® may also have a role in expanding combination therapy for HCV. *Mycophenolate mofetil* is a new *immunosuppressant* that blocks an important enzyme called inosine monophosphate dehydrogenase (IMPDH). However, it appears to a have a very weak effect on HCV replication and has not shown any benefit in the treatment of HCV.

HCV attaches to liver cells and other cells through the *CD81 receptor* (an attachment site on the cell surface).[21, 22] Molecules that block the attachment of the virus to the human cell would prevent the virus from entering the cell. This is another area of active research.

Many scientists were excited to hear that currently available drugs may aid in the treatment of hepatitis C. These drugs include *amantadine* (an antiviral agent used to treat influenza), over-the-counter non-steroidal anti-inflammatory drugs (NSAIDs) such as ibuprofen, and COX-2 inhibitors. Although studies to date have not found these medications to be effective in reducing viral levels in the *serum* or liver, they remain an area of great interest to researchers.

FUTURE NON-WESTERN TREATMENTS

One of the goals of *complementary and alternative medicine (CAM)* is to prove that CAM therapies have a role in the treatment of hepatitis C. This is important for both people whose lives are affected by HCV and health care providers who treat them. The role of herbal and other therapies in controlling *arthralgia, myalgia*, mental fogginess, and *fatigue* is clear to individual patients. However, large, controlled trials are required to prove that these agents have a role in *symptom* management across diverse populations.

Large studies would also be able to define which type of therapy is best and most beneficial to specific subgroups of HCV patients. For instance, herbal therapy may benefit patients with joint pain. Acupuncture may benefit patients with pain in the liver area. Studies could clarify whether the use of CAM approaches may be beneficial and safe in combination with western therapies such as *interferon-based treatment*. Such studies could also determine if CAM therapies may be useful to control side effects of western therapies.

Safety is an issue that needs to be addressed since many CAM therapies have been *anecdotally* reported to cause side effects that may be serious. We need to discover the actual incidence of these reported side effects and document their severity with carefully designed clinical studies.

Proving the presence or absence of direct antiviral effects of non-western therapy is also important. Certain practitioners have claimed cures with many therapies, but these cases are poorly documented. Larger studies are needed to discover which, if any, CAM agents have *clinical* benefit. Herbal remedies may actually decrease liver inflammation, the early component of liver disease that can lead to scar tissue and eventually cirrhosis. Prevention of the development of cirrhosis would be of great benefit to patients with chronic HCV who cannot be cured with interferon or *combination therapy*.

Chapter Nine

AYURVEDIC MEDICINE

Shri K. Mishra MD, MS, Bharathi Ravi, BAMS (Ayurveda)
and Sivaramaprasad Vinjamury, MD (Ayurveda)

INTRODUCTION

Ayurveda is a natural system of medicine that has been practiced in India for more than 5,000 years. It was developed by the seers (*rishis*) through centuries of observation, experiments, discussion, and meditation. For several thousand years, Ayurvedic teachings were passed down orally from teacher to student. The origins of Ayurvedic medicine are recorded in the *Atharva Veda,* one of the four Vedic scriptures.[1] The first summary of these teachings was put into writing around 1500 B.C. The main sources of knowledge are the three Vedic classics: *Charaka Samhita, Susruta Samhita,* and *Ashtanga Hridaya.*[2]

Ayurveda is a Sanskrit word made up of two components, *ayush* meaning life and *veda* meaning knowledge or science. Hence, Ayurveda is the 'science of life.' The teachings of this ancient system of medicine are written in Sanskrit, the ancient language of India and Hinduism. It is based on Indian or Vedic philosophy. Ayurveda was the first holistic system of diagnosis and treatment integrating nutrition, hygiene, rejuvenation, and herbal medicine. Ayurvedic medicine considers the human body to be in balance with nature. The body is believed to be a dynamic and resilient system that can cope with all stresses from its environment while maintaining the ability to heal itself.[3,4]

The main objectives of Ayurveda are to maintain and promote health by preventing physical, mental, and spiritual ailments, and to cure disease through natural medicine, diet, and a regulated lifestyle. Ayurveda tries to help us live a long and healthy life, achieve our fullest potential, and express our true inner nature on a daily basis.[4] The Ayurvedic classic Charaka Samhita defines Ayurveda as "the knowledge that indicates the appropriate and inappropriate, happy or sorrowful conditions of living, what is auspicious or inauspicious for longevity, as well as the measure of life itself." [5]

BASIC CONCEPTS OF AYURVEDA

It will be helpful to understand a few important concepts and some Ayurvedic terminology before you decide whether you want to include Ayurveda in your hepatitis C treatment plan. The next few pages will provide a brief review of Ayurvedic concepts on which the diagnosis and treatment of any ailment are based.

Pancha-Maha-Bhoota Theory

According to Ayurvedic philosophy, the entire cosmos is made up of the energies of five elements: earth, water, fire, air, and ether (space). Even the human body and herbs are made up of these elements. Collectively, these elements are called *pancha-maha-bhootas,* or material particles. The material particles and the anti-material particles (the spirit) form the cognitive aspect of a living being. The predominance of a particular element(s) determine the characteristics of a thing, whether it is an animal, a person, or an herb. The medicinal properties of a drug or herb are determined by the characteristics it exhibits. Similarly, depending upon the relative amounts of the elements, each of us exhibits a unique set of physical and mental characteristics. A disease state changes these characteristics. This change is the basis for the diagnosis and treatment of disease. In prescribing a remedy, the doctor chooses a treatment with the opposite characteristics of the disease to counteract the *symptoms*.

Tri-Dosha Theory

According to Ayurvedic theory, there are three humors in the body called *doshas*. These determine the constitution of a person and also the life processes of growth and decay. The doshas are genetically determined. The three doshas are *vata*, *pitta,* and *kapha*. Each dosha is made up of the five fundamental elements. Each dosha is responsible for several body functions. When the doshas are healthy and balanced, this is the state of good health. Imbalances cause disease. Ayurveda recognizes that different foods, tastes, colors, and sounds affect the doshas in different ways. For example, very hot and pungent spices aggravate pitta. Cold, light foods such as salads calm it down. This ability to affect the doshas is the underlying basis for Ayurvedic practices and therapies.

Vata

Vata is composed of space and air. It is the subtle energy associated with all voluntary and involuntary movement in the human body. It governs breathing, blinking, muscle and tissue movement, and the heart beat. It is also responsible for all urges. Creativity, flexibility, and the ability to initiate things are seen when vata is in balance. Indecision, restlessness, anxiety, and fear occur when vata is out of balance. Vata is the motivating force behind the other two humors. In modern medicine, the *physiological* role of vata is in the central and peripheral nervous systems.[6,7,8] Vata has a tendency to expand indefinitely and to disturb the nervous activity or the vital forces in the body.

Pitta

Pitta is composed of fire and water. It is responsible for all digestive and metabolic activities. It governs body temperature, complexion, visual perception, hunger, and thirst. In a balanced state, pitta promotes intelligence, understanding, and courage. Out of balance, pitta produces insomnia, burning sensations, inflammation, infection, anger, and hatred. Pitta is the humor involved in liver disorders.[6,7,8] Pitta has a tendency to become more liquid and to weaken the digestive and biochemical processes in the body.

Kapha

Kapha is composed of water and earth. It provides the strength and stability for holding body tissues together. Kapha is the hydrodynamic aspect of the body. It also provides lubricants at the various points of friction in the body. In balance, kapha is responsible for wisdom, patience, and memory. Out of balance, kapha causes looseness of the limbs, *lethargy,* greed, and generalized sluggishness or *hypoactivity*. This dosha maintains body resistance to disease.[6,7,8] Kapha has a tendency to thicken and obstruct the passages of the body and damage the process of lubrication.

Sapta-Dhatu Theory

Ayurvedic theory states the human body is composed of seven tissues called *dhatus*.

1   plasma and *interstitial* fluids (*rasa*)
2   blood (*rakta*)
3   muscle (*mamsa*)
4   fat or adipose tissue (*medas*)
5   bone (*asthi*)
6   *bone marrow* (*majja*)
7   reproductive tissue (*sukra*)

Kapha is specifically responsible for plasma, muscle, fat, marrow, and semen. Pitta creates blood. Vata creates bone. Diseases of the humors are usually reflected in the tissues they govern. When out of balance, the humors can enter any tissue, in addition to those they govern, and cause disease.[6,7,8]

Malas

The quantities and qualities of the three excreta from the body, sweat (*sweda*), feces (*mala*) and urine (*mutra*), and other body waste products play an important role in the diagnosis and treatment of disease. The Sanskrit word for these waste products is *malas.* [6,7,8]

Tripod

Tripod includes the doshas, dhatus and malas. They maintain health when they are in equilibrium and produce disease when they are not.

Srotas

The human body has numerous channels to allow the flow of energy, nutrients, and waste products. These channels are called *srotas*. Some of the srotas such as the alimentary canal (the digestive channel that runs from the mouth to the anus) are very large. Some are small such as arteries and veins. Others are very minute such as the capillaries, nerve terminals, and the lymphatics. Some srotas carry nutritional materials to the tissues of the body. Other srotas carry waste materials out of the body. The three doshas are present in every part of the body and move through every srota. Blockage or improper flow within the srotas produces an ailment. The physical channels are similar to the different systems of western medicine such as the digestive system, respiratory system, and cardiovascular system. Diseases are classified according to the systems they involve.[9]

Agni and Aama

Poor functioning of the digestive system leads to many diseases. The digestive fire or *agni* controls the activities of digestion. According to Ayurveda, digestion is the cornerstone of good health. Good digestion nourishes the body. Eating the correct foods makes a big difference in your well-being. Agni helps the body produce secretions and generates the metabolic processes necessary to create energy, and maintain and repair the body.[10] Agni is also part of the immune system since its heat destroys harmful organisms and *toxins*. There are 13 agnis. The activity of agni varies throughout the day. A natural ebb and flow of your digestive fire is necessary for good digestion, good immune function, and resistance to disease.[11]

The opposite side of this process is *aama*. Aama is defined as imperfectly metabolized food or drugs. In other words, an aama is a toxin that needs to be eliminated from the body. Aama is usually generated in the body because of weak digestive fire or *jatharagni*.[12] It is also believed that aama is produced by out of balance doshas. Aama gets mixed up with the tissues and causes disease by clogging the channels. Out of balance pitta, dosha, and poor agni play important roles in the symptoms liver disorders.

Ojas

Ojas is the essential energy of the immune system. It is a unique concept of Ayurveda that embodies a subtle essence of all the tissues in the body. In other words, ojas is the glue that cements the body, mind, and spirit together, integrating them into a functioning individual. Proper agni is required for proper production of ojas. Ojas decreases with age. Low ojas levels cause chronic degenerative and immunological diseases.[13] In western medicine, ojas would be similar to *immunoglobulins* and other *immunomodulators* like *cytokines*. Abnormalities of ojas lead to decreased immunity, making a person more vulnerable to infections including hepatitis.

Prakruti and Gunas

The proportion of the humors varies from person to person. One humor is usually predominant and leaves its mark on a person's appearance and disposition. Based on the predominant humor, every person is born with a unique mind-body constitution called *prakruti*. *Gunas* denote a person's mental make up and are of three types: *satva* (perfect), *rajas* (semi-balanced), and *tamas* (unbalanced). A person's prakruti is determined at the time of conception. Every person has specific physical, mental, and emotional characteristics. These characteristics are called a person's constitution. Prakruti must be considered in determining natural healing approaches and recommendations for daily living.[14]

DEFINITION OF HEALTH

Ayurveda defines health as "the equilibrium of the three biological humors [doshas], the seven body tissues [dhatus], proper digestion, and a state of pleasure or happiness of the soul, senses, and the mind." [15] This definition dates back to 1500 B.C. and is described in Sushruta Samhita, the surgical compendium of Ayurveda.

A balance among the three doshas is necessary for health. Together, the three doshas govern all metabolic activities. When their actions in our mind-body constitution are balanced, we experience psychological and physical wellness. When they go slightly out of balance, we may feel uneasy. When they are more obviously unbalanced, symptoms of sickness can be observed and experienced.[16,17]

PATHOGENESIS OF DISEASE

Ayurveda asserts that each person is unique, made up of specific characteristics that are his or her own. This means that in order to protect or preserve your health, you need to follow a diet and lifestyle that will create balance with **your** constitution or internal environment. Such a lifestyle keeps the humors at normal levels. Aggravating factors such as diet, climate, seasons, emotions, and lifestyle can make the humors go out of balance. Imbalance weakens the digestive fire and increases the production of toxins. The toxins along with the out of balance humor(s) block the channels and disrupt the energy and nutrition flow to that particular tissue. The result is that the tissue involved in the process becomes diseased.[17] This happens in six stages: accumulation, aggravation, overflow, relocation, manifestation, and diversification.[18]

Classification of Diseases

Various diseases are produced by imbalances of specific humors in specific tissues. Diseases are classified as vata, pitta, or kapha disorders, and combinations of these three. Based on the predominant humor, 80 vata, 40 pitta, and 20 kapha disorders have been identified. There is further classification of the disorders based on the physiological systems or srotas involved. Most diseases of the organ systems are further sub-classified and are named after the predominant humor, tissue, or organ involved in the disease process.[19]

Diagnosis of Disease

Diagnosis in Ayurveda is done in eight parts. Disease is diagnosed by taking a detailed history of the causative factors, *prodromal symptoms, cardinal signs* and symptoms, and the aggravating and relieving factors.[20] The affected humor and tissue are identified for treatment. Various methods are used to help acquire information during an assessment. These methods are very similar to other medical disciplines and include questioning, observation, *palpation,* direct perception, and inference. Techniques such as taking the pulse, observing the tongue and eyes, noting the physical symptoms, and examinations of urine and stool are employed during an assessment.[21] The pulse is one of the important tools in diagnosing the constitution of an individual and the humors involved in a disease. In some cases, the pulse can identify the *stage* of the disease. Pulse diagnosis gets more accurate as the Ayurvedic practitioner gains experience.[22]

Prognosis of Diseases

Ayurveda is not a cure for all ailments and all stages of disease. Diseases are classified based on their *prognosis.*

- Easily curable: recent onset, one humor involved; example - digestive disorders
- Difficult to cure: chronic, one or two humors involved; example - most skin disorders
- Chronic with maintenance therapy: two or more humors involved, or chronic and metabolic diseases; examples - diabetes and *hepatitis C*
- Incurable: all three humors involved with associated complications; example - cancer
- Terminally ill: the chance of continued life is very bleak

If the first two stages of a disease are not treated properly, they can progress to become a chronic disease with maintenance therapy or could end up as incurable.[23]

PRINCIPLES OF AYURVEDIC TREATMENT

The first goal of Ayurveda is health promotion and disease prevention. The second goal is to treat physical, mental, and spiritual illness. Ayurveda teaches that separating mind and spirit from the body creates physical imbalance, the first step in the disease process. It naturally follows that reintegration of mind, spirit, and body is the first step toward healing. The goal of treatment for any disease is to restore the balance of the humors to reestablish a person's original constitution. This is achieved by adjusting the factors responsible for causing disease. A combination of herbs, bodywork, and lifestyle changes are suggested for the treatment of a disease or ailment. Dietary advice is also an important component of Ayurvedic treatment. The practitioner will suggest a specific diet that helps eliminate or slow the progression of disease. Finally, yoga and meditation are advised because they are integral to Ayurvedic treatment. Treatment recommendations are based on a person's constitution, current health imbalances, and the time of year.[15, 24]

The humors are balanced and toxins are eliminated from the body through cleansing therapies known as *panchakarma.* Panchakarma is another hallmark of Ayurvedic treatment. Panchakarma is comprised of five parts: emesis, purgation, cleansing enemas, retention enemas, and cleansing nasal medication.[2]

After panchakarma, *rasayana* (rejuvenation therapy) is recommended. This helps enhance immune function and also helps the person have a longer, healthier life.

AYURVEDIC MEDICINE AND HEPATITIS C

The liver is called *yakrit* in Ayurveda. Pitta is the predominant humor of the liver. Most liver disorders are aggravated conditions of pitta. Excessive *bile* production or a blockage in the flow of bile usually indicates high pitta, which in turn affects the agni or *enzyme* activities responsible for absorption, digestion, and metabolism.

Diet and lifestyle activities that aggravate pitta include:

- alcohol abuse
- red meat
- spicy, oily, heavy foods
- lack of sleep
- too much direct exposure to the sun, and
- smoking.

Aggravation of the pitta causes such liver diseases as fatty liver, *cirrhosis*, and hepatitis. All types of viral hepatitis are of relatively recent discovery, so there is obviously no mention of them in the classic Ayurvedic texts. Nevertheless, one can find similar symptoms described under *kaamala*.[26,27]

Ayurveda describes two basic types of kaamala (hepatitis or jaundice).

- *Shakhasrita* is caused by the minimal aggravation of pitta and kapha, and is easily curable.
- *Kumbha kaamala* results from very high pitta and is difficult to cure. It can become incurable if not attended to immediately.

Panaki and *haleemaka* are two other types of hepatitis or *jaundice* that are explained in Ayurvedic texts. Panaki is late stage kaamala. Haleemaka is an advanced stage of *anemia* that occurs when both the vata and pitta are out of balance.[26]

Pathogenesis

Excessive intake of alcohol, and hot, spicy, sour, or contaminated food or water aggravate pitta. When pitta is out of balance, the liver causes disease in the blood, muscle tissue, and biliary system. This manifests as kaamala or jaundice. It is believed that an anemic and/or immunocompromised person is more prone to this ailment.

Symptoms of kaamala include:

- loss of appetite and taste
- generalized weakness
- yellowish discoloration of the eyes, nails, oral cavity, and urine
- vague body pains
- burning sensation, and
- weakness in all sensory organs.

In extreme cases, *emaciation* is also seen. All these symptoms signify the involvement of the immune system in infectious hepatitis. Ayurveda teaches that hepatitis involves the gastrointestinal system, cardiovascular system, musculoskeletal system, and the skin.[26, 27, 28]

Symptoms such as generalized *edema* (shotha), excessive thirst (atitrishna), bloody stools (*krishna varna mala mutra*), vomiting blood (*rakta yukta chardi*), red eyes (*rakta netra*), dizziness (*bhrama*), drowsiness (*tandra*), total loss of appetite (*teevra agni mandya*), and *hepatic* coma (*nashta sanjna*) indicate that the liver disease is at an incurable stage, and the patient is believed to be terminally ill.[29]

Diagnosis of Liver Disorders and Hepatitis C

A diagnosis of liver disease is suggested by *signs* and symptoms such as loss of appetite, fatigue, jaundice, occasional vomiting, and mild fever. The determination of the type of liver disease is made according to the severity of the symptoms. The magnitude of pitta aggravation is diagnosed through pulse reading, observing the eyes and tongue, and palpating the abdomen. Important parts of the examination include assessments of the person's constitution, physical strength, and mental state. Other information is also gathered such as whether the person lives or has lived on the coast, far inland, or in the mountains, and his or her lifestyle.[29, 30]

Treatment of Liver Disorders and Hepatitis C

Ayurveda advocates a specific treatment for every ailment. The objective of any treatments is to return balance to the affected dosha. Reestablishing a person's constitution is always an important component of therapy. The method used to achieve constitutional balance could be elimination, palliation, or both.

The treatment of liver disorders usually involves a combination of herbs, bodywork, dietary advice, lifestyle changes, yoga, and meditation. It is important to follow a specific diet and curtail excessive activities. Depending on the physical state of the person, the treatment begins with a mild laxative either limited to the start of treatment, or taken daily. If the person is unable to tolerate the laxative, it is stopped and treatment proceeds to the next step. After cleansing, oral medications are given two or three times a day. These medications can be herbal concoctions, powders, pills, fermented syrups, and/or herbs processed in clarified butter (ghee). The dosage, form, and combination of medications are selected depending upon the patient's constitution, stage of disease, and physical condition. Only an experienced Ayurvedic health care provider can make appropriate medication recommendations. Though special emphasis is placed on agni in all instances, it is given more importance when treating liver disorders.[26, 27, 28, 31]

For descriptions of the herbs used to treat liver disorders in Ayurvedic medicine, see *Appendix IV: Ayurvedic Medicine.* The appendix also contains sample panchakarma and rasayana protocols for patients with liver disease. However, recall that Ayurvedic therapy is individualized according to each person's unique characteristics. If you are interested in pursuing Ayurvedic therapy for your hepatitis C, you are urged to see a qualified Ayurvedic practitioner.

Dietary Guidelines for Liver Disorders

Pitta is the primary humor involved in liver disorders. It influences digestion, metabolism, and biological transformations in the body. Therefore, it is important to follow a diet and lifestyle that reestablishes the balance of pitta.

In general, Ayurvedic medicine promotes a vegetarian diet for liver disorders. Bitter, sweet, and astringent tastes are favored. It is recommended that you consume starchy foods such as vegetables, grains, and beans. Salads are also good.

Excesses of salty, sour, and/or spicy food items are harmful. Avoid processed and fast foods as they tend to have excessive salt and sour tastes. You are urged to reduce your consumption of oil, butter, and fats. Avoid doughnuts, fried foods, pickles, yogurt, sour cream, cheese, egg yolks, coffee, alcohol, and fermented foods. Try to avoid vinegar in salad dressings by using lemon juice. A detailed list of recommended food items for people with liver disorders is given below.

Dietary Recommendations by Food Group

Food Group	Favor	Reduce or Avoid
Vegetables - sweet and bitter vegetables	asparagus, broccoli, Brussels sprouts, cabbage, cauliflower, celery, cucumbers, green beans, green sweet peppers, leafy green vegetables, mung beans	beets, carrots, eggplant, garlic, hot peppers, mushrooms, okra, onions, radishes, parsley, peas, potatoes, sprouts, squash, spinach, sweet potatoes, tomatoes, tofu, zucchini, other soy products
Fruits - all fruits should be sweet and ripe	apples, avocados, cherries, coconut, figs, dark grapes, mangoes, melons, oranges, pears, pineapples, plums, prunes, raisins	apricots, bananas, berries, sour cherries, cranberries, grapefruit, papayas, peaches, persimmons, green grapes*, oranges*, pineapples*, plums*
		*unless they are sweet and ripe
Grains	barley, oats, wheat, white rice (preferably basmati rice)	brown rice, corn, millet, rye
Dairy	butter, buttermilk, egg whites, ice cream, milk	cheese, egg yolks, sour cream, yogurt

Herbs and Spices

Spices should generally be avoided as they aggravate pitta. In small amounts, cardamom, cilantro (green coriander), coriander seed, dill, fennel, mint, saffron, and turmeric are good for protecting the digestive fire and for helping remove blockages.[28]

Lifestyle Changes and Yoga

Your lifestyle is as important as your diet in preserving health. Our changing lifestyles have been a major cause of many ailments. If you have a liver disorder, you should avoid sleeping in the afternoon, exposure to hot sun, exertion, anxiety, alcohol abuse, smoking, eating at irregular intervals and times, and staying up late at night.

Yoga

The literal translation for yoga is "union." Yoga is an excellent way to take care of both your body and your mind. Yoga helps improve your energy level, improves immune function, calms mood swings, and helps alleviate the "brain fog" that some HCV-infected people experience. A yoga posture or *asana* is a dynamic position in which the person is perfectly poised between activity and inactivity. A corresponding mental balance exists between movement and stillness. In yoga, each posture reflects a mental attitude. Yoga strengthens the elimination system and helps to detoxify the body. A few stimulating postures help disperse stagnation and congestion, and get energy flowing again to strengthen the digestive system and liver function.[32]

Vajraasana, shalabhasana, halasana, padahastasana, savasana, abdomen lift and stomach lift are some of the yoga postures that are very helpful in liver disorders.[32] Yoga postures cause a squeezing action on a specific organ or gland resulting in the stimulation of that body part. While holding the yoga posture, breathe slowly and deeply, moving only the abdomen. This increases the oxygen and prana (life force) supply to the target organ or gland. While breathing slowly and deeply, focus attention on the target organ or gland. This brings the mind into play and greatly increases the circulation and prana supply to the organ or gland.

It is best to practice yoga in the early morning or early evening. However, yoga can be practiced at any time. You should not eat right before practicing yoga. However, it is a good idea to eat something about thirty minutes after finishing your yoga session. Wait at least one hour after getting out of bed before doing yoga because you will be too stiff. Avoid taking a hot shower or bath immediately after yoga because it draws blood away from the internal organs and glands. A shower that is just warm will not counteract the benefits of yoga. It is important to drink plenty of water after yoga practice. The water will help flush the toxins released by the body during yoga.

Yoga is advised only for individuals who can withstand mild exercise and whose liver function is not compromised. If you are interested in adding yoga to your hepatitis C treatment protocol, you should first talk it over with your primary care practitioner to be certain it is safe for you. If your health care provider gives permission to proceed, we urge you to look for a well-trained, experienced yoga instructor. Be sure to tell your instructor that you have hepatitis C, and let him or her know if you have any other medical conditions.

Pranayama is a systematic breathing exercise that helps increase blood supply and oxygen to the affected part of liver and helps liver regeneration.[32] There is no restriction for this exercise unless you are very weak and/or suffer from fluctuations in blood pressure. Pranayama provides relaxation and relieves anxiety. There are various methods for pranayama which consists of inhalation, retention, and exhalation.

A simple method for performing pranayama is to close the right nostril using the right thumb and close the left nostril using the right little and ring finger. Breathe in through the left nostril while closing the right nostril. Hold the breath as long as you can tolerate. Exhale through the right nostril thus completing one cycle. Next, breathe in through the right nostril and breathe out through the left nostril. Repeat this process ten to twelve times.

Meditation

Meditation is an important part of yogic practice. It has various stages. The first stage is *Dharana,* meaning concentration. It is accomplished by sitting in a quiet place, closing your eyes, and chanting mantras. Focus your mind on an inner object, look at the tip of your nose, or focus on a picture of your choice. Continue this process until you are able to focus your mind. You try to concentrate by bringing your mind to the desired object.

The second stage of meditation is *Dhyana,* which means contemplation. During this stage, you attempt to advance to a deeper stage of meditation. In this stage, you increase your concentration for a longer period through practice.

The third stage of meditation is only for very advanced practitioners. It is known as *Samadhi.* This form of meditation has the ability to control vital functions such as the heartbeat, breathing, etc. This is beyond the scope of the majority of yogic practitioners.

REASONS FOR USING AYURVEDIC MEDICINE AND WHO MAY BENEFIT

Ayurvedic medicine is a system of health care that emphasizes disease prevention and health promotion. Periodic cleansing of the system and a review of lifestyle practices and diet are the most important parts of treatment.

Ayurvedic treatments support liver function, and have some *antiviral* properties. The use of antiviral and time-tested *hepatoprotective* herbs, and cleansing provide additional benefit to a person with hepatitis C.

People newly diagnosed with hepatitis C whose liver function is not compromised and whose liver enzymes are not highly elevated may derive great benefits from Ayurvedic treatment. Non-alcoholics and those in younger age groups who are otherwise healthy respond well to the Ayurvedic approach. Because the mind and body are interconnected, people with a positive attitude toward Ayurveda benefit more from this approach than those who are skeptical.

Anecdotal Story of Treatment Success with Ayurvedic Medicine

A 54-year-old male presented to our clinic for evaluation. He was an alcoholic and a diabetic on oral diabetes medicine. He was diagnosed with hepatitis C in July 1999. He was being evaluated for painful swelling in the abdomen, legs, and feet. On physical exam, an inflamed left lobe of the liver was felt which was associated with mild tenderness. Ultrasound revealed a moderately enlarged liver. Laboratory tests showed a moderate increase in liver enzymes, but were otherwise normal. *Liver biopsy* showed *grade* II *inflammation* and *stage* II *fibrosis*. The man was treated with *interferon* plus *ribavirin* for more than two months, but he did not respond to treatment. Liver enzyme levels did not drop significantly and other liver blood tests were unchanged.

The patient's hepatitis C infection and associated changes in liver biochemistry were treated as an excess of pitta humor. However, because this patient had edema and abdominal discomfort, the involvement of kapha humor was also considered. After analyzing the man's physical constitution, it was decided that he was a vata prakruti person.

The following treatment plan was designed in three stages for five, one, and 45 days, respectively. The selection of herbs for this patient was based on the assessment of his unique condition.

- Elimination of toxins with *panchakola choornam* in a powder formula.
- Elimination of aggravated pitta through purgation, after preparation of the patient with *avipatti choornam* in a powder formula. This was repeated every two weeks as long as the patient could tolerate it.
- Rejuvenation of the liver with herbs and diet with *Piper longum* in a powder formula, and in a graded dose called *vardhamana pippali rasayana*.

A diet free of fat with softly cooked old rice, porridge, non-citrus fruits, sugar cane juice, boiled vegetables, lentils, and freshly made buttermilk was advised for the patient. The patient was also advised to avoid non-vegetarian foods including fish, eggs, and ice cream. The patient was told to avoid cold drinks and sleeping for long periods of time during the day to prevent aggravating the humors.

At the end of 56 days, the patient experienced reduced symptoms. His abdomen became soft and without tenderness. Ultrasound revealed the liver was of normal size. His alkaline phosphatase (a liver enzyme) level, which had been high, returned to normal. The patient was advised to continue the rejuvenating herbs. His *viral load* could not be measured because of financial constraints.

REASONS FOR NOT USING AYURVEDIC MEDICINE

People with *acute hepatitis* C or chronic hepatitis C with multiple complications and a severely cirrhotic liver may not benefit from Ayurvedic medicine. Those who cannot tolerate bitter medicines and/or who have reservations about Ayurvedic medicine are also unlikely to benefit. *Ascites* (an accumulation of fluid in the abdomen) is an incurable condition according to Ayurveda. People presenting with that complication due to hepatitis C cannot be helped by Ayurvedic medicine, nor can those who are highly debilitated.

Anecdotal Story of Treatment Failure with Ayurvedic Medicine

A 70-year-old male came to our clinic with mild jaundice, elevated liver enzymes, ascites, loss of appetite, shortness of breath, and *fatigue*. He had been diagnosed with HCV five years earlier when he developed jaundice after a blood transfusion during abdominal surgery. His liver blood tests were consistently abnormal. *Serum bilirubin* remained between 1.5-3.5mg/dL. He had no major symptoms and was able to carry out his normal activities. He had been treated with rest and polyunsaturated fatty acids for the first two years of his illness, perhaps due to lack of awareness of other treatments. Later, his viral load was tested and he was put on interferon plus ribavirin. He completed his drug therapy but did not improve. A year later, he developed ascites. This is when he approached an Ayurvedic doctor for help.

Given this man's presenting symptoms, particularly his ascites, the Ayurvedic treatment options were limited. Detoxification and cleansing procedures, which are mandatory in Ayurveda, could not be used in this patient because of his poor health and nutrition. A symptomatic treatment was planned and he was put on concoctions of liver protecting herbs such as *Tinospora cordifolia*, *Picorrizha curroa*, *Vitis vinifera*, and *Piper nigrum*, and others. Mild laxatives such as *avipatti choornam* were given in small doses, and a pitta-pacifying diet and lifestyle were recommended. Initially, his appetite improved and his serum bilirubin returned to normal. His other liver blood tests remained abnormal. His shortness of breath came down from class three to class one. His abdomen became soft and he was able to pass normal stools. Ultrasound showed cirrhosis and ascitic fluid in abdomen. Viral load testing was not repeated, as the patient could not afford it.

Though the patient is continuing treatment after more than six months, there has been no significant improvement in his liver health. This is not unexpected because of this patient's cirrhosis and ascites. According to Ayurveda, the onset of ascites indicates a poor prognosis. Age, time, and complications could also have worked against this patient.

FUTURE RESEARCH POSSIBILITIES — PREVENTION AND TREATMENT

Chronic hepatitis C presents in a number of different ways. The liver damage is due to both the direct effect of the virus, and the inflammatory changes created by activation of the immune system. The effectiveness and potential liver *toxicity* of botanicals (herbs and other plant-derived supplements) used to treat chronic hepatitis have not been adequately studied. Research needs to continue on a large scale. Multi-center trials are needed to determine the role of botanicals in the prevention and treatment of hepatitis. We also need studies to determine the best dosage forms for botanicals. Finally, research is needed on the use of the total plant, rather than just what is believed to be the active ingredient(s).[33]

Double blind, randomized, controlled studies, the gold standard of clinical research, should be the ultimate goal of all future research.

SUMMARY

Hepatitis C poses unique challenges for both patients and health care providers. Ayurveda, the holistic Indian system of medicine, provides a ray of hope. It emphasizes prevention of disease and promotion of health. There is a great deal of historical information about the drugs and plants used in Ayurveda. We have descriptions of how these treatments work to improve the health of people with liver disorders. Ayurvedic texts describe how treatments protect and detoxify the liver. To validate this traditional knowledge, Ayurveda is undergoing scientific inquiry to establish its efficacy in the treatment of liver disorders.

Chapter Ten

HOMEOPATHIC MEDICINE

Sylvia Flesner, ND

INTRODUCTION

Homeopathy is a nontoxic form of medicine that was developed approximately 200 years ago by Dr. Samuel Hahnemann. The word homeopathy is derived from two words: *homoios* meaning similars and *pathos* meaning suffering. Homeopathy is a form of medicine that uses highly diluted *pathogens* or other potentially *toxic* substances as remedies. These remedies provoke healing responses in a person's *immune system*, or provoke other body responses to treat the root causes of illnesses.

The theory behind homeopathy is based on the law of similars. "Like cures like." In the 1700's, Peruvian bark (also known as *chincona* or *china*) was used to treat malaria. The healing power of Peruvian bark was thought to be due to its bitter taste. Dr. Hahnemann disagreed with this conclusion and experimented on himself. He ingested the bark to evaluate its effects. Eventually, he developed fevers and chills, *symptoms* typical of malaria. Dr. Hahnemann theorized that because the bark produced symptoms similar to malaria, taking a small amount of the bark would stimulate the body to heal itself of malaria. The law of similars dates back to the time of Hippocrates, but it also has present-day applications. For example, many *vaccines* involve giving a small dose of the *microorganism* that causes a specific disease. This stimulates an immune response against that microorganism thereby protecting the person from the disease.

The theoretical basis of the homeopathic approach is as follows. Symptoms of a disease that result when large doses of a homeopathic drug are given to healthy subjects under controlled conditions (called provings) will be eliminated when the homeopathic drug is given in extremely small doses to someone who actually has the disease.

Practitioners of homeopathy come from a variety of health care disciplines, as well as the lay public. Naturopaths, chiropractors, psychologists, nurses, and even some western doctors practice homeopathy. A homeopath can also be a layperson who has knowledge of homeopathy. Currently, there are no certification or licensure requirements to practice homeopathy. However, because homeopathic remedies are safe and nontoxic when used appropriately, there is virtually no danger in using them.

PRINCIPLES OF HOMEOPATHY

Homeopathy requires that drugs be tested, or proved, in healthy subjects. Proving is necessary because the homeopathic drug can only express itself in its pure form in a healthy person, unaffected by interactions with a disease process. The quest for knowledge about homeopathic drugs through provings on healthy subjects has yielded a fascinating body of literature. This is particularly true in Europe where homeopathy is a more common form of therapy than in the United States.

One double-blind study that evaluated the effect of a homeopathic remedy on people with the flu found almost twice as many flu sufferers recovered within 48 hours after receiving the homeopathic remedy compared to patients who received *placebos* (inactive pills).[1] In another study, hay fever sufferers experienced six times as much symptom relief after taking a homeopathic remedy compared to those who took placebos.[2] An evaluation of 89 *clinical trials* of homeopathic remedies was recently conducted by seven health professionals in the United States and Germany.[3] They found homeopathic medicines were more than twice as effective as placebos in the evaluated trials.

Symptoms as the Basis for Homeopathic Treatment

One of the biggest differences between the homeopathic medicine and western medicine is the emphasis on making a diagnosis.

Western medicine groups patients according to the diagnosis they share. Patients who have the same diagnosis generally receive the same or similar treatments, even if there are striking differences in their symptoms. One of the major goals of western treatment is to suppress symptoms. This has resulted in a large market for products that reduce pain, fever, and other common symptoms.

Homeopathic treatment is determined by looking at the whole patient as a unique individual rather than categorizing his or her illness based on symptoms that are similar to those of other patients. According to homeopathic thought, the body's symptoms of illness are an expression of the body trying to heal itself and should not be suppressed. This individual expression of symptoms is of utmost importance in determining homeopathic prescriptions, since the remedy must perfectly match the symptoms. It is like finding the correct key for a specific lock. Homeopathic treatment can begin based on symptoms alone even if an underlying diagnosis has not been made. For record-keeping purposes and/or to make it easier to discuss a person's ailment, homeopathic practitioners might say that a person is suffering from a certain kind of flu or ulcerative disease. However, such names by themselves do not determine a patient's treatment.

Homeopathic remedies do not eliminate the cause of disease, nor do they cure disease. They do not provide immediate relief of symptoms. Rather, homeopathic remedies help establish balance in the body, and promote its ability to heal itself. In order to treat seriously ill people, the practitioner must effect a profound change at the deepest levels. Homeopathy intervenes at the level of a person's reactive, self-curative powers, with or without the person's fully conscious cooperation. The goal is to bring about a change in the total functioning of the body. Although homeopathic treatment can be supplemented by other holistic therapies, practitioners believe such a change can be brought about by homeopathic treatment alone.

HOMEOPATHY AND HEPATITIS C

Hepatitis C is a very serious disease. Everyone who has hepatitis C should be under the care of a western doctor (an MD or DO) on a regular basis. If you are experiencing any of the symptoms listed below, you should consult an MD or DO who can provide appropriate testing and treatment as these symptoms may indicate disease progression.

- extreme *fatigue*
- low-grade fever
- disinterest in food and queasiness
- heavy, painful, and/or tender liver
- very light-colored stools or very dark-colored urine

Homeopathic Treatments for Symptoms of Liver Disease

Some homeopathic medicines require a prescription while others can be purchased over-the-counter. While homeopathy is ideal for self treatment of conditions that are generally self-limited such as colds, influenza, and headaches, the treatment of chronic hepatitis C is best accomplished by a trained professional.

Aconite is sometimes used to treat the high fever, restlessness, and fearful anguish that can occur in the earliest *stage* of acute liver disease. Belladonna, chelidonium, lycopodium, mercurius, nux vomica, and the herb china may be used to treat shooting pain in the region of the liver.

The herb china is also useful for treating symptoms such as sensitivity to pressure in the liver, the tendency to become chilled, and sensitivity to open air. It is also used to treat feelings of heaviness or fullness in the stomach and abdomen, especially after eating.

I use an immune stimulator in my practice to help patients handle viral infections such as hepatitis C more effectively. The stimulator is a combination remedy that includes *Triffolium pratense, Echinacea purpurea, Asclepias tuberosa, Ferrum lodatum, Vaccinum, Euphrasia off., Thuja occidentalis, Camphora, Calcarea arsenica, Ichthyolum, Vaccinotoxinum, Morbillinum, Variolinum, Influenzinum, Vincetoxicum, Coxsackievirus, Encephalitis, Calmette-Guerin, Cy-tomegalovirus,* and isotonic plasma.

INSURING THE SAFETY OF HOMEOPATHIC REMEDIES

According to federal law, homeopathic remedies are considered drugs. To be considered an official homeopathic medicine, a product must meet the guidelines described in the *Compliance Policy Guide* (CPG) developed by the American Homeopathic Pharmacists Association and the Food and Drug Administration (FDA). A remedy must have known homeopathic provings and/or known effects that mimic the symptoms, syndromes, or conditions for which it is given. It must also meet the manufacturing specifications established by the Homœopathic Pharmacopœia of the United States (HPUS). HPUS is the official compendium of homeopathic medicines recognized by the FDA. The HPUS contains all of the official manufacturing procedures for homeopathic medicines. This includes procedures for dosing, labeling, and administration information for users. Currently, there are over 1,300 official HPUS substances. The HPUS initials on a product label identify that product as a homeopathic medicine, and insures that the legal standards for strength, quality, purity, and packaging have been met for that product.

The standards applied to products seeking HPUS approval are established by the Homœopathic Pharmacœpœia Convention of the United States (HPCUS). HPCUS is a nongovernmental, non-profit, scientific organization. HPCUS members are experts in the fields of medicine, art, biology, chemistry, and *pharmacology* who have appropriate training and demonstrated knowledge, and an interest in homeopathy.

THE ROLE OF DIET IN HOMEOPATHIC MEDICINE

A good diet that stimulates your immune system is an important companion to homeopathic remedies. Good nutrition can help you obtain and maintain good health. It can also help improve the health of your liver.

The following yeast-free diet was designed to help clean your system, reduce stress on your liver, and maintain good health.

Recommended Foods and Liquids

Fish, Lamb, Wild Game	• preferably organic, not smoked, and without the skin
Poultry	• chicken and turkey – preferably organic, not smoked, and without the skin
Dairy Products	• butter - preferably brands that are pesticide and hormone free such as Horizon® • eggs • sheep and goat milk yogurts and cheeses • rice cheeses
Fresh Vegetables	• preferably organic, if possible • wash thoroughly
Starchy Vegetables	• potatoes • sweet potatoes • yams • pumpkin • acorn and butternut squash
Fresh Fruits	• citrus fruits • kiwi • melons • apples • pears • peaches
Beverages	• unsweetened juices • filtered water • soy drinks such as Eden Soy Original® • herbal teas such as Take-a-Break® • Pero Coffee® is a good, caffeine-free substitute for coffee • it is very important to drink at least eight glasses of water each day

Foods To Be Eaten in Moderation

Legumes	• pumpkin seeds
Rice and grains Limit white flour and wheat products.	• air-popped popcorn • muffins • biscuits • cornbread • pancakes (made with soymilk or water and honey) • pastas • potatoes • rice and rice cakes • grains (such as couscous, quinoa, millet) • tortillas and tortilla chips (not fried) • homemade mayonnaise - made without vinegar or sugar • grits • yeast-free breads made with baking powder and limited white flour • tortillas and tortilla chips (not fried)
Condiments	• homemade mayonnaise - made without vinegar or sugar • guacamole - made without mayonnaise or vinegar • honey, maple syrup, apple butter - all in moderation and in very small quantities • nuts and nut butters such as peanut butter and almond butter

Some suggested food substitutes include:

- Crispini® crackers for crackers made with yeast
- Eden Soy Original® for animal milk
- Bragg's Liquid Amino® for soy and teriyaki sauces, and
- Rice Dream® for ice cream.

After 21 days on the yeast-free diet, you can add the following foods.

Fresh Fruits	• strawberries – in moderation
Legumes	• lentils • lima beans • pinto beans • split peas • black eyed peas
Rice and grains Limit white flour and wheat products.	• sourdough rye • Essene bread
Condiments	• carob • Jeannie Macaroons®

Foods and Liquids To Avoid on This Diet

Red Meats	• beef • veal • pork
Fruit	• grapes • raisins • bananas • plums • all dried fruits glazed with sugar
Vegetables	• mushrooms
Cow Dairy Products	• milk • milk products: cheese, margarine, yogurt, cottage cheese, ice cream, etc. • Butter is acceptable if it is pesticide and hormone free.
Rice and grains	• breads made with yeast
Specific Condiments	• ketchup • mustard • mayonnaise (unless homemade) • vinegar (except apple cider vinegar) • yeast • pickles • olives • soy, Tabasco® teriyaki, and barbecue sauce • margarine
Sweeteners	• sugar • artificial sweeteners such as Sweet-N-Low® and NutraSweet®
Beverages	• alcohol - including all beer, wine, hard liquor, or anything fermented • caffeinated or decaffeinated coffee • tea • soft drinks
Other Food Rules	• no fried foods • no chocolate • no canned fruits or vegetables • no chemicals or preservatives, including MSG

Read all labels. Many products contain yeast, sugar, vinegar and/or preservatives that you should eliminate from your diet.

All artificial sweeteners, such as NutraSweet® and Sweet-N-Low® should be permanently eliminated from your diet. Margarine should also be permanently eliminated from your diet.

Antibiotics, birth control pills, prescription drugs, steroids, and hormones should be avoided unless you and your doctor believe they are necessary.

REASONS FOR USING HOMEOPATHIC MEDICINES AND WHO MIGHT BENEFIT

Homeopathic medicine can be very effective for treating some of the symptoms of hepatitis C. It can also be effective for some of the side effects from western drug-based treatments. Homeopathic remedies are safe when taken as directed because they are virtually nontoxic. However, hepatitis C is a very serious disease. Homeopathic remedies are best provided under the direction of a trained *complementary and alternative medicine (CAM)* practitioner.

Anecdotal Story of Success Using Homeopathic Medicine

David J. is a 36-year-old husband and father of two. He was overweight and a heavy drinker when he came to me for care of hepatitis C. I started him on the yeast-free diet, liver detoxification, and homeopathic remedies. I advised him to eliminate the use of alcohol. He followed all of my instructions. One month after his initial visit, his *ALT* and *AST* levels were almost normal. One year later, he experienced a *relapse* when his liver *enzymes* became elevated again. A *liver biopsy* was done and showed normal liver tissue. We decided he needed to resume the yeast-free diet. He also began taking a different group of homeopathic drugs. His liver enzymes returned to and remain at normal levels. He is currently in *remission*.

REASONS FOR NOT USING HOMEOPATHIC MEDICINES

Homeopathy does not claim to be able to eliminate the hepatitis C virus (HCV). If your primary treatment goal is to eliminate HCV, homeopathic remedies are not the right choice for you.

Unless they are also MDs or DOs, homeopathic practitioners cannot conduct certain tests such as liver biopsies that are needed to monitor HCV disease progression. Only MDs or DOs can do these tests.

Homeopathic medicine requires a significant commitment from the patient to make necessary lifestyle changes. Many people find they cannot make the commitment and/or required changes if they are drastically different from their current lifestyle.

Anecdotal Story of Treatment Failure Using Homeopathic Medicine

Joe S. is a 42-year-old Vietnam veteran. He is married with children and has a stressful job. When he came to see me, he smoked cigarettes, drank moderate amounts of alcohol, and large quantities of coffee daily. He had been diagnosed with hepatitis C and consulted me to see how I could help him. He had elevated liver enzymes, moderate *viral load*, and some *fibrosis* on liver biopsy. I advised him to stop smoking cigarettes, and to give up alcohol and coffee. I prescribed a yeast-free diet to cleanse his liver. After completing the liver cleansing process, I planned to prescribe some homeopathic remedies to help improve the health of his liver. He was able to make most of the changes I recommended, but did not give up drinking coffee. Rather than put a greater effort into eliminating coffee from his diet, Joe chose to return to many of his previous behaviors. His liver health has not improved.

SUMMARY

Homeopathy has the potential to alleviate the symptoms of hepatitis C and to help the body reestablish internal balance at the deepest levels. When cure is possible, homeopathy may help the body maintain a lasting cure.

If you have hepatitis C, get as much rest as you feel you need and eat a well-balanced, lowfat diet with moderate amounts of protein. Try to eat well even if you are not hungry. Avoid eating irritating spices, oily foods, and coffee. You should also avoid unnecessary drugs. You must abstain entirely from drinking alcohol.

Homeopathic medicines are inexpensive and often do not require a prescription. Over-the-counter homeopathic medicines are available in health food stores, pharmacies, grocery stores, and other outlets. Product labels that contain the HPUS initials mean that the products were manufactured according to the guidelines of the Homœopathic Pharmacopœia of the United States.

As with all forms of medicine, no one *modality* is right for everyone all the time. We need to continue to conduct research into the causes and cures of illness, and to use the least toxic and most effective systems of treatment.

Chapter Eleven

MIND-BODY MEDICINE AND SPIRITUAL HEALING

Peggy McCarthy, MBA

INTRODUCTION

Medical research has clearly shown there are connections among the body, mind, and spirit. The mind is the conscious and unconscious processes of the brain that manifest themselves in how we think, perceive, imagine, and exhibit emotion. The spirit is the vital animating force that exists in all of us. This chapter is about the connections among the mind, body, and spirit, and how those connections affect your well-being.

Spiritual healing and mind-body medicine have been practiced for centuries in many cultures. These healing traditions became less common as science and western medicine developed. Recently however, western researchers have focused once again on these age-old approaches to health care. Today, most health care providers acknowledge that mind-body-spirit connections can have direct effects on our health.

Many areas of mind-body medicine and spiritual healing are currently being studied. Though the results of these studies are varied, they are interesting enough to encourage a significant increase in funding for such research. Many of the studies on mind-body medicine and spiritual healing in the U.S. are supported and/or funded by the National Center for Complementary and Alternative Medicine (NCCAM). Most studies focus on people with chronic illnesses such as cancer and *HIV*/AIDS. No study to date has focused solely on people with *hepatitis C*.

HOW THE MIND-BODY-SPIRIT CONNECTIONS WORK

Though there are many theories about how mind-body-spirit connections work, there are no certain answers. Physics experiments have shown that energy is not destroyed, but rather changes from one form to another. The same transformation of energy that takes place throughout the universe also takes place in our bodies. An estimated 6 million energy transforming reactions take place every second in our bodies. This transformation leads to some remarkable changes. The lining of the stomach is replaced every five days. Our fat stores are replaced every three weeks. We are covered by brand new skin every four to five weeks. The cells of the liver are replaced every six weeks. Even our bones are continually replaced. Studies at Oak Ridge Laboratories show that 98% of the chemicals that make up our bodies are replaced every year.[1]

Our brains and bodies are fully connected, and their energy is continually transformed and recycled. Researchers believe this connection and interchange is how the mind is able to affect the rest of the body.

Mind-body connections can be influenced by what we do, how we think, and what we eat. They can also be influenced by environmental factors such as our ethnic and cultural habits, where we were born and raised, and the family situation in which we grow and develop. Mind-body connections play a part in our lifestyle choices, how we cope, our decision-making processes, our sensitivity to pain and other discomforts, and our outlook on life.

The following discussion examines the relationships among the mind, body, and spirit and how those relationships can affect your experience of living with hepatitis C. There is an overview of the kinds of goals mind-body medicine practitioners and spiritual healers try to accomplish with their treatments. There is also a review of reasons for and against the use of these healing techniques.

TREATMENT GOALS OF MIND-BODY MEDICINE AND SPIRITUAL HEALING

You may use mind-body medicine and spiritual healing in addition to other treatments, or you may use these approaches alone. If and how you use mind-body medicine and spiritual healing in your health care is a decision only you can make.

Mind-body medicine and spiritual healing can be used for a number of purposes.

- Managing disease *symptoms* and/or treatment side-effects such as body temperature fluctuations, *depression*, loss of appetite, nausea/vomiting, pain, and sleep disturbances
- Helping clear the hepatitis C virus (HCV)
- Enhancing other treatments
- Promoting well-being and general health
- Gaining an understanding of what having hepatitis C means to you

There are growing numbers of health care professionals trained in western medicine who practice an approach called *integrated medicine*. Integrated medicine involves using western medicine along with mind-body medicine and/or other *complementary and alternative medicine (CAM)* treatments.

Whatever treatments you decide to use, it is very important to inform each of your health care providers about all of treatments you are using. If you decide you might like to try one or more CAM therapies, talk with your primary health care provider first. This is important because:

- unexpected side effects can occur with certain combinations of therapies, and

- unexpected benefits may provide your health care practitioners with new information that can be shared with others.

TYPES OF MIND-BODY MEDICINE AND SPIRITUAL HEALING

There are many kinds of mind-body medicine and spiritual healing. Many such as yoga, meditation, and *tui na* (Chinese massage) originated from traditional folk medicines that have been used in other cultures for centuries. Others such as biofeedback and therapeutic touch have been used by various cultures for many years but have been renamed by western researchers.

We have tried to include in this chapter the most common mind-body medicine and spiritual healing practices used in North America. However, there are other approaches that are not included here because of space limitations. The inclusion or exclusion of any approach should not be considered in any way to affirm or deny the usefulness of that approach. The included mind-body practices are arranged alphabetically.

Acupuncture

Acupuncture is an ancient technique that uses very thin needles inserted into the skin at specific points on the body called acupoints. These points lie along invisible *meridians* that serve as channels for the flow of vital energy called *qi* (or *chi*). Insertion of the needles at these points can promote energy flow to reduce or eliminate the symptoms of a disease or condition.

The use of acupuncture in the United States is widespread with over 10,000 licensed acupuncturists. In the United States, acupuncture is used to treat common conditions such as addiction, headache, arthritis, and carpal tunnel syndrome. In Asia, acupuncture has a wider variety of uses such as alleviating the symptoms associated with chronic and infectious diseases, and for anesthesia and/or pain control.

There are no known studies on the use of acupuncture specifically among people with hepatitis C. However, there have been many clinical studies on the use of acupuncture to relieve symptoms such as pain and nausea.[2, 3]

Aromatherapy

Aromatherapy uses extracts of essential oils from herbs and other aromatic plants to influence health and well-being. There are over 40 essential oil extracts that are believed to have medicinal or health benefits. Essential oils should never be taken internally because many are poisonous. Oils should only be used in small amounts either directly on the skin or placed close enough to smell the fragrance. You should test any essential oil to determine if you are allergic to it before using it on your skin.

Aromatherapy is used alone or in conjunction with massage. Each oil extract has its own use and benefit. Oils can be obtained from a naturopath, homeopath, or other CAM provider. They can also be purchased at health food stores or on the Internet.

There are no reported studies on the effects of aromatherapy among people with hepatitis C. There is also no evidence that aromatherapy cures or prevents disease. However, studies have shown that aromatherapy can reduce anxiety, tension, depression, and pain. Citrus extracts seem to be particularly good at alleviating depression.[4] Peppermint, ginger, and cardamom extracts appear to relieve nausea in cancer patients receiving therapy.[5] Black pepper extract appears to reduce the craving for nicotine.[6]

Art, Music, and Dance Therapies

Art, music, and dance or movement therapies have been used to treat patients with a variety of diseases. These therapies appear to reduce stress, anxiety, and depression.[7]

Art therapy involves using artistic expression to explore what having a disease means to you. Music therapy involves listening to music or playing musical instruments. Music therapy may be especially helpful for reducing pain, controlling nausea, lowering the heart rate, and reducing blood pressure.[8, 9] Many people who combine music therapy with movement or dance therapy find it helps calm the mind. Music therapy can promote the production of *endorphins* that help reduce depression.[10]

There are no scientific data to support the notion that these approaches help reduce the incidence of side effects due to disease or treatment. However, they may help you more clearly identify what is going on in your body and mind, and the potential for harm is extremely low.

Biofeedback

Biofeedback was first studied in the 1970's. Researchers found that with training, people could learn to do such things as raise the temperature of the hands or feet, raise or lower blood pressure and heart rate, and control specific muscles by focusing mental concentration on these activities. Biofeedback trainers use equipment such as temperature gauges, blood pressure monitoring devices, and heart rate monitors. These tools provide immediate feedback to the person attempting to use this technique to produce a biological response.

Biofeedback studies have shown it can be effective in reducing stress and muscle tension, relieving migraines and other types of headaches, and relieving anxiety.[11, 12, 13] No studies have been performed specifically among people with hepatitis C.

Chiropractic Therapy

Chiropractors provide treatment by manipulating the spine. Chiropractic theory states that blockages in the spinal cord nerves that lead to all areas of the body can cause illness, pain, or other distress. Moving the spine in certain ways is intended to reduce or clear these blockages. Chiropractic therapy has been shown to be effective in reducing low back pain and other pain due to muscle or bone injury.[14, 15, 16]

There have been no studies involving the use of chiropractic therapy for patients with hepatitis C. Chiropractic therapy is considered to be relatively safe, however if you have a chronic condition such as cancer or heart disease, we suggest you check with your health care provider to make sure there are no *contraindications* to this form of therapy.

Craniosacral Therapy

Craniosacral therapy is based on the theory that many people who have experienced the normal birthing process or have had head, neck, or back injuries retain residual stresses in the skull and lining of the brain. Therapists treat these stresses by applying gentle pressure to the skull, jaw, and areas in the mouth to produce movement of the bones of the head and neck. There are no known controlled studies of this therapy. However, therapists claim craniosacral therapy is effective in treating headaches, and neck and back pain. It is also used to treat TMJ (temporomandibular joint dysfunction), eye problems, mental disturbances such as attention deficit disorder, and to stimulate the *immune system*.[17]

As with chiropractic therapy, this method of treatment is considered low risk and it may be helpful. However, if you have any medical condition, check with your health care provider to make sure there are no contraindications to this therapeutic approach.

Crystals

The use of healing crystals is quite popular in the United States, however there is no scientific proof of its effectiveness.[18] A variety of crystals are used to treat a number of conditions and diseases. Some believe that the light held by or passed through a crystal has healing powers. Crystals are generally placed on the parts of the body affected by a disease or condition, or are worn as a necklace or bracelet.

Energy Manipulation

Many mind-body treatments are believed to shift energy patterns in the body. You may encounter these treatments if you seek the services of a CAM therapist. Some of the most common forms of energy *manipulation* are Reiki, therapeutic touch, tui-na, reflexology, and watsu. With all of these treatments, the therapist applies gentle touch to the body. Watsu is done with the patient floating in warm water. None of these therapies is likely to cause harm. They may be helpful for reducing stress, anxiety, tension and pain.[19, 20, 21, 22] There have been no studies done specifically among people with hepatitis C.

Humor

Norman Cousins, former editor of *The Saturday Review*, has written about his use of humor to cure himself of a debilitating illness.[23] A number of studies have been conducted evaluating the therapeutic use of humor. The studies indicate that laughter can cause a release of endorphins in the same way exercise does.[24] Endorphins can reduce depression and stress, sensitivity to pain, and produce a feeling of well-being.[25, 26, 27] While no studies have specifically focused on hepatitis C, there is no reason to think laughter would not have the same effects on people living with hepatitis C as it has on other people.

There are a number of ways to bring humor into your life: movies, cartoons, books, jokes, and television shows are just a few. There are even Internet sites devoted to spreading humor.

Hypnosis, Self-Hypnosis, Hypnotherapy

Hypnotherapy has been effectively used to treat a variety of conditions including tobacco and other addictions, migraine headaches, sleep and eating disorders, pain, and nausea and vomiting. Hypnosis involves deep relaxation that can be induced by a trained therapist or self-induced. Hypnosis usually involves suggestions to be carried out by the person after the hypnosis session ends. Some examples of such instructions are, "Remain calm in a stressful situation," or "Remember to take ten deep breaths before responding verbally." Hypnosis requires the mind to be relaxed, calm, and free from extraneous thoughts to be effective. Some studies have shown hypnosis may be helpful in stimulating the immune system.[28, 29, 30, 31] Hypnosis produces a feeling of calm, reduces stress, and imparts a sense of well-being.

Hypnotherapy may be helpful for people living with hepatitis C. If you decide to try hypnotherapy, it is important to find a good hypnotherapist to work with you. You may want to ask your health care provider for a referral.

Massage

Massage involves rubbing and kneading the body's soft tissues and muscles. Massage has been used for centuries to ease muscle tension, reduce pain, provide relaxation, and reduce anxiety and depression. It is also used to increase alertness, relieve joint pain and stiffness, and to help heal injured muscles. It can reduce blood pressure and the frequency of migraine headaches. It can also help induce sleep, and increase the flow of blood and oxygen to body tissues.[32, 33, 34]

There are many types of massage. With shiatsu, the therapist focuses the massage on acupressure points. Shiatsu is generally considered a gentle form of massage. Swedish massage is considered a deep tissue massage. Rolfing is a form of massage in which the therapist uses his or her elbows and knuckles to provide a very deep tissue massage that may at times be painful. Bowen massage focuses specifically on soft tissue manipulation to stimulate the *lymphatic system*.

It is likely that massage can be as beneficial to people with hepatitis C as it is to other people. However, there have been no studies to prove this assumption. The risk of harm from massage is low. However, we advise you to check with your health care provider before beginning this form of therapy.

Meditation/Imagery/Visualization

Meditation, imagery, and visualization are mental techniques that can be self-taught with the aid of books or instructional videos, or can be learned from an experienced practitioner. Although some initial training is needed, once these techniques are learned, you will need no additional outside assistance.

There are many different forms of each of these techniques. However, all of these techniques share in common a form of deep breathing called abdominal breathing or belly breathing. Abdominal breathing uses the diaphragm, one of the body's strongest muscles, along with the abdominal and pulmonary muscles to completely fill and empty the lungs. When you exhale using abdominal breathing, the diaphragm contracts and literally pushes the air from the lungs.

For many people, meditation is more of a spiritual practice than a therapeutic one. Some practice simple meditation by clearing the mind of all extraneous thoughts, and speaking, chanting, or thinking a single word or short phrase. You might choose a word like health, happiness, joy, or any other word or phrase that has personal meaning. Some people use the word *ohm*, a word used in traditional East Indian meditation. Meditation has been shown in a number of studies to be effective in reducing blood pressure, anxiety, and cholesterol levels, and for pain control. It is also an effective tool for treating substance abuse.[35, 36] It may even be effective in preventing diseases such as cancer.[37, 38, 39]

Visualization or guided imagery involves allowing your thoughts to guide you, or to be guided with the assistance of a spoken message. Self-guided imagery is similar to self-hypnosis in that you plan what you want to think about ahead of time. Visualizing the image of a healthy you can be a very powerful tool.

Moxibustion and Cupping

Moxibustion and cupping are sometimes used as companion treatments to acupuncture. Professionals trained in Chinese or Ayurvedic medicine sometimes use both techniques.

Moxibustion involves placing an ignited cone of mugwort or wormwood leaves over an acupuncture point where an energy blockage is believed to exist. The cone is left in place just long enough for the skin under the cone to feel warm. Moxibustion has been shown to be helpful in a number of conditions including asthma and ulcerative colitis. It can also help control diarrhea.[40]

Cupping involves the placement of a glass cup on the skin over an acupuncture point. The air in the cup has been heated so that vacuum occurs when the cup is placed on the skin. The cup is left in place or moved gently over the area for a few minutes. This procedure is done to help realign the energy or qi.

Many Chinese studies have evaluated the use of moxibustion and cupping. However, no studies of these techniques have been conducted in the west.

Prayer

Prayer is used in almost every world culture. Prayer is perceived as communication, either silent or spoken, with a spiritual force. This force is called by many names depending on the culture, religion, and belief system of the person praying. God, the Great Spirit, and Yahweh are a few examples. Prayer involves an external focus as opposed to the internal focus that practices such as *tai chi* or yoga involve.

Many studies have evaluated the effects of spirituality and prayer. Analysis of a number of studies showed that in over 90% of these studies, participants derived positive mental health benefits.[41] Studies focused on the practice of prayer have been done among people with heart disease, cancer, and other diseases.[42, 43, 44, 45] These studies included people praying for themselves and people who were prayed for by others without their knowledge. The overwhelming majority of these studies showed benefits including reduced incidence of disease, and improvement in the quality of life for those living with disease. No studies have been done specifically among people with hepatitis C.

Patients with life-threatening illnesses have spontaneously recovered in countless cases worldwide. The question most often asked is whether these are cases of spiritual healing or merely happy coincidences. More studies on the use of prayer and spiritual healing are reported every year in an effort to answer this question. However, even if prayer has not been *clinically* proven to cure disease, you may find its benefits significant if its practice fits with your lifestyle and belief system.

Psychosocial Support/Support Groups

One of the early studies in mind-body medicine conducted during the 1980's focused on *psychosocial* support. The study involved women with late-stage breast cancer. Half of the study participants attended a weekly psychosocial support group in addition to receiving their usual treatment. The other participants received their usual treatment, but no psychosocial support. The women who received support survived significantly longer than the women who did not receive support.[46]

Another study examined immune cell function in cancer patients who received psychosocial support compared to those who received no support. Those receiving support had significantly greater immune function up to one year after the support ended compared to those who received no support.[47]

Support groups or group therapy can be formal or informal. In formal groups, a trained professional usually leads the group. However, support groups are also formed by people who share a common concern such as hepatitis C. Many of these groups are participant directed.

There are no published studies on the effects of psychosocial support among people living with hepatitis C. However, group support has been shown to be effective in helping people with other chronic, and/or life-threatening diseases such as cancer and heart disease.

The skill of the group leader can play a major role in the support group experience. Facilitators who place blame on the participants are not helpful and should be avoided. If you find a certain group or facilitator is not providing the help you seek, try another group.

Psychotherapy

There are many forms of psychotherapy and many different types of practitioners who provide these services. Psychiatrists are medical doctors and are the only providers who can provide both psychotherapy and prescription drugs such as antidepressants and anti-anxiety medication. Psychologists, social workers, chaplains, and other religious professionals can also provide psychotherapy.

Psychotherapy usually involves regularly scheduled appointments. Therapy often focuses on helping people make the most of the healthy coping strategies they have, and limiting the use of coping strategies that can cause problems. Psychotherapy is often useful for people who are dealing with alcoholism and/or drug abuse. Studies have shown it is also effective in helping people deal with crisis situations such as being diagnosed with a life-threatening disease.[48] No studies have been done specifically among people with hepatitis C.

Qi gong

Qi gong (*chi gong*) is an ancient Eastern mind-body practice that involves exercises done standing, sitting, or lying down. Qi gong should initially be learned from a trained practitioner. However, once the practice is learned, it can be performed alone or as part of a group. There are several types of qi gong. The gentle form is the type that promotes and preserves health. There are specific routines to help reduce blood pressure and cleanse the liver, kidneys, and lungs.

Qi gong has been studied in *clinical trials*, though not among people with hepatitis C. Studies have shown that qi gong can reduce pain, improve the immune system, increase appetite, reduce the frequency of diarrhea, and help maintain normal weight.[49, 50] Caution should be taken when practicing qi gong to prevent any discomfort in the muscles and joints.

Spiritual Healing

Almost every culture has its own form of spiritual healing with its own unique rituals. However, many rituals are common to all forms of spiritual healing, such as the use of prayer.

The basic premise of spiritual healing is that the healer has the power to heal and cure those who seek their services. Usually, healers participate in many years of training. Healers are known by different names in different cultures. Indian cultures call their healers shamans. Western Hispanic cultures refer to healers as *curanderos*. Many Native American tribes refer to their healers as medicine men or women.

Western medicine usually uses remedies that have been tested in scientific studies to prove their benefit. On the other hand, spiritual healers use remedies that have been passed down from generation to generation. The proof of benefit of these remedies comes from history and experience rather than science. Interestingly, many of the drugs prescribed today by western doctors were originally used by healers of other cultures.

There have been spontaneous cures as the result of spiritual healing, just as there have been spontaneous cures in western medicine. There have been no studies to determine if spontaneous cure rates increase if spiritual medicine is used either instead of or combined with western medicine.

Spiritual healers often use herbs or other substances to be ingested, inhaled, rubbed on the skin, or used another way. Treatments can involve participation in healing rituals such as the Native American sweat lodge. Healing rituals and herbs have been shown in clinical trials to reduce stress and relieve symptoms such as nausea and *fatigue*.[51] A clinical trial involving people with asthma, diabetes, depression, cancer, chronic pain, and other conditions found Native American healing benefited more than 80% of participants.[52] To date, no studies on spiritual healing have been done specifically among people with hepatitis C.

Tai Chi

Tai chi is an ancient Eastern mind-body practice. It is a series of specific movements performed in a standing position. Tai chi is best learned from an experienced practitioner. Once learned tai chi can be done alone, with the aid of a videotape or CD, or in a group. Each movement in tai chi is very slow, specific, and meditative. The goal of tai chi is to move the good energy (chi) into and through the body while getting rid of the bad or depleted energy that may be trapped in the body.

Clinical studies have shown that tai chi is especially helpful for older adults and people with chronic illnesses such as arthritis, chronic obstructive pulmonary disease (COPD), *osteoporosis*, and heart disease.[53, 54, 55] Tai chi can improve balance and flexibility, increase muscle mass, and reduce blood pressure and pulse rate.[56, 57, 58] No studies specifically involving people with hepatitis C have been done to date.

Yoga

Yoga uses controlled breathing, mental focus, and specific body positions to induce inner calm. There are many different forms of yoga. Some are very gentle, others are more strenuous. Yoga positions stretch and strengthen the muscles of the body, including the facial muscles. The positions should be maintained only as long as is comfortable for you. The practice of yoga should never produce pain. Though yoga practice can provide cardiovascular exercise and improve fitness, yoga originated as a mind-body practice, not an exercise program.

You can gain strength, flexibility, and endurance from practicing yoga. Yoga has been shown in a number of medical studies to be effective in helping control blood pressure, heart rate, body temperature, *metabolism*, brain waves, and many other body functions.[59] It is particularly helpful in the treatment of musculoskeletal problems such as arthritis and carpal tunnel symdrome.[60, 61] Yoga can also help reduce disease symptoms and treatment side effects.[62]

Yoga is best learned from a skilled and trained instructor, but can also be learned from instructional videotapes or CDs. Once learned, yoga can be practiced either alone or in a group.

REASONS FOR USING MIND-BODY MEDICINE AND SPIRITUAL HEALING AND WHO MAY BENEFIT

The mind-body medicine and spiritual healing therapies presented here include those most commonly used by health care practitioners trained in both western medicine and CAM. Because the mind plays an important part in how you feel, mind-body medicine and spiritual healing therapies may be helpful in adjusting to your diagnosis. They may also be beneficial parts of your treatment plan.

Mind-body medicine and spiritual healing may have a role in your perception of the many challenges hepatitis C presents. Such challenges might include giving up alcohol, making treatment decisions, maintaining treatment compliance, adjusting to living with the disease, and managing treatment side effects.

REASONS FOR NOT USING MIND-BODY MEDICINE AND SPIRITUAL HEALING

Mind-body medicine and spiritual healing approaches may not be useful for people who do not wish to make the lifestyle and/or philosophical changes that may be needed to incorporate them into your life. In many states, practitioners of some of these therapeutic approaches must be certified or licensed. Examples include acupuncturists, chiropractors, massage therapists, and psychotherapists. While licensure or certification does not guarantee skill or ability, it generally indicates the practitioner has completed a supervised training program. Practitioners of many of the other forms of mind-body medicine or spiritual healing are not certified or licensed. This means there can be great practice variation from one therapist to another.

SUMMARY

If you are interested in incorporating mind-body medicine and/or spiritual healing into your health care plans, it is important to find qualified practitioners who work well with you. Check with your health care provider to see if he or she can refer you to skilled practitioners. You might also ask friends and/or other people with hepatitis C for referrals. If you do not like one practitioner's approach, you can always try someone else. Just as with your other health care providers, you need to find people whose skills you believe in and trust. This form of healing is very personal. Therefore, your relationship with your practitioner is extremely important.

Chapter Twelve

MODERN AND TRADITIONAL CHINESE MEDICINE

Qing Cai Zhang, MD (China), LicAc

INTRODUCTION

More than 30 million people in China are infected with the *hepatitis C* virus (HCV).[1] For the most part, China is still a developing country. Expensive drugs such as *interferon* and *ribavirin* are not readily available, nor are they affordable. In addition, the success rate of these drugs is not satisfactory and the side effects can be severe. All of this has prompted most Chinese hepatitis patients to use traditional Chinese medicine (TCM), or integrated Chinese and western medicine known as modern Chinese medicine (MCM).

TCM serves more than one billion people in China and Southeast Asia. There are more than one million TCM practitioners in China alone. Five years ago, the Chinese government conducted a national survey on Chinese medicinal substances and found that 11,146 species of plants, 1,581 species of animals, and 80 minerals have been used as TCM remedies.[2] One-fourth of the world's population uses TCM, the second largest medical system in the world today. In Japan, there are more than 200,000 health care providers prescribing Chinese herbal medicines for their patients. TCM is used to treat almost every disease identified by western medicine. TCM is used in Europe, Canada, and the United States, especially in the western, eastern and northern parts of the U.S.

There is increasing interest and discussion in the United States about TCM and MCM as treatment options for people living with hepatitis C. Doctors in China have a great deal of experience treating hepatitis with TCM since one-third of the world's hepatitis carriers are in China.

WHAT IS TRADITIONAL CHINESE MEDICINE?

TCM is a very old, but still vital health and healing system. It is based on harmony or balance. A healthy person is in complete balance, both with him or herself and with nature. TCM theory states that disease is a deviation from balance, and the purpose of treatment is to restore it. TCM focuses on maintaining health rather than managing disease. TCM is an empirical medicine, which means it was developed mainly through *clinical* observation over a long period of time. It is a logical system that uses observation and clinical experience to determine what actions need to be taken.

TCM has developed unique diagnostic and therapeutic methods such as tongue diagnosis, pulse reading, herbal formulas, acupuncture, *tui na* (Chinese massage), and *qi gong*. TCM treats patients holistically, that is as a whole, rather than treating individual parts. This ancient medical system is continuously developing.

WHAT IS MODERN CHINESE MEDICINE?

During the past four decades, there has been a new development in TCM. Practitioners have begun integrating TCM and western medicine. This combination of TCM and western medicine has created a new version of integrated medicine, modern Chinese medicine. The marriage of TCM and western medicine has brought great benefits to every patient it serves.

Since the late 1950's, a modernization movement brought TCM into every medical school in China. TCM is taught along with western medicine. Many Chinese health care providers include both TCM and western medicine in their practices. For most clinical conditions, these two medical approaches are used together and the results are usually better than if either approach was used alone. As part of this movement, many western health care providers have devoted large amounts of time and energy to the scientific study of TCM.

Today, there are three kinds of medical practice in China: TCM, western medicine, and MCM.

HOW WAS CHINESE MEDICINE MODERNIZED?

One method used to modernize TCM was the creation of special terms for western mental and physical diagnoses to match the terms TCM uses when referring to herbs. This allowed the language barrier between these two medical systems to be overcome.

This modernization made it possible for TCM and MCM to treat some of the new diseases affecting humans such as hepatitis C, *HIV*/AIDS, and Lyme disease. Although these diseases are not discussed in the traditional TCM literature, their descriptions can be used to find suitable TCM diagnoses and treatments.

With the modernization of TCM, we now use herbs based on both TCM principles and *pharmacology*. We now know the active ingredients of the herbs and their actions in the body. We have learned more about possible *toxicities* and side effects, proper doses, and treatment courses. These new abilities make MCM a more effective medical approach than TCM. MCM can treat some diseases that are difficult to treat with western medicine, often avoiding the severe side effects that may be caused by many western drugs.

Most states in the U.S. require licensure to practice acupuncture. However, a license is not required to practice herbology, the dispensing of medicinal herbs. Any person with knowledge of herb usage can call him or herself an herbalist. Furthermore, the Food and Drug Administration (FDA) does not regulate herbal products. Their quality, safety, efficacy, and potency are in the hands of the manufacturers, with no governmental oversight. For these reasons, anyone considering the use of herbs should be very careful to find a qualified practitioner and to use reputable products. One way to do this is to ask friends or relatives for referrals. You can also check with professional associations and ask for referrals to qualified practitioners in your area.

CHINESE MEDICAL APPROACH TO CHRONIC VIRAL INFECTIONS

Chinese medicine's approach to chronic viral infections is called *fu zheng qu xie*. The translation of this phrase is, "dispelling evil [the virus] by supporting righteous *qi* [normal function of the body]."

The *immune system* is a major part of the righteous qi (pronounced chee). Therefore, supporting the immune system is an important part of Chinese medical treatment for hepatitis C. There are many Chinese therapies to help regulate and support the immune system. Chinese medicine asserts that the body itself is the major healing force. Medications and procedures can help the body heal, but they cannot replace the healing function of the body itself. In treating *chronic hepatitis* C, Chinese medicine focuses first on normalizing liver functions and restorating overall health. With improving health, the body's immune function is strengthened. With the help of *antiviral* herbal remedies, the hepatitis C virus (HCV) will be suppressed and kept at bay, causing no further harm. The TCM and MCM therapies discussed in this section are based on these principles.

Diagnosing Chronic Viral Hepatitis

TCM diagnosis is based on four basic techniques: inspection (observation), auscultation and olfaction (smelling and listening), interrogation (questioning), and palpation (physical examination). According to TCM, the body is a whole whose parts are both interconnected and interactive. Because of this interconnection, a condition in one part of the body may affect the entire body. Therefore, signs of disease in one organ can be seen in many different parts of the body. The four diagnostic methods are used to look for *symptoms* and *signs* of disease, and to determine their cause. The TCM diagnosis is the basis for both determining the cause of an illness and deciding the appropriate treatment.

Inspection

The TCM doctor inspects (observes) the patient's mental state, complexion, physical condition, and behavior. The practitioner observes the person's vitality (*qi*), face and skin color, body figure, hair, eyes, lips, teeth, throat, and other features. The most important observation is of the tongue to see its color, size, and coating or fur.

Auscultation and Olfaction

Auscultation (listening) and olfaction (smelling) are used to detect the health status of the patient. The practitioner listens to the voice, breathing, and coughing. The odors of the patient are also noted. TCM considers these sounds and odors to be reflective of the health status of the various body organs.

Inquiring

Inquiring involves asking the person and his or her relatives about such things as the person's history, symptoms, family history, and previous therapies. Typically, the practitioner will ask the person about the presence of chills and/or fever, excessive perspiration, pain, sleep, diet, thirst, alcohol consumption, other beverage consumption, urination, bowel movements, menstruation, and childhood illnesses.

Palpation

Palpation is a physical examination that includes pulse reading and the use of the hands to touch and press certain areas of the body. Pulse reading is one of most important Chinese diagnostic methods. There are 24 different pulses that can be read from a person's wrists.

Based on all the data obtained from the four diagnostic methods, a differential diagnosis is made according to the eight principal syndromes: yin or yang, exterior or interior, cold or heat, and deficient or excessive.

According to TCM theories, treatment is based on an overall analysis of symptoms and signs. The doctor considers four characteristics in deciding on a treatment.

- the cause of the illness
- the nature of the illness
- location of the illness
- the patient's overall physical condition

In this way, treatment is individualized. It may be changed according to changes in the patient's condition during the course of the disease.

TRADITIONAL CHINESE MEDICINE THERAPIES FOR CHRONIC VIRAL HEPATITIS

Through numerous clinical observations, major symptom patterns in chronic viral hepatitis have been identified and treatment methods have been developed. In 1990, the National Hepatitis Conference of China developed the TCM Scheme for Chronic Viral Hepatitis Prevention and Treatment. According to this scheme, chronic viral hepatitis is categorized into the following five TCM symptom patterns:[3, 4]

- *Gan dan shi re* - liver-gallbladder damp-heat
- *Gan yu pi xu* - depressed liver-energy and spleen deficiency
- *Gan shen yin xu* - liver-kidney yin deficiency
- *Pi shen yang xu* - spleen-kidney yang deficiency, and
- *Yu xue zu luo* - stagnant blood blocks collaterals.

Gan Dan Shi Re (liver-gallbladder damp-heat)

Symptom pattern:

- dull pain in the right *hypochondrium* (area below the ribs)
- stomach *flatulence* (gas)
- nausea
- aversion to oil
- *jaundice* or no jaundice
- dark urine
- difficulty eliminating feces
- wet, thick, yellowish tongue coating
- fast, slippery pulse

Treatment method:

Clear the heat and eliminate the dampness. Cool the blood and resolve the toxin.

Formula:

Capillaris Combination plus blood cooling and toxin resolving herbs

Gan Yu Pi Xu (depressed liver-energy and spleen deficiency)

Symptom pattern:

- *distended* sensation in the hypochondrium (area below the ribs)
- *depression* and/or anxiety
- withered and yellowish complexion
- poor appetite

- stomach flatulence (gas)
- loose stools or diarrhea
- pale tongue with white coating
- submerged and tight pulse

Treatment method:

Disperse the depressed liver energy and alleviate the depression. Invigorate the spleen, and regulate the stomach.

Formula:

Modified formulas of Bupleurum and Tang-kuei Formula and Bupleurum and Peony and Six Major Herb Combination

Gan Shen Yin Xu (liver-kidney yin deficiency)

Symptom pattern:

- *vertigo* (dizziness)
- *tinnitus* (ringing in the ears)
- dry eyes
- thirst
- dry mouth
- insomnia and dreamy sleep
- feverish sensation in palms and soles
- *lassitude* of the *loins* and legs (a heavy feeling)
- menstrual problems
- red and flaccid tongue with little dry coating
- fast, fine, and weak pulse

Treatment method:

Nourish the blood, liver, and yin, and invigorate the kidney.

Formula:

Modified Glehnia and Rehmannia Formula

Pi Shen Yang Xu (spleen-kidney yang deficiency)

Symptom pattern:

- intolerance to cold
- cold pain in the lower abdomen, loins, and legs
- poor appetite
- loose stools and/or diarrhea
- indigestion
- leg and ankle *edema* (swelling)
- pale and puffy tongue
- submerged and fine, slow pulse

Treatment method:

Invigorate the spleen and nourish the *qi*. Warm the kidney and support yang.

Formulas:

Modified Aconite, Ginseng, and Ginger Combination, and Gardenia and Hoelen Formula, or Four Major Herb Combination and Rehmannia Eight Formula

Yu Xue Zu Luo (stagnant blood blocks collaterals)

Symptom pattern:

- dim and grayish complexion with rashes or reddish spots
- enlarged and hardened liver and spleen
- liver palm
- spider moles
- painful and dark menstruation with blood clots
- dark purple tongue with *petechia* (red or purple spots)
- submerged and uneven pulse

Treatment method:

Activate the blood circulation and dispel the stasis. Disperse the accumulation, and dredge the meridian passage.

Formulas:

Modified Persica and Achyranthes Combination and "Persica and Cinidium Combination, or Persica and Eupolyphaga Combination

TREATMENT OF CHRONIC VIRAL HEPATITIS WITH MODERN CHINESE MEDICINE

Different treatment methods and herbal formulas for each of the symptom patterns have been developed. Treatments are changed if the symptom pattern changes. The herbal composition of the formulas can be found in the *Appendix V: Modern and Traditional Chinese Medicine.*

The protocols described below were reviewed by me, and are generally used in Zhang's Clinic in New York, NY. It is important to note that, because of differences in education and training, every qualified practitioner develops his/her own way of practicing TCM or MCM. This approach is only one example of how TCM or MCM can be applied to the treatment of people with chronic hepatitis C. Anyone considering TCM or MCM should compare different practitioners' approaches, and then make an educated decision about whom they should see for treatment.

Hepatitis C is a newly defined disease. The pathology is similar to chronic *hepatitis B*, so many treatment methods were borrowed from those used to treat chronic hepatitis B.

During the course of HCV infection, many changes occur in the body. Some of these changes are immune system abnormalities, liver *inflammation, fibrosis*, and *portal vein* hypertension. All of these changes can have significant effects on disease progression and your *prognosis*. Therefore, it is not enough to treat only the virus. Chinese medicine emphasizes restoring liver function and overall health (supporting the righteous *qi* of the body). A healthier body is better able to control the virus, prevent it from causing further harm, and possibly eradicate it (dispelling the evil). In treating chronic hepatitis C, MCM uses western medical knowledge about diagnosis, the cause of disease, and how the virus causes harm. This knowledge is combined with TCM diagnostic tools and herbal treatments to derive the best from both systems of medicine.

Treatment Protocol for Chronic Hepatitis C

The following *protocol* for treating chronic hepatitis C has several goals.

- heal liver inflammation and restore liver function to halt disease progression
- reduce the *viral load* and/or suppress viral replication
- regulate the immune system
- improve *microcirculation* (blood flow to organs and tissues)
- promote liver cell regeneration
- suppress *fibroblastic* activity (reduce scarring)
- promote *bile* flow
- treat hepatitis C related symptoms and complications to improve quality of life

The protocol consists of seven parts. See *Appendix V: Modern and Traditional Chinese Medicine* for the pharmacology of the major herbs used in the treatment protocol for chronic hepatitis C.

Part 1. Improve or normalize liver enzyme levels and liver functions

Inflammation causes fibrosis, which leads to *cirrhosis*. To stop this progression, inflammation must be controlled. If the liver is not actively inflamed, the time it takes for cirrhosis to develop is estimated to be 80 years, the approximate length of the human life span.[5] The following herbal remedies are used to control inflammation.

- Hepa Formula No. 2 Capsule
- Ligustrin Tablet
- Glycyrrhizin Tablet
- Circulation No.1 Tablets

ALT is an important marker of liver inflammation. After treatment, if three consecutive ALT tests (done 2-3 months apart) are normal, liver inflammation is considered to be under control.

The active ingredients of schizandra and schisandrin B and C have been tested in *clinical trials* in China. Studies involving 4,558 patients showed schisandrin B and C reduced and/or normalized ALT levels in 75% of the cases within 2-3 months.[6] Schizandra and schisandrin B and C are the major ingredients in Hepa Formula No. 2.

Oleanolic acid, the active ingredient of *Ligustrum fructus*, has also been studied. Out of 153 patients treated, 110 (70%) experienced normalization of their ALT within 50 days.[7] Glycyrrhizin, a licorice root extract, has been used to treat chronic viral hepatitis in China and Japan. Studies have shown it to be effective in normalizing ALT in 64% of patients in Japan, and 84.5% of patients in China.[8]

Part 2. Lower and stabilize the HCV viral load

Suppressing HCV is achieved by strengthening the immune system and using antiviral herbal remedies. Herbal treatments may be able reduce HCV viral load, but cannot eliminate the virus. Antiviral therapy is the weak point of MCM. More research needs to be done to develop more effective anti-HCV herbal remedies.

Most herbal antiviral studies were done with the hepatitis B virus (HBV), not HCV. The herbs *Polygni cuspidati rhizoma, Houttuyn herbaiae, Rhei rhizoma,* and *Blechni rhizoma* have been found to suppress HBV in the laboratory. Another group of herbs, *Salviae miltiorrhziae radix,*

Prunellae spica, *Gardeniae fructus*, and *Montan radicis cortex*, have been found to reduce HBV replication by over 50% in the laboratory.[9] Studies of HBV patients treated with this herbal combination found 30-40% became negative for HBV antigens (laboratory indicators of HBV in the body).[10]

Most patients' viral load can be reduced and/or stabilized below one million. The following herbs have been used to lower viral load.

- Glycyrrhizin Tablet
- Olive leaves *Decoction*
- Olivessence Capsule

Part 3. Regulate the immune system

HCV causes liver damage in two ways. It can directly damage or kill liver cells, or it can cause damage by causing the immune system to react abnormally. An inadequate immune response allows HCV to invade and damage or kill liver cells. This is how most liver damage from HCV is done. Without an adequate immune response, HCV infection becomes chronic.

The other mechanism of HCV damage comes from an overactive *antibody* response to the virus. The immune system makes large quantities of *proteins* called gamma globulins. These proteins form larger molecules called soluble immune complex (SIC). When SIC is deposited in the liver, joints, skin, and other areas, it causes inflammation. Other abnormalities in the immune system allow this inflammation to persist. Ongoing inflammation can eventually lead to fibrosis and/or cirrhosis.

Glycyrrhizin and AI #3 Capsule are used to suppress autoimmunity. Blood activating and stasis expelling herbs such as Circulation No. 1 Tablet are used to clear SIC. *Cordyceps sinensis*, *Sophorae subprostratae radix*, and *Polyporus umbellatus pers* are used to regulate other immune functions.

- Glycyrrhizin Capsule
- AI #3, Capsule
- Circulation No. 1 Tablet
- Cordyceps Capsule

Part 4. Improve microcirculation, promote liver regeneration, and suppress fibroblastic activity

Patients with chronic hepatitis C often have microcirculation disorders. This means blood flow to organs and tissues is abnormal. In MCM, a microcirculation disorder is called blood stagnancy. Typically, patients with blood stagnancy have liver palms, spider moles, cold hands and feet, purplish tongue, dark lips, a dark ring around each eye, and/or an enlarged spleen. Studies in China found the severity of a person's microcirculation disorder is a good indicator of the severity of liver inflammation and damage.[11] Microcirculation disorders in the liver can keep it from getting the proper oxygen and nutrients. This promotes the process of fibrosis. If microcirculation in the liver is improved, liver cell regeneration will be promoted and the progression of fibrosis will be suppressed. To improve all of these symptoms, a blood activating and stasis expelling herbal formula such as Circulation No. 1 Tablet is used.

Part 5. Facilitate secretion and excretion of bile

People with chronic viral hepatitis can have thickened bile that may become blocked by inflamed liver tissue. This often causes jaundice, gall bladder inflammation, and gallstones. Bile blockage can also injure the liver and promote fibrosis. This leads to an increase in liver *enzymes* and *bilirubin* in the blood. Therefore, improving bile secretion is very important. The following formulas can effectively release blocked bile and clear jaundice. These formulas can also be used for gallbladder inflammation and gallstones.

- Gall No. 1 Tablet

- Capillaris Combination

Part 6. Lower portal vein pressure and suppress fibroblastic activities

Portal vein hypertension is the main cause of many of the complications of advanced liver disease. *Portal hypertension* is usually present only in people with cirrhosis. It can cause *ascites* (the accumulation of fluid in the abdomen), spleen enlargement, *varices* (the ballooning of veins), hemorrhoids, and edema (abnormal swelling, especially in the feet and lower legs). Reducing portal pressure is very important for people with advanced liver disease because this condition can cause severe bleeding.

In China, herbs used to treat the fibrosis seen with the disease miner's lung have also been used to treat early-stage cirrhosis. Controlled animal studies found cirrhotic animals treated with these herbs had lower levels of liver *collagen* (the material that makes up fibrotic tissue) than untreated animals.[12]

Cordyceps sinensis, Persicae semen, Salvia miltiorrhziae, and glycyrrhizin have been found to soften the liver, promote the breakdown of collagen, and enhance liver cell regeneration.

- Circulation No.1 Tablets
- Cordyceps Capsule
- Glycyrrhizin Capsule

Part 7. Treatments for Hepatitis C Related Conditions

Herbal treatments to alleviate HCV-related symptoms can improve patients' quality of life. Some of these symptoms and their herbal treatments are discussed in this section.

A. Fatigue

The liver is the major powerhouse of the body. When liver function deteriorates, *fatigue* often results. The elimination of fatigue relies mainly on the improvement of liver function. If fatigue is the major problem, it can be treated with the following formula.

- Cordyceps Capsule

B. Insomnia

Sleep disorders are a common complaint among people living with hepatitis C. Prescription sleep medications can be addictive and cause side effects such as morning drowsiness. They may also be *toxic* to the liver. The following herbal formula addresses this problem successfully.

- HerbSom Capsules

C. Joint pain, skin rashes, vasculitis, psoriasis, Sjogren syndrome

Many people with hepatitis C also have autoimmune symptoms and syndromes such as those listed above. These are the *extrahepatic* (outside the liver) symptoms of the abnormal immune response caused by HCV infection. Since the underlying cause of these different problems is the same, so is the treatment.

- AI #3 Capsule
- Circulation No. 1 Tablet

D. Diabetes

One of the liver's many functions is regulating blood sugar. The amount of sugar in the blood increases after eating. Excess sugar is turned into *glycogen* and is stored in the liver. When the blood sugar drops, the glycogen in the liver is broken down into sugar again and is released into the blood. This process is sometimes disrupted in people with chronic hepatitis C causing blood sugar abnormalities. HCV can also cause blood sugar abnormalities by damaging the cells of the pancreas that produce *insulin*, the hormone that controls blood sugar levels. HCV-related blood sugar abnormalities can often be controlled with an herbal remedy.

- BM (Bitter Melon) Capsule

E. Infections

During the course of chronic hepatitis C, people may get other infectious illnesses such as sore throats, sinusitis, colds, and bronchitis. Many health care providers use antibiotics to treat these conditions. However since many of these illnesses are caused by viruses, antibiotics are often ineffective and may injure the liver. Herbs can be used to fight these infections. The most important herbal remedy for infections is Allicin, which is the essence of garlic. Coptin and Rhubarbin Tablets may also be used to fight infections.

- Allicin Capsule
- Coptin Tablet
- Rhubarbin Tablet

F. Ascites and edema

Ascites (fluid in the abdomen) and edema (swelling of the feet, legs, and hands) can occur with cirrhosis and liver failure. If these symptoms occur, salt and protein intake should be limited. At the same time, an herbal formula can be used to expel excess water.

- Tiao Ying Yin Formula

G. Bleeding

Cirrhotic patients may be at risk for *bleeding varices*. This is bleeding from abnormally large and thin-walled veins around the stomach and the esophagus (the food pipe leading to the stomach). This kind of bleeding is accompanied by vomiting blood and/or passing black, tar-like stools. Bleeding from varices is a medical emergency. If this happens, you need to go to an emergency room immediately.

Bleeding from the gums or nose are more common and less serious forms of bleeding that can occur with liver failure. The following herbal formula is used to treat these less serious types of bleeding.

- Yunan Pai Yao Capsule

H. Diarrhea

Diarrhea is a common complaint of people with chronic hepatitis C. Diarrhea often improves as liver function improves. If diarrhea lasts and becomes severe, the following formula can be used.

- Ginseng and Atractylodes Formula

I. Nausea and vomiting

Nausea is more common than vomiting in people with chronic hepatitis C. It can occur when bile secretion is blocked as this affects digestion. If these complaints become persistent, the following formula can be used.

- Pinellia and Hoelen combination

Clinical Outcomes of the Protocols

More than 900 patients at Zhang's Clinic in New York City have used these protocols. In January 2000, we had test results on file for over 400 patients. A scientific analysis was conducted on 75 patients for whom both pre- and post-treatment ALT levels were available. ALT was used to determine whether the protocols were effective. The average before treatment ALT level was 128 (±114), and the average after-treatment ALT level was 47(±42). Of these 75 patients, 77% experienced normalization of their ALT, and 93% experienced ALT improvement. All patients reported improvement in their symptoms.

INTENDED ENDPOINTS OF CHINESE MEDICAL TREATMENT: HOW TO DEFINE CURE WITH TCM AND MCM

Chinese medicine defines cure as the body's return to balance and normal functioning. The ultimate goal of Chinese health care is to restore a person's health, full function, and a normal life expectancy. Eliminating the virus and controlling inflammation are methods for reaching this goal. The goals of Chinese medical treatment for hepatitis C are to arrest the virus, and reverse of the impact of the virus. This results in improved or normal liver function. In turn, quality of life improves and there is a reasonable expectation for a normal life span. However, long-term ongoing treatment may be required. By utilizing this approach, we can buy sufficient time for patients to wait for new developments and better treatments for hepatitis C.

IS IT POSSIBLE OR NECESSARY TO COMPLETELY ERADICATE HCV?

The most frequently asked question about MCM treatment is, can it eradicate the hepatitis C virus? Many patients are concerned about having the virus in their body. They worry about not having been 'cured' even after their liver functions have been normalized and they have a normal, or near normal, quality of life.

While they are two different infections, it may help to compare HIV treatment to HCV treatment. HCV was identified eight years after the identification of HIV. Western medical treatment approaches for HCV followed closely behind those for HIV (approximately ten years later). The main goal of western medical treatment for HIV has been to aggressively attack the virus and eradicate it with powerful antiviral medications. So far, however, this method has not worked as expected.

Virologist Robert Siliciano of Johns Hopkins University found that HIV hides inside resting cells to form stubborn reservoirs of virus. He states, "Pools of latent HIV, lurking in the cells of infected people, remain untouched even by powerful drug combinations."[14] These reservoirs make many researchers doubt the possibility of eliminating HIV from the body, and forces them to rethink strategies for fighting the virus. This discovery also raised a more basic question, does the 'hit hard' method really work? As Dr. Anthony Fauci said, "The concept of a reservoir is of paramount importance to the whole philosophy of what we wish to accomplish therapeutically."[13]

Faced with this challenge, it seems that HIV/AIDS researchers have a difficult task ahead of them. While the growing realization of the importance of viral reservoirs has dashed most researchers' hopes of completely eradicating HIV from the body, elimination may not be necessary to manage the disease. HIV co-discoverer Dr. Robert Gallo asked, "If you could have a therapy that was easy, inexpensive, not toxic, not inconvenient, worked without side effects, could work life-long, but you didn't eradicate [the virus], is that OK?" The article concludes with, "Sure it's OK."[14]

It appears that more and more HIV experts are granting the right for the virus to exist within the body, and acknowledging that it does not necessarily need to be eradicated.

People may argue that HCV is different from HIV. Whether HCV has reservoirs in the body is still unknown. However, between 1-5% of people who have a *sustained response* to treatment for over 6 months eventually *relapse*. This suggests there is a possibility that HCV resides in a reservoir that has not yet been detected. Currently, only *blood serum* (the liquid part of blood) is tested for viral load, but testing whole blood (blood liquid plus the blood cells) is more accurate. Undetectable viral load in serum does not necessarily mean undetectable viral load in blood cells and tissues. HCV PCR testing is still not sensitive enough to determine total virus eradication. However, the newer whole blood tests may help answer this important question.

REASONS FOR USING TCM OR MCM THERAPIES AND WHO MAY BENEFIT

Chinese herbal treatments for HCV have many positive features. They are:

- effective
- time-honored
- easy to take
- affordable (15-20 times less expensive than western medication)
- virtually nontoxic
- largely side effect free, and
- work life-long.

However, Chinese remedies do not necessarily eradicate HCV. Chinese herbal treatments provide an alternative for people who are unwilling or unable to use western medicine treatment options. Some examples of situations in which TCM may be chosen are listed below.

- Many people are afraid of the side effects of prescription medicines. For them, TCM or MCM may be a viable alternative. "In the US, it is likely that more patients with hepatitis C use nonprescription agents of unproven effectiveness than use *interferon-based therapy*." [15]
- For the approximately 50% of people who do not respond to western treatment, TCM or MCM can be used to help improve liver function and overall quality of life.
- For those who cannot take interferon and/or ribavirin, TCM or MCM may provide an alternative treatment option. Conditions that may make the use of interferon or ribavirin

impossible include *decompensated* cirrhosis, persistently normal ALT, active alcohol or illicit drug use, a history of major depression, cytopenia (low white blood cell count), *hyperthyroidism*, *renal* transplant, and/or evidence of autoimmune disease.

- For those who cannot tolerate western treatment, TCM or MCM may provide an alternative.
- Individuals who initially respond to interferon and/or ribavirin but then relapse may have a recurrence of liver disease. TCM and MCM can be used to treat this recurrence.
- TCM or MCM therapies can be used to treat damage already caused by chronic hepatitis C.

REASONS FOR NOT USING TCM OR MCM

Common reasons given for not using TCM or MCM are described below.

- It is not intended to eradicate HCV, so it is not a 'cure.'
  As stated above, the concept of 'cure' in TCM and MCM is different than it is in western medicine.
- TCM or MCM herbal remedies are unproven and have not gone through rigorous scientific testing.

  Most TCM and MCM remedies are customized to meet the specific needs of the client, taking into account other conditions and limitations. It is very difficult to conduct clinical trials with herbal remedies because TCM and MCM do not subscribe to the 'one size fits all' approach of western medicine. In many cases, this means clinical trials would be invalid because they would be comparing 'apples to oranges.'

  The National Center for Complementary and Alternative Medicine (NCCAM) Internet page "Hepatitis C: Treatment Alternatives" labeled TCM and MCM as having "no research to a limited amount of research." Because most of the published research on TCM and MCM is in Chinese, this issue is further complicated.

- The FDA does not regulate herbal products, so using herbs can be dangerous. You may not get what you are supposed to get.

  This can be true, especially if the herbalist is not well versed in *phytopharmacology* and *toxicity* data. Because of this potential danger, it is important to verify the credentials of any herbalist you decide to consult.

  The Internet site at www.consumerlab.com is privately owned, and monitors the quality of nutritional supplements and herbs. You may find this site useful. If you choose to take herbal products, it is very important to confirm the quality of the herbs or products.

- Herbal medicines are not stable with respect to their active essence because species, collecting seasons, and production sites vary.

  The method of preparation (drying, steaming, and decocting) can dilute the active essence of an herb. It is also argued that herbal medicines are inconvenient to prepare for ingestion. Finally, herbal medicines can be perceived to be bitter and unpleasant to ingest.

  These drawbacks can be alleviated through scientific preparation procedures to achieve a consistent amount of active ingredients. In addition, herbal extracts can be concentrated so that the daily dosage is small and requires no special preparation.

Since capsule, tablet, and granular forms of herbal preparations are placed on the tongue and swallowed with a large glass of water, poor taste need not be a deterrent.

- The numbers of different chemicals in herbs make it hard to control their interactions with conventional drugs.

    If you are taking any herbal products, you need to tell your western doctor. He or she will be able to advise you about any possible interactions. Your herbalist can also advise you about this.

ANECDOTAL STORIES OF TREATMENT SUCCESS WITH TCM AND MCM

An *anecdotal* story is one that is not based on a controlled, clinical trial, but on an individual's personal experience. Whether or not the results of anecdotal stories have value is up to you.

Below are two stories of success and two stories of failure based on real cases from my clinic in New York City. Patient names have been changed.

Joseph V.

Joseph V. is a New Jersey firefighter. He was diagnosed with hepatitis C in 1996. When he saw me in 1997, he was on disability and his ALT was quite high (above 300). He felt tired and could not work. Two months after herbal treatment, his liver enzyme levels normalized and he went back to active duty as a firefighter.

His western health care provider suggested he try interferon, and he did not want to lose the chance to try this FDA-approved therapy. He stopped taking herbs and went on interferon for eight months. During this time, he went back on disability and felt very sick. When the treatment was finished, his ALT went up to 380. At that point, his western doctor suggested the combination of interferon and ribavirin. He refused. He came back to me for treatment and resumed herbal therapy. Within two months, his liver function tests normalized. He has since returned to active duty as a firefighter and has married. He told me the herbal treatment helped him to put his life together and gain the confidence to build a family.

Lorraine D.

Lorraine D., 41, works for a large pharmaceutical company that produces interferon. She was diagnosed with hepatitis C in 1997. She might have contracted the virus seven years earlier. In March 1998, she stopped a seven-month course of interferon treatment. At that time, her liver function tests were normal. However, the side effects of interferon forced her to discontinue treatment. Her *platelet* count dropped to a dangerously low level. She often had bruises on her skin. She was diagnosed with idiopathic thrombocytopenic purpura (ITP), an autoimmune disease. She was put on steroids to treat the ITP. Her thyroid gland was also not functioning well. She was given synthetic thyroid hormone to correct her thyroid function. The steroids helped her platelet count increase in two months, but they triggered a relapse of liver inflammation. She came to see me in May 1998 after this relapse. Her ALT and *AST* were both abnormal. Her viral load was at 27 million, much higher than before interferon treatment. Lorraine was very tired and had pain in her liver area and joints, dark urine, and occasional diarrhea with pale stool. Her skin and *conjunctiva* (the skin around the inside of the eyes) were yellowish. In addition, she had a *pituitary* tumor as an underlying condition, which made her situation quite complicated. Her western health care provider recommended interferon and ribavirin, but she refused.

I first focused on her liver inflammation. Her ITP and thyroid gland abnormality showed that her liver inflammation had autoimmune involvement. I emphasized anti-autoimmune therapy. She began taking Hepa Formula No. 2, Glycyrrhizin Capsule, Ligustrin Capsule, AI Capsule No. 3, Circulation Tablet No. 1, and Formula R6379 (for hypothyroidism). One month later, her blood tests showed that all liver enzyme levels had normalized. Her platelet count increased and her thyroid tests also normalized. She was ecstatic because the treatment had normalized her ITP and rid her of *hypothyroidism* and liver inflammation in only one month.

Her liver enzyme levels have been normal since that time, except once in reaction to a drug treatment for edema in her ankles. She is now on a maintenance protocol. All of her symptoms are gone.

ANECDOTAL STORIES OF TREATMENT FAILURE WITH TCM AND MCM

About 10% of the patients using Chinese medicine protocols do not get favorable results.

Doug F.

Doug F., 50, visited my office in August 1999. He was first diagnosed with non-A, non-B hepatitis (hepatitis C) in 1977 after a blood transfusion. He was a heavy drinker from age 17 to 29. His liver enzymes were very high (ALT 426, AST 155). His viral load was 48,000. He had *genotype* 1a HCV. He occasionally felt fatigued, his urine was golden yellow, and he sometimes had diarrhea. After approximately one month on the herbal treatments Hepa F. #2, Ligustrin, Glycyrrhizin, AI #3, and Circulation #1, his ALT and AST decreased, but his viral load went up to 200,000. He was very happy with these results. On the next test approximately one month later, his ALT and AST levels went back up. Although his ALT level went back down approximately one month later, his AST continued to rise. He was very depressed and felt more fatigued. From then on, the results on his liver enzyme tests were continuously worse. In January 2000, he had a *liver biopsy* and found *grade* II inflammation and stage II fibrosis. His ALT and AST continued to be markedly elevated, and his viral load was greater than one million. I tried using second line herbal remedies and switched the Hepa F. #2 to Hepa F. #1a. In March 2000, his ALT and AST dropped, but he lost confidence in herbal treatment and went on western therapy.

Bruce D.

Bruce D., 61, was diagnosed with hepatitis C in 1984 as non-A, non-B hepatitis. He might have become infected in 1975. His HCV genotype was 1b. Before he started an herbal protocol in December 1998, his baseline liver function tests were ALT 389, AST 192, and viral load 2.6 million. His liver biopsy showed stage II-III fibrosis with marked, active, ongoing inflammation (grade III). His blood clotting studies were slightly abnormal. He had been an alcohol drinker, but stopped drinking four years earlier. Clinically, he had a gassy stomach, loose stools, and slightly yellowish skin, but no other obvious symptoms.

He started a first line protocol of Hepa F. #2 Capsule, Ligustrin Capsule, Glycyrrhizin Capsule, AI#3 Capsule, and Circulation #1 Capsule. In the first year (1999), his ALT levels improved.

Once in July 1999, when his ALT went up to 276, I added a new herb, Paniculate Tablet, which brought the ALT back down. His viral load was sometimes very high. In 2000, his ALT shot up again. Beginning in March 2000, I switched him to a second line protocol, which included using Hepa F. #1a to replace Hepa F. #2. This change did not generate any significant positive effect.

SUMMARY

TCM has been used for thousands of years by millions of people to promote health and provide therapy when health is impaired. TCM and MCM use observation and deduction to identify those areas of the body that are out of balance. TCM and MCM use a variety of therapeutic approaches such as herbs, acupuncture, and massage to help the body overcome the effects of disease and regain a healthy balance.

Each practitioner of TCM or MCM uses his or her own herbal formulations, and approaches the treatment of disorders such as hepatitis C based on his or her training and background. If you are currently seeing a TCM practitioner or are considering TCM as a treatment option, be sure to check your practitioner's training and qualifications. The *Resources Directory* at the back of this manual provides information on locating a TCM practitioner.

Regardless of what options you decide to pursue in the treatment of your hepatitis C, be sure to inform all of those in whom you entrust your health care of all the approaches you are using.

Chapter Thirteen

NATUROPATHIC MEDICINE

Lyn Patrick ND

INTRODUCTION

The philosophy of naturopathic medicine can best be described as the utilization of the healing power of nature. A number of basic thoughts are at the core of this philosophy. Naturopathic health care providers approach health with prevention and education foremost in their minds. If disease enters the picture, the approach is to treat the whole person so that the natural healing powers of the body can rid it of the root cause of the illness.

THE NATUROPATHIC APPROACH

Naturopathic health care providers use many different tools in the care and treatment of patients. These include botanical medicines (herbs), acupuncture, *nutritional supplements*, traditional Chinese medicine, homeopathic remedies, nutrition counseling and diet therapy, massage and/or spinal *manipulation*, exercise, and other forms of therapy.

There are four accredited naturopathic medical colleges in the United States. If you choose to include naturopathic medicine in your treatment of *hepatitis C*, it is important that you see a licensed naturopathic doctor. The American Association of Naturopathic Physicians can provide information on well-trained, naturopathic doctors in the United States (see the *Resource Directory*).

THE PRINCIPLES OF NATUROPATHIC TREATMENT FOR HEPATITIS C

The following is a discussion of the naturopathic approach to treating hepatitis C and the options a naturopathic doctor might consider when treating someone with hepatitis C.

The Liver as an Organ of Detoxification

The liver is a large organ. It weighs about 3° pounds. It requires approximately one-third of the heart's output of blood to do its many jobs. The liver filters almost two quarts of blood every minute. This filtration is essential to the body's survival because the liver receives blood directly from the intestines. It has to filter *proteins* and other nutrients and chemicals absorbed from the food we eat. The liver regulates blood sugar levels, stores fat soluble vitamins, activates and breaks down hormones and drugs, and aids in the elimination of pollutants and *toxins* from disease causing *microorganisms*. The liver also manufactures nutrients, *enzymes*, and *hormones*.

For the liver to function well, it needs certain nutrients for the detoxification system and immune cells. The liver requires B vitamins (B_2, B_3, B_6, B_{12}, and folic acid), magnesium, zinc, copper, choline, betaine, and the *amino acids* methionine, taurine, and cysteine in order to break down medications, pollutants, and chemicals found in air, water, and food.[1]

Glutathione

Glutathione is one of the most important chemicals needed for liver health. Glutathione is an *antioxidant*, a chemical that protects the liver from damage by other chemicals called *free radicals* and oxidants. Glutathione is produced in the liver and elsewhere in the body from some of the nutrients listed above. Glutathione is a sulfur-based *peptide* (a protein precursor) that helps the liver eliminate free radicals and *metabolize* (break down) medications and chemicals. Glutathione is used by other cells in the body as the main antioxidant defense against *oxidative stress* (an overabundance of free radicals). It is also a crucial activator of certain cells in the *immune system* called cytotoxic *T-cells*. Cytotoxic T-cells kill viruses and cancer cells.[2]

The body cannot function without glutathione. Loss of glutathione causes liver and kidney failure, and ultimately death. Low glutathione levels are found in people with cataracts, *HIV* infection, *chronic hepatitis* C, and *cirrhosis*.[3] People with cirrhosis of the liver can have difficulty making glutathione. This may explain why glutathione levels are 30% below normal in people with cirrhosis.[4]

Because glutathione acts as an antioxidant and prevents damage from oxidants like iron, it may actually slow the *fibrosis* process. Damage from liver iron in chronic hepatitis C is a contributing factor in the process of fibrosis. Levels of the most important form of glutathione, called reduced glutathione, are significantly below normal in people who have alcoholic hepatitis or hepatitis C.[5, 6] Studies have shown that people with hepatitis C who had the lowest glutathione levels also had the highest *viral loads* and more evidence of liver damage.[6] Glutathione has been shown to have direct *antiviral* effects. Although no research has been done with the hepatitis C virus (HCV), glutathione has been shown to inhibit HIV in the test tube.[7] Although this research does not prove that raising glutathione would automatically lower viral load, it does indicate that optimal levels of glutathione may be an important factor in controlling HCV infection.

Limiting Exposure to Liver Damaging Substances and Situations

If you have hepatitis C, it is important to avoid exposure to anything that can cause additional damage to your liver. Following are some of the things that can place additional stress on and possibly damage your liver.

Alcohol

Chronic alcohol consumption is a significant risk factor for liver cirrhosis. Chronic alcohol drinkers who do not have HCV are actually at a **higher** risk of developing cirrhosis than those who **do** have hepatitis C but do not drink.[8] We know the risk of developing cirrhosis is about 16 times higher in people with HCV who are chronic drinkers than in those with HCV who do not drink alcohol. It is important to remember that even low levels of alcohol consumption (less than 6 ounces per week) are related to higher HCV viral loads and increased liver fibrosis.[9] National consensus conferences of doctors and scientists in both France and the United States have recommended that all people with hepatitis C refrain from drinking <u>any</u> alcohol.[10, 11]

One way alcohol damages the liver is by depleting it of glutathione. Even in people who have hepatitis C without *symptoms* and only mild elevations in *liver enzymes*, liver damage may still exist and the damage is worsened by loss of glutathione due to alcohol use.

Acetaminophen

Acetaminophen is a drug that can deplete the liver of glutathione.[12] Because glutathione levels may already be low in people with hepatitis C, risking even lower levels with long-term acetaminophen use may be unwise. Using acetaminophen for a headache every now and then is not enough to affect the level of glutathione in the liver, but daily use of this medicine over months can deplete the liver's store of glutathione. Acetaminophen is the active ingredient in many over-the-counter pain relievers such as Tylenol®. It is also found in many cold medications. If you need a pain reliever, ask your health care provider about alternatives to acetaminophen that provide similar pain relief. Naturopathic doctors prescribe botanical medicines for pain relief such as food extracts and herbs. Examples include Bromelain (an enzyme extracted from pineapples), *Picrorhiza kurroa* extract, *Boswellia serrata* extract, *Curcuma longa* (a tumeric root extract), and *Salix alba* (white willow bark).

Tobacco and Recreational Drugs

The liver must break down all the toxic and *carcinogenic* compounds found in tobacco, marijuana, and other recreational drugs. Tobacco and marijuana use (marijuana contains many of the same carcinogenic compounds as tobacco) increase the risk of *liver cancer* for people infected with HCV.[13] If you feel you need to use marijuana for pain relief or to stimulate your appetite, try alternative pain relievers and other strategies for increasing your appetite. If you feel you must use marijuana, use as little as possible.

Coffee

Although caffeine appears to pose no problem for the liver in chronic hepatitis C, there are other substances in coffee that have been shown to raise liver enzyme levels in healthy people. Research has been conducted on two compounds found in coffee beans, cafestol and kahweol (called diterpenes). The research showed these compounds raised *ALT* levels (the most important liver enzyme in monitoring chronic hepatitis C) by 80% in 46 healthy subjects who were drinking 5-6 cups of strong, French press (unfiltered) coffee daily.[14] ALT levels dropped to 45% above normal 24 weeks after the study participants stopped drinking coffee. However, the authors concluded they could not rule out the possibility that the coffee had caused subclincal (something that happens but cannot be seen through blood analysis or symptoms) injury to participants' liver cells.

Other studies have shown that cafestol and kahweol raise blood cholesterol, *triglyceride*, and low-density *lipoprotein* (a harmful fat) levels, and increase other risk factors for heart disease.[15] Filtering coffee eliminates both cafestol and kahweol. However, because they are not filtered, espresso or French press coffee contain both of these compounds. If you are a coffee drinker, make sure you drink filtered coffee. Drinking water-processed, decaffeinated, filtered coffee decreases any potentially harmful effects coffee may have.[16]

Occupational Exposures

We know that exposure to pesticides, *herbicides*, and other chemicals can cause liver damage and elevation of liver enzymes.[17,18,19] If your job exposes you to chemicals, solvents, fumes, pesticides, or herbicides, it is very important that you use *OSHA*-approved protective gear to prevent breathing the fumes or having physical contact with these chemicals. This includes exposure to paint and lacquer, solvents such as dry cleaning fluid, glues and epoxy, and fabric coatings among many others. If you have a history of chemical exposure and are concerned about the effects on your liver, there are proven ways to reduce the burden of these toxic compounds on your body. Elimination of these toxic compounds requires the supervision of a trained doctor. Naturopathic doctors and medical doctors trained in environmental medicine can supervise programs designed to eliminate these substances from the body. The *Encyclopedia of Natural Medicine* was written by licensed naturopathic doctors, and is a good resource for information about naturopathic support for detoxification.[20]

Diet and Hepatitis C

One of the basic concepts of a naturopathic diet is the inclusion of only minimal amounts of processed foods and simple sugars (sucrose, *glucose*, corn syrup, etc.). This recommendation is based on research that examined the effect of large amounts of simple sugars on the body's immune system. Eating 75-100 grams (approximately 2.5-3.5 ounces) of white sugar, honey, or fruit juice appears to reduce the ability of specific white blood cells to attack foreign organisms such as viruses and bacteria by 50%.[21, 22] This immune suppressing effect starts 30 minutes after eating, and lasts for five hours afterward. Since the average American eats and drinks 175 grams of sugar daily, the potential effect on the immune system is considerable. The immune system is an important factor in hepatitis C because we know that those who clear HCV appear to have *lymphocytes* (white blood cells) that are better able to kill the virus than those who go on to become chronically infected.[23]

Dietary Fat

The only available research on diet that relates directly to HCV infection is a study that examined how dietary fat, *carbohydrate*, and protein levels affect the risk for disease progression to cirrhosis. The study indicated a high-fat diet coupled with low amounts of protein and carbohydrates increases the risk of progressing to cirrhosis.[24] However, the study did not indicate what specific types of fat may be dangerous.

As explained in *Chapter 7: Nutrition and Hepatitis C*, not all fats are bad. The omega-3 fatty acids actually have helpful immune regulating effects and should always be included in a nutritional plan for optimizing the immune system. Some types of fat actually appear to be beneficial for people with hepatitis C. Studies of *phosphatidylcholine*, a type of fat found in fish and soybeans, showed it has a beneficial effect in reducing liver enzymes and increasing the response rate to *interferon*.[25] People who were given polyunsaturated phosphatidylcholine (1.8 grams/day) during treatment with interferon and for six months following treatment had significantly fewer *relapses* than those who did not take the fat supplement. Forty-one percent of the patients in the phosphatidylcholine group had a sustained response compared to 15% who received only interferon. Different forms of phosphatidylcholine have been used in hepatitis resulting from alcoholism, and have been effective in decreasing fibrosis.[26]

For a thorough discussion of the fundamentals of a naturopathic approach to eating a healthy diet, see *Chapter 7: Nutrition and Hepatitis C*.

Nutritional Supplementation

A nutritious diet, nutritional supplementation, and botanical medicines are the foundations of the naturopathic approach to treating chronic hepatitis C. The nutritional supplements listed in *Chapter 14, Nutritional Supplementation* are mostly antioxidants. They work to decrease liver *inflammation* and raise glutathione levels. Glutathione is an important antioxidant and immune system regulating protein. The supplements listed in *Chapter 14: Nutritional Supplementation* are meant to be taken together as a total *protocol*, not as substitutes for each other or as choices that can be taken individually. As stated in *Chapter 7: Nutrition and Hepatitis C*, neither diet alone nor supplements alone are enough to help the body effectively manage chronic hepatitis C.

Botanicals Used To Treat Hepatitis C Liver Problems

Silybum marianum (Milk Thistle)

Silybum marianum (milk thistle) has been used medicinally in Europe since the 13th century to treat liver related diseases. It is available in Germany in both injectable and oral forms.[27] A recent survey evaluated the use of *complementary and alternative medicine (CAM)* among hepatitis C patients in liver clinics. The survey found 42-73% of all patients who used other alternative therapies were also taking milk thistle. All participants who used only herbs to treat their liver disease (63%) identified milk thistle as one of the herbs taken.[28]

The active ingredients in milk thistle are contained in the extract silymarin. Silymarin is a mixture of active plant materials that includes silybinin, a plant compound known as a *flavinoid*. Although silybinin has not been shown to have any antiviral activity against HCV, some flavinoids do have antiviral properties.

Silymarin has specific effects on liver cells that have been seen in laboratory animal studies. Silymarin appears to stabilize or strengthen liver cells' ability to withstand the effects of substances that are toxic to the liver including recreational drugs, some medications, poisonous mushrooms, and chemicals. It prevents the damage that occurs when free radicals attack the fatty layer of liver cell membranes.[29] Silymarin also appears to inhibit the process of inflammation of liver cells that eventually leads to cirrhosis.[30] Silymarin increases glutathione levels in the liver. Some studies of hepatitis C patients have found abnormally low levels of glutathione.[31, 32, 33]

There are no published studies on the effects of silymarin among large populations of hepatitis C patients, though there have been several studies on the effects of silymarin among people with liver disease. In people with *acute hepatitis* (both A and B), silymarin was found to decrease the number of complications, speed recovery time, and improve liver function test scores.[34] In chronic liver disease (both alcoholic and chronic hepatitis), silymarin has been shown to decrease symptoms of *fatigue* and abdominal pain, and to significantly decrease liver enzyme levels.[35] Silymarin has also been shown to improve the survival rates of people with cirrhosis. Those with histories of alcohol related liver damage fared better than those who had cirrhosis from drug use.[36] Because these studies were done prior to widespread testing for hepatitis C, it is not known how many of the patients in these studies were actually infected with HCV.

Not all studies with silymarin have shown a clear benefit in liver disease. A study of 125 patients with alcoholic cirrhosis who took 450 mg of silymarin per day for two years did not find any improvement associated with silymarin use.[37] Whether these results were influenced by the effects of alcohol abuse is not known.

Another form of silymarin called silipide or silybin-phosphatidylcholine has also been studied. This form is more easily absorbed than forms of silymarin. In a small study with eight patients (five had hepatitis C), liver function tests and markers that reflect cell damage in the liver were significantly improved in patients who had been taking the equivalent of 120 mg of silybin twice daily between meals for two months.[38]

Milk thistle is available over-the-counter in standardized extracts that contain 70% silymarin. Because the active ingredients are not water soluble, a tea made from milk thistle seeds is not useful. If the label for milk thistle does not list the silymarin content, there is no guarantee that there is any silymarin in it. Standard dosages used in studies range from 400-1,140 mg per day of the standardized extract. The common dosage for active liver disease is 200 mg of standardized extract (containing 70% silymarin) taken three times daily. Silipide (the phosphatidylcholine form) is commonly dosed at 100 mg taken three times daily. Silymarin is very safe and has no known *toxicity*, though high doses (over 1,500 mg per day) may cause diarrhea because of increased *bile* secretion. It is safe to use in pregnancy and while breast feeding.[39]

Glycyrrhiza glabra (Licorice Root)

Glycyrrhiza glabra (licorice root) preparations have been used in Japan to treat both *hepatitis B* and *C* for over 20 years.[40] Glycyrrhizin, an extract made from the *Glycyrrhiza glabra* plant, is used as an intravenous injection on a daily basis for eight weeks. The preparation can be given at that frequency or reduced to several times a week, and can be continued for as long as 16 years.[41]

A study of 193 hepatitis C patients being treated with intravenous glycyrrhizin for 2-16 years showed decreased risk of developing cirrhosis. Those on treatment were about half as likely to develop cirrhosis compared to those not on the treatment (21% compared with 37%).[41] The rate of liver cancer was also less than half in those who were treated compared to those who were untreated. Twelve percent of the treated patients and 25% of the untreated patients developed liver cancer. German studies with intravenous glycyrrhizin showed that, when given daily, glycyrrhizin was as effective an antiviral agent as interferon, without the side effects.[42]

The intravenous form of glycyrrhizin is not readily available in the United States, but the oral form is easily available over-the-counter. The effectiveness of the oral formulation of glycyrrhizin against hepatitis B was studied in China. Significant numbers of patients who had taken 7.5 grams of licorice root (concentrated to 750 mg licorice root extract) twice daily for 30 days experienced a normalization of liver enzyme levels. Twenty-five percent of the patients fully recovered from hepatitis B, while no one in the control group recovered.[43]

Licorice root does have one potentially problematic side effect. A breakdown product of glycyrrizin alters the production of the hormone aldosterone. This can cause increased blood pressure, water retention, and a reduction in blood potassium. The injectable form of glycyrrhizin has two amino acids (glycine and cysteine) added to prevent this side effect, but pure licorice root does not. If you are taking doses higher than 400 mg of glycyrrhizin daily, have your blood pressure monitored regularly. If you have a history of high blood pressure and/or have kidney failure, you should avoid taking licorice root.

Other Botanical Medicines

Catechin is an extract of the *Unicaria* (cat's claw) plant that has been researched extensively in England for its ability to improve liver function in people with hepatitis B.[44] Although study results were positive, the research on catechin was discontinued in the late 1980's because the use of the synthetic form of catechin resulted in a serious form of *anemia* in six patients.[45]

Recently, research in Africa has identified plant compounds in the *Garcinia* species that have antiviral activity and are used by native people to treat hepatitis.[46] The active compound is a flavinoid (a vitamin-like compound found in many plants, fruits, and vegetables) and will continue to be the subject of research in treating both hepatitis B and C.[47]

Other plant medicines used by native people in areas where hepatitis is common, such as those from the *Phyllanthus amarus* plant, have been shown to have direct antiviral effects on the hepatitis B virus.[48] *Picrorhiza kurroa* also has activity against hepatitis B, though neither of these plants have been tested specifically with hepatitis C.[49]

Botanicals Used To Treat Extrahepatic Hepatitis C Problems

The serious effects of HCV on the liver are well known. We now know HCV also has serious effects on other parts of the body. Recently, it has been shown that the fatigue, depression, and lack of energy reported by hepatitis C patients (not on *interferon-based therapy*) may be related to an effect of HCV on the central nervous system.[50] In one study, researchers found that problems with memory and concentration were not necessarily due to a history of intravenous drug use, *depression*, or fatigue, but were more closely related to HCV infection and some changes in brain function that were measured by a brain scan. This study brings to light what hepatitis C patients have long been describing as 'brain fog.' The changes seen in the brain scans were similar to changes seen in the brains of people with HIV infection. Although the way that HIV can damage the brain is still being studied, one of the mechanisms seems to involve the immune system found in the brain. When immune cells in the brain are stimulated by HIV infection, they produce free radicals that damage brain cells.[51] Treating the HIV infected brain cells with vitamin E stopped damage and death in the affected brain cells.

Although we have little information about the effects of HCV on brain function, symptoms of forgetfulness and 'brain fog' are common complaints of people with hepatitis C. Research data showing that changes can be seen in the brain tissue of people with hepatitis C is evidence that HCV infection has an effect on brain tissue. Although we do not know if these changes occur in the same way as HIV induced brain cell damage, we do know that free radical damage is a factor in many brain diseases such as Parkinson's disease[52], Alzheimer's dementia[53], and many others. While it is reasonable for a person with HCV to take antioxidants for liver health, there are antioxidants that have been tested specifically for treating damage to brain cells and the symptoms of memory loss and lack of attention that result.

Gingko biloba

Gingko biloba extract has been shown to protect brain cells from damage due to aging and oxidative stress. It has been the subject of over 400 published studies in the last 30 years. In human trials, *Gingko biloba* extract has been shown to be effective at improving blood supply to the brain. It also has a beneficial effect on attention span and brain function in elderly patients, resulting in significant improvements in memory, alertness, and mood.[54] Studies in those with Alzheimer's dementia have shown beneficial effects on alertness, concentration, and memory.[55] When *Gingko biloba* extract was compared to four medications called cholinesterase-inhibitors that are used to treat mild to moderate dementia from Alzheimer's disease, gingko was as effective as all four drugs with very few side effects.[56]

Depression is another common symptom of hepatitis C, even among people who are not being treated with western drug therapy (see *Chapter 4: Signs and Symptoms That May Be Associated with Hepatitis C*). In one study, 28% of people being seen in a clinic for hepatitis C were diagnosed with depression.[57] *Gingko biloba* was used in a study about depression in older adults who had not responded to standard antidepressants.[58] The group that stayed on their antidepressant medication experienced little improvement in their depression, however the group that took antidepressant medication plus gingko experienced significant improvements. Gingko is an approved prescription drug in Europe, and has been proven safe and nontoxic.[59] All of the published studies with gingko used an extract that contains 24% gingko heterosides. The extract was given in doses of 40-80 mg three times daily. There have been a few case reports in the medical literature of people who were diagnosed with bleeding in the brain who were also using high amounts (up to 1200 mg per day) of gingko. It is not clear if the gingko was related to the bleeding. There are no *contraindications* (situations in which it should not be used) to ginko use stated by the German Commission E (a group that studies the uses and safety of herbs and nutritional supplements) if it is taken in prescribed doses of 120-240 mg per day.

Hypericum perfoatum (St. John's Wort)

St. John's Wort (*Hypericum perfoatum*) is a plant product that has been studied for its antidepressant action. A review of 27 human studies indicated St. John's Wort is effective for mild-to-moderate depression. All of the St. John's Wort in these studies was given as a 0.2% hypericin-based preparation (one of the active ingredients).[60] The studies examined St. John's Wort alone and in comparison to the popular antidepressants fluoxetine (Prozac®) and imipramine (Tofranil®). These studies clearly demonstrated that St. John's Wort was equally effective with significantly fewer side effects than the standard antidepressants. However, it was also clear that St. John's Wort is not effective for severe depression. Prescription drugs work better in this case.

There have been a very small number of harmful side effects reported from use of St. John's Wort. Over eight million people were given prescriptions for St. John's Wort in Germany over the past decade. In this same time period, only 70 people complained of negative side effects which included allergic reactions, stomach complaints, rashes after sunlight exposure, breakthrough bleeding on birth control pills, prolonged *prothrombin* (clotting) *time*, and interactions with the drug cyclosporin (given to transplant recipients).[61] St. John's Wort has been shown to affect the speed at which the liver breaks down certain drugs. It may lower levels of certain drugs in the bloodstream. Following is a list of drugs that are known to interact with St. John's Wort. If you are taking any of these drugs, you should consult your health care provider <u>before</u> taking St. John's Wort.

Drugs that interact with St. John's Wort:
- Prescription antidepressants
- Oral contraceptives
- Anticoagulants (Coumadin)
- Theophylline
- Indinavir
- Digoxin
- Cyclosporin

REASONS FOR USING NATUROPATHIC MEDICINE AND WHO MAY BENEFIT

Naturopathic treatment options may benefit those who are motivated to adopt the following healthy lifestyle practices.

- following a nutritious diet that is low in sugar, red meat, and processed foods
- not smoking

- avoiding alcohol and recreational drugs
- exercising often
- managing daily stress

While these practices will be helpful with any therapeutic approach, they are vital to the success of naturopathic treatment. If you choose a naturopathic approach, you need to be willing to take nutritional supplements and botanicals suggested in this chapter and in the chapter on nutritional supplementation (*Chapter 14: Nutritional Supplementation*), or those prescribed by your naturopathic doctor. You must also be willing to eat a healthy diet (see *Chapter 7: Nutrition and Hepatitis C*). If cost is a concern, you need to be aware that most health insurance policies do not cover nutritional supplements and botanicals.

Anecdotal Story of Treatment Success with the Naturopathic Approach

Helen had been diagnosed with hepatitis C after a slight elevation of her liver enzymes led to testing six years prior to coming into our office. She had no idea how she had been infected, and had not experienced any symptoms that she knew were related to hepatitis C. Although her viral load was in the low range (300,000 copies) and her *liver biopsy* showed only mild inflammation, her gastroenterologist encouraged her to start interferon-based treatment. Helen was resistant because she was a single mother of three children, had a demanding job, and was supporting an ailing mother. She was afraid the side effects of treatment would make it hard for her to keep up with her responsibilities. She worried about being able to care for her children and provide financial support for her mother. She did not have a strong support system of friends and family who could step in and take care of her children if treatment made her tired and depressed.

Helen was willing to change her diet and she had given up alcohol when she was first diagnosed. She was also willing to find time to exercise with her children several times per week. She agreed to take the antioxidant protocol and botanicals faithfully. Her gastroenterologist agreed to follow her liver enzymes for six months and repeat the liver biopsy to see if any improvement had occurred. Helen was relieved that she could do something other than watch and wait, and that the treatment approach she was taking fit into her belief system.

REASONS FOR NOT USING NATUROPATHIC MEDICINE

If you are in end-stage liver failure, the appropriate treatment for you is western medical care, including possible liver transplantation. Alternative medicine, including naturopathic medicine, cannot effectively treat end-stage liver failure.

If you are unwilling or unable to make the necessary lifestyle changes, you probably will not benefit from a naturopathic approach. From the naturopathic perspective, it is difficult for the liver to heal when it is under siege from cigarette smoke, alcohol, recreational drugs, and/or the chemicals found in processed foods. For a naturopathic treatment to work, you need to be willing to 'clear the way' before you can expect any changes from of a naturopathic treatment protocol.

Anecdotal Story of Treatment Failure with the Naturopathic Approach

Robert is a 43-year-old lawyer who contracted hepatitis C during a brief period of intravenous drug use when he was in his twenties. He was diagnosed when a yearly physical showed that his liver enzymes were elevated 10-15 times above the normal level. His viral load was also high (over 30 million) and his liver biopsy revealed cirrhosis. Robert had not experienced symptoms other than some intestinal bloating and a little fatigue after work. He blamed these symptoms on his heavy work schedule, eating on the run, and the stress of his demanding job. Robert was interested in treating his hepatitis C, but wanted to use an alternative approach. He wanted to take an herbal pill that would 'get rid of the virus once and for all without the side effects that the drugs have.' He wanted to continue working full time. He also drank alcohol often, usually after work to wind down, and smoked a pack of cigarettes per day. He was quite willing to take supplements and antioxidants, but when it came to lifestyle changes, Robert was not so sure. He did not want to make any drastic changes, though he was willing to cut down on his alcohol and nicotine use and "maybe start eating a little better." However, he was not willing to give up anything altogether. He was aware that he was not dealing with stress very well. He had high blood pressure and daily tension headaches. He did not have time to exercise or do anything that would take him away from his work. Robert was also seeing a gastroenterologist who had warned him that his condition was serious and he needed treatment, but Robert wanted an "easier" route to recovery.

It was suggested to Robert that he pursue western antiviral therapy in addition to a naturopathic approach for several reasons. It was crucial that Robert quit drinking and his naturopathic doctor knew that. She also knew that Robert would not be able to get western treatment if he continued to drink. She hoped that with the support of Robert's gastroenterologist, they could convince Robert to stop using alcohol and begin treatment. Robert's situation was dangerous. He had a high viral load, significantly elevated liver enzymes, and cirrhosis. He was at risk for advanced hepatitis C including the possibilities of liver transplant and/or liver cancer. With a combined treatment approach, he could have a positive response to treatment. This would stabilizes his liver and prevent the complications of advanced cirrhosis. Robert did not want to make the lifestyle changes that his naturopath suggested: working less, making drastic changes in his diet, getting exercise, using stress management tools, and giving up nicotine and alcohol. The naturopathic approach requires lifestyle changes in addition to taking supplements and botanical medicines. Robert really did not have a lot of time to waste, so a combined approach was probably the best approach for him. This would allow him to use supplements and some botanicals to help his liver while undergoing western treatment for the hepatitis C.

SUMMARY

Naturopathic medicine offers people infected with HCV another tool in their efforts to treat their infection. Many people infected with HCV who include naturopathic medicine in their treatment protocol use it primarily as a way to enhance the body's ability to heal itself. Many feel that by doing this, they can keep the virus under control until more is known about it and/or better treatment options are available. Other people infected with HCV use naturopathic medicine as their primary care option. If and how naturopathic care fits into your treatment protocol is up to you.

If naturopathic care is something you are interested in, it is important that you find out as much as you can about it. There are many books and Internet sites that can help you better understand what naturopathic medicine has to offer. Some of these resources are listed in the *Resource Directory*.

Chapter Fourteen

NUTRITIONAL SUPPLEMENTATION

Lark Lands, PhD and Lyn Patrick, ND

INTRODUCTION

There are two sources of liver damage with *chronic hepatitis* C. One is from the infection itself. The other is from the *immune system's* attempt to fight the virus. Even if you eat a healthy, balanced diet that provides a broad spectrum of nutrients, there is still an important role for *nutritional supplements*. *Antioxidants, amino acids,* and fatty acids help moderate liver damage and improve the health of people with *hepatitis C.*

Researchers have found that a process called *oxidative stress* plays a role in the progression of chronic hepatitis C. Oxidative stress occurs when *free radicals* (unstable electrons and oxygen molecules) move through the liver causing *inflammation* and scarring. The formation of free radicals happens naturally in the body, especially when the immune system attacks an invader. The process is accelerated in chronic viral infections. The amount of damage caused by oxidative stress is linked to both the *grade* of liver *fibrosis* and to the overall level of liver damage.[1, 2]

Researchers have also found that the level of *glutathione* (an antioxidant) in the blood and in cells is significantly depressed in many people with hepatitis C.[1] Insufficient amounts of glutathione can reduce the liver's ability to break down drugs, chemicals, and other *toxins*. This can result in liver damage.

INDIVIDUAL SUPPLEMENTS

A study of people chronically infected with the hepatitis C virus (HCV) found their blood levels of the antioxidants glutathione, vitamin A, vitamin C, vitamin E, and selenium were much lower compared to people of the same age and sex who did not have HCV.[3] The finding of low levels of antioxidants was accompanied by high levels of blood markers that indicate oxidative stress (damage from free radicals). The levels of these markers were closely correlated to the amount of liver fibrosis. The higher the level of oxidative stress, the more advanced the fibrosis. Fibrosis was also related to low blood levels of the same antioxidants.

These findings applied not only to those with significant fibrosis and *cirrhosis* on *liver biopsy*, but also to those with minimal fibrosis and no cirrhosis (Ishak scores of 0-2). Higher levels of oxidative stress were associated with lower levels of antioxidants and more severe liver damage. The most important information this research revealed is that even in the beginning stages of hepatitis C, antioxidants are important. Although this information does not prove that antioxidants will prevent liver damage, the authors of this research suggested that antioxidants might play an important role in slowing the progression of HCV disease and delaying the onset of cirrhosis.

Nutritional antioxidants can counteract the damage caused by oxidative stress and low levels of glutathione. There are many different kinds of antioxidants working in many different ways in the body. These include vitamins A, E, and C, the family of carotenoids (including beta-carotene), the minerals zinc and selenium, alpha-lipoic acid, N-acetyl cysteine, and SAMe.

The antioxidants vitamin E, N-acetyl cysteine, SAMe, and selenium have been studied in people with hepatitis C to determine their effect on liver inflammation. The process of inflammation involves the accumulation of fat in the liver. Fatty cells are susceptible to damage, which can cause fibrosis and, ultimately, cirrhosis.[4,5]

The antioxidants vitamin E, selenium, zinc, and N-acetyl cysteine (NAC) have been studied for their potential to inhibit the process of fibrosis in chronic hepatitis. Of particular importance are the antioxidants and nutrients that work together to increase glutathione. The use of supplements to normalize glutathione levels may be very important for preventing liver damage. The nutrients that contribute to glutathione production are alpha-lipoic acid, vitamin C, vitamin E, NAC, and glutamine. The B vitamins and the mineral selenium also contribute to the antioxidant defense system.

Following are descriptions of several nutritional supplements, their effects in the body, and their roles in maintaining or improving liver health.

Alpha-lipoic acid (ALA)

Alpha-lipoic acid is a fatty acid and antioxidant. It is very important in liver cell *metabolism*. ALA is rapidly depleted when the liver is under stress. ALA has a long history of use in Europe where it is used to treat liver disorders because of its apparent ability to help the liver repair itself.[6] ALA's effectiveness in raising cellular glutathione levels is thought to be very important for liver repair with diseases like hepatitis C and *HIV* since both cause glutathione deficiency.

Unlike most other antioxidant nutrients that work in either the fatty parts of the body (including the outer layers of cells) or the watery parts (including the blood), ALA works in both. This ability allows ALA to provide protection to cells throughout the body. ALA also helps recycle and regenerate other antioxidants including vitamins E and C. This helps maintain optimal levels of these nutrients in the body. ALA has been given to humans in doses up to 1,200 mg intravenously without *toxicity*. The only side effect reported was nausea and vomiting, and this was reported infrequently. No side effects have been reported with oral doses up to 1,000 mg daily.[7,8] Oral ALA doses of 500-1,000 mg have been well tolerated in *placebo* controlled studies.[9]

Glutamine

Glutamine is an amino acid normally found in greater abundance in the body than any other free amino acid. It is crucial to many healthy body functions including maintenance of optimal antioxidant status, intestinal health, and immune function. Glutamine powers immune cells and is therefore in high demand in the bodies of people living with viral infections.

Researchers believe that among people with chronic hepatitis C, the body's demand for glutamine can exceed the amount that can be supplied in the diet.[10] Lack of glutamine can result in inadequate production of glutathione, which is needed to counteract the oxidative stress of chronic hepatitis C. The reason is somewhat complex, but simply stated, glutamine is the factor that determines how much glutathione the body can produce if a sufficient amount of cysteine is available (see the discussion of NAC and cysteine production for additional information).

If glutamine stores are depleted by ongoing immune system demands, glutathione production will be inadequate. This situation is particularly important for people coinfected with HCV and HIV because their immune systems are fighting two chronic infections instead of one.

Glutamine is an important nutritional supplement. It is given to support the liver and its glutathione production. Research suggests doses of at least 10 grams of powdered glutamine daily for people coinfected with HCVand HIV (Shabert J, personal communication).

N-acetyl cysteine (NAC)

NAC is a form of the amino acid cysteine found in plants and animals. Like all amino acids, cysteine is a building block of *proteins*. NAC has been used to treat lung diseases and *acetaminophen* poisoning. It is used in acetaminophen poisoning to increase glutathione in the liver. NAC has been shown to increase blood glutathione levels in HIV infected patients who have low levels of glutathione because of their chronic infection.[11] One study of 24 hepatitis C patients who had low glutathione showed that 600 mg of NAC taken three times daily along with *interferon* led to a normalization of *ALT* in 41% of patients.[12] The viral loads of patients who were on NAC were significantly lowered. NAC appeared to have the important effect of bringing glutathione levels back to normal inside white blood cells after six months of the combined therapy. NAC alone had no effect.

However, the results of studies using NAC in hepatitis C are conflicting. A study of low dose NAC (1,200 mg per day) along with 600 IU per day of vitamin E and interferon found no effect on *liver enzymes*.[13] Similar studies using 1,800 mg daily doses of NAC and interferon also found no effect on liver enzymes. Researchers found no changes in glutathione levels in the blood or white blood cells.[14] A separate study that included NAC at 1,800 mg per day had no effect when it was given along with selenium and interferon.[15]

It is not clear whether NAC does not influence the effectiveness of interferon, or if it is a matter of needing larger doses. The doses necessary to raise glutathione levels in studies with HIV infected people appeared to be 3,200-8,000 mg daily.[11] Unfortunately, doses that high often cause nausea. The authors of this research have speculated that doses of approximately 2,000 mg may be capable of achieving the same effect. However, the study dose of 1,800 mg in hepatitis C patients was very close to that amount and still had no effect.

Studies of HIV infected people who improved on a combined antioxidant protocol of NAC, glutamine, vitamin C, vitamin E, selenium, and beta carotene indicate that antioxidants may need to be given together to have an effect.[10]

NAC should always be taken with meals. It should be avoided if you have active stomach ulcers.

Selenium

Selenium is a mineral that has been investigated for its potential to improve immune function and decrease cancer risk. Selenium provides powerful antioxidant protection to the body via the selenium-containing *enzyme* glutathione peroxidase. This enzyme helps the body maintain sufficient levels of glutathione in the liver and all other glutathione containing cells of the body. Selenium is one of the most crucial of all nutrients for maintaining effective immune responses. Many cancer researchers believe it is one of the most important nutrients in preventing cancer. [16]

Selenium is one of the antioxidant nutrients found in significantly reduced levels among people with hepatitis C.[3] People with hepatitis C who did not have cirrhosis had selenium levels 20%

below normal, and those with cirrhosis had levels 40% below normal. Selenium is very important both as an antioxidant and as a cancer prevention agent. Therefore, low selenium levels in people with hepatitis C could contribute to progressive liver damage and the development of liver cancer. A recent study looked at blood selenium levels in 7,342 men with *chronic hepatitis B* and C and their risk of developing *liver cancer (hepatocellular carcinoma)*.[17] For analysis, the participants were divided into four groups based on their selenium levels. The study found selenium levels were lowest in the men with chronic hepatitis C. Participants in the group with the highest selenium levels were 38% less likely to get liver cancer than those in the group with the lowest selenium levels. This decreased risk of liver cancer was greatest in the men with chronic hepatitis C who smoked and had low levels of vitamin A or carotenoids. Carotenoids are vitamin A-like compounds and include beta-carotene. Although this study does not prove that selenium is the direct reason people developed less liver cancer, other studies have shown that selenium does play a protective role against liver cancer in people with chronic hepatitis.

Another selenium study conducted in China, an area with high rates of chronic hepatitis B and liver cancer, involved 130,471 people. Participants were given table salt that had been supplemented with selenium and were followed for eight years.[18] The rate of liver cancer in people taking supplemental selenium was found to be one-third lower than the usual liver cancer rate observed in that area. The same study included 226 people from the same area with chronic hepatitis B. Participants were given either 200 mcg of selenium daily or placebo (an inactive substance), and were followed for four years. No one in the group that took selenium (113 people) developed liver cancer. Of the 113 who took placebo, seven developed liver cancer. The selenium was then taken away, and both groups were followed for another four years. The incidence of liver cancer in people no longer taking selenium rose to a rate similar to those who never took selenium. This indicates the supplemental selenium may have had a preventive effect on the development of liver cancer in this particular group of chronic hepatitis B patients.

A study that examined selenium levels in HIV positive people showed that people who were coinfected with HCV and HIV had lower levels of selenium than those who had only HIV.[19] Whether this occurs because the virus uses selenium or because these people were selenium deficient before they became infected is not known. However, HIV infection is more likely to be fatal in a person who is selenium deficient.[20] Clearly, having HCV, HIV, and low selenium is not a good combination. We know coinfected people experience an accelerated rate of disease progression. Although we do not have proof at this time that selenium deficiency is a cause for this accelerated progression, having a sufficient amount of selenium appears to be helpful.

Studies on selenium supplementation have used 50-400 mcg (micrograms) daily of different forms of selenium. Research is currently underway at the University of Miami with HIV positive patients taking 400 mcg of selenium per day (M. Baum, MD, and E.W. Taylor, personal communication). Selenomethionine, a well-studied form of selenium, appears to be one of the safest and most absorbable forms of selenium. Other forms of selenium can be *toxic* at high doses.[1]

Selenium provides general antioxidant protection and immune defense. Selenium in doses of 200-400 mcg daily may also provide protection against the development of potentially life-threatening liver cancer.

S-adenosyl-L-methionine (SAMe)

S-adenosyl-L-methionine (SAMe) is another compound that aids glutathione production in the liver. SAMe is an amino acid that can be made in the liver. It helps cell membranes (the outside layer of a cell) function normally. It also assists in the process of detoxifying drugs and other compounds the liver needs to break down.[21]

SAMe is used as a medication to treat liver disease in Europe. SAMe is usually called AdoMet in Europe. SAMe has been shown to delay the need for liver transplantation in people with alcoholic cirrhosis.[22] Recent research revealed that SAMe has the ability to protect normal liver cells while causing liver cancer cells to die.[23] Although this research does not mean that SAMe alone can prevent or treat liver cancer, it does indicate that SAMe may provide some protection against developing liver cancer.

Other research involving liver disease and SAMe centers around its ability to normalize *bile* secretion by the liver, a process commonly affected by chronic liver diseases. SAMe has been used in multiple studies to treat the chronic skin irritation and resulting itching (pruritus) that is a common *symptom* of hepatitis C and many other chronic liver diseases. Studies in hepatitis B and C, and other chronic liver conditions found that SAMe helps reduce the symptoms of itching, *jaundice*, and *fatigue*, and lowers liver enzymes and *bilirubin* levels in as little as 16 days.[24, 25] Doses of SAMe in these studies were either 800 mg intravenously, or 800-1,600 mg by mouth. No side effects were reported in any of the studies with SAMe in chronic liver disease. It is clear more studies with SAMe need to be done in the United States since all of the current studies were done in Europe or Russia.

SAMe is sold over-the-counter. It is usually packaged in bottles or vacuum-sealed containers known as blister packs because it oxidizes (loses its potency) easily. SAMe is expensive, therefore some people take a combination of the amino acid methionine, tri-methyl glycine (betaine), vitamin B_{12} and folic acid to help the body make its own SAMe. The dosages for this combination are 500 mg methionine, 500 mg betaine, 800 mcg folic acid, and 500-3000 mcg of vitamin B_{12} daily. Whether this combination results in the same effect as taking supplemental SAMe is unknown. However betaine, folic acid, and vitamin B_{12} are nontoxic and do not have any harmful side effects at these doses.

Vitamin C

Vitamin C (ascorbic acid) is a powerful antioxidant and natural anti-inflammatory agent. Both characteristics are crucial for people with hepatitis C since much of the damage caused by HCV comes from a combination of oxidative stress and inflammation in the liver. Vitamin C is also very important for optimal immune function. The white blood cells that perform many of your immune functions are dependent on vitamin C. Therefore, vitamin C is a crucial nutrient for control of any viral infection. Individual needs for vitamin C seem to vary. For this reason, recommended dosages can range from 1,000-6,000 mg or more per day. Amounts in excess of individual tolerance can result in gas and/or diarrhea.

Vitamin E

Vitamin E is an antioxidant that works in the fatty parts of the body, including the outer layers of cells called cell membranes. It is crucial for the protection of liver cell membranes.

In one study, 24 people with hepatitis C undergoing *interferon therapy* were divided into three treatment groups. Group one took interferon alone. Group two took interferon plus 1,800 mg of

NAC and 400 mcg of selenium per day. Group three took 544 IU of vitamin E per day in addition to interferon, NAC, and selenium.[15] Liver enzyme levels, HCV *viral load*, and response to interferon were similar in the first two groups. Those who received the complete combination that included vitamin E had a significantly greater response to treatment, and achieved significantly greater drops in viral load. Even though the study was small and the *relapse* rate was equal in all groups, the effect of vitamin E was significant and deserves more research.

Another study of 23 hepatitis C patients on 800 IU of vitamin E, almost half of the participants experienced improvement of liver enzyme levels.[26] Liver enzymes went back up almost immediately after stopping the vitamin E. This indicates that vitamin E was neither combating the viral infection nor permanently stopping the process of inflammation in the liver, but was directly affecting inflammation in the liver while it was being taken. In other words, vitamin E only works while you take it. Other studies looking at the use of vitamin E and other antioxidants along with interferon have found similar results. It appears that vitamin E taken with interferon does not reduce viral levels long-term and therefore, does not make interferon more effective.[13] However, it may slow the process of fibrosis.[1] Vitamin E appears to work by interrupting the biochemical pathway that leads to fibrosis in the liver. Fibrosis can lead to cirrhosis. A study of six patients on 1,200 IU of d-alpha tocopherol (a form of vitamin E) per day for eight weeks resulted in a complete interruption of this pathway, but had no effect on viral loads.[27] Animal studies have shown d-alpha tocopherol inhibits the genetic mechanisms that lead to cirrhosis.[28] A dose of 800-1,200 IU of vitamin E is safe, unless you are on a blood-thinning drug such as coumadin, or suffer from a vitamin K deficiency.[29]

Zinc

Patients with chronic liver disease have low levels of several minerals including zinc.[30] Zinc is an effective *antiviral* agent against herpes and influenza viruses. Zinc deficiency is known to suppress the immune system. In studies of people with chronic hepatitis C, zinc supplementation was found to increase the effect of interferon therapy.[31] A recent study looked at the effect of zinc in people with HCV *genotype* 1b. Participants were given interferon either alone or in combination with daily zinc supplements. The supplement used was polaprezinc. It is a combination of zinc and the amino acid L-carnosine. The amount of elemental (pure) zinc used for this study was 34 mg per day. The study was small (75 patients) but the findings were impressive. Forty percent of people with viral counts less than 500,000 had a complete response to treatment. A complete response in this study meant no measurable viral load and a normal ALT for six months after the end of treatment. The study response rate was considered significant because it was markedly higher than what had been previously documented with interferon monotherapy among people with HCV genotype 1b. More studies are needed with much larger numbers of patients who have HCV genotype 1b to determine if zinc can augment response to western therapy for HCV. Although polaprezinc is not available in this country, there are other well-absorbed forms of zinc available. Zinc picolinate is one example and is available over-the-counter.[32]

NUTRITIONAL SUPPLEMENT COMBINATIONS

Antioxidants and other nutrients interact with each other in positive ways. Therefore it comes as no surprise that positive results occur in trials in which people are given a combination of nutrients rather than any single nutrient. A combined antioxidant approach has been used in research conducted at the Integrative Medical Center of New Mexico in Las Cruces, New Mexico.[33] Three patients with progressive hepatitis C and moderate to severe cirrhosis were treated with a daily combination of 600 mg of ALA, 400 mcg of selenium, 900 mg of silymarin, 100 mg of vitamin B complex twice, 400-800 IU of vitamin E, 1,000-6,000 mg of vitamin C, 300 mg of coenzyme Q, and one multiple vitamin and mineral supplement. In addition to taking the supplements, participants were advised to eliminate alcohol, sugar, and caffeine, to decrease their meat intake to a few times weekly, to increase intake of purified water to eight glasses daily, and to begin a modest exercise program. The nutrients in this protocol were chosen because of their ability to protect the liver from free radical damage, to increase the levels of other important antioxidants, and to interfere with the progression of HCV infection. The results were very impressive. There were reductions in ALT of at least 60% in all three patients, and even more significant improvements in overall health and well-being. After 5-12 months on the protocol, all three patients achieved sufficient improvement in liver function to avoid liver transplant. The yearly cost of this nutrient therapy is very small compared to the cost of liver transplant surgery. According to the researcher, treatment with a combination of nutrients is a reasonable approach during the evaluation process prior to liver transplant so that if significant improvement can be achieved, surgery can be avoided.

SUMMARY

There is strong evidence that nutritional supplements such as antioxidants can play a very important role in limiting the damage HCVcauses in the liver. Antioxidants can counteract the damage caused by increased free radical activity in the body. Other nutrients such as glutamine are important in the production of glutathione, an antioxidant that is used by the liver to break down toxins, drugs, and chemicals. Adding appropriate nutritional supplements may have a significantly positive effect on the health of your liver and on the progression of hepatitis C.

Chapter Fifteen

PRODUCTS MARKETED TO PEOPLE WITH HEPATITIS C

Lyn Patrick, ND

INTRODUCTION

There are many over-the-counter products marketed to people living with *hepatitis C*. Many claims are made about these products. At times, it can be very hard to determine what to believe. Your western doctor may not be able to provide you with guidance because he or she may not be familiar or experienced with these products. Making a decision about whether to use one or more of these products can be quite difficult. In addition, there is no way to be sure how any one person will react to any one product.

One of the most common complaints from western health care providers about alternative products is that there is little or no data to support their claims of effectiveness. The data that does exist is often from studies that were not well designed. Claims based on such studies are not considered valid by most western doctors. While for the most part it is true that many alternative products have not been adequately studied, this situation is beginning to change. Many manufacturers of alternative products are realizing that in order to gain credibility in the western medical community, they need valid evidence that proves their products are safe and useful.

PRODUCTS TARGETED TO PEOPLE WITH HEPATITIS C

Some of the products targeted to people with hepatitis C are reviewed in this section. Many more are available that do not appear here. The inclusion or exclusion of any product should not be considered to deny or affirm its existence or effectiveness. The products we have selected are those people with hepatitis C seem to be most aware of and therefore ask about most frequently.

Ultimately, it is up to you to do whatever research is necessary to make an informed decision about whether to try a certain product. This is especially important in deciding whether to take an product that has little or no test data available. We have included references to trial data where applicable. We independently researched each product discussed. We also contacted the manufacturers of the products discussed to request information directly from them. In some cases, we did not receive the information we requested. Therefore, the following information may not be complete.

Bee Propolis

Propolis is a resinous material produced by bees from plant parts. It is used as sealing material for the hive. Because it has significant antibacterial and antifungal activity, it has been used as a topical medicine for skin, ear, nose, and throat problems.[1] Propolis also has *antiviral* activity, specifically to influenza and herpes viruses.[2] This antiviral activity is thought to be due to the *flavinoid*s in propolis. These vitamin-like substances come from the plant materials picked up by the bees. Flavinoids also appear to be the active ingredients in the plant based folk remedies used by traditional African medicine practitioners for the treatment of *hepatitis*.[3] There have been no animal or human studies on propolis as a treatment for hepatitis.

God's Remedy

God's Remedy is a group of products advertised to treat hepatitis C. The products are alcohol based liquid extracts of plants. Products in the group include Pure Herbal Remedy™, Milk Thistle™, Hepacure™, Immune Booster™, and Energy Formula™.

The Pure Herbal Remedy™ formula is advertised as an *antioxidant* supplement. It is said to contain burdock root, nettle, red clover blossom, ginseng root, echinacea root, yellow dock root, gingko leaf, dandelion root, blessed thistle, schizandra, astragalus root, olive leaf, plaintain, and milk thistle. The text explains that the phytochemicals found in the plants are potent anti-oxidants and stimulate the human *immune system*. Although this statement is true in that phytochemicals called flavinoids are highly potent antioxidants, more potent than nutrients like zinc, vitamin E and vitamin C, not all plants contain flavinoids. With the exception of schizandra, astragalus, and milk thistle, the plants contained in Pure Herbal Remedy™ are not known for their high flavinoid content. Unfortunately, there are no published studies looking at the effects of the flavinoids contained in these plants among people with hepatitis C. Hopefully, these studies will be done in the future.

The milk thistle product is also a liquid extract. No information about the silymarin or silybin content of the product is mentioned, so it is difficult to know the potency of this extract. Silymarin is the active ingredient in milk thistle, and all the clinical trials involving milk thistle used a specific amount of silymarin. See *Chapter 13: Naturopathic Medicine* for additional information on silymarin.

Hepacure™ is another product sold by this producer that is claimed to be similar to Hepatico™. (See Hepatico™ in this chapter for information about this product.) The text explaining this product refers to clinical trials with Hepatico™ in Russia quoting, "a 91% success rate" in hepatitis and some degree of reversal of *cirrhosis* in 1-7 months. The text goes on to say the product has been researched and is safe for treatment of acute and chronic forms of hepatitis A, B, and C, and cirrhosis and *liver cancer*. However, there is no reference to the source of this information. It is also unclear where this product was researched and how it was determined to be safe. As mentioned in the section under Hepatico™, none of the references mentioned were published studies. The only published study we found was an animal study looking at the *toxicity* of the plants in Hepatico™. The ingredients listed for Hepacure™ are very different from the original Hepatico™ formula. The ingredients given for Hepacure™ are nettle, plaintain, horsetail, yarrow, golden rod, chamomile, feikhoa batsu, fern, ekala, pau d'arco, cleaver, black Indian hemp, and mayapple in a base of milk thistle, dandelion, and turmeric root.

The Immune Booster™ formula contains goldenseal root, red clover blooms, yellow dock root, burdock root, witch hazel, wild American ginseng, capsicum, pau d'arco, and echinacea. The Immune Booster™ formula text states, "Numerous studies have shown that these remarkable natural substances stimulate our immune system's ability to recognize and surround foreign matter and eliminate it at a cellular level." The only actual published data looking at the immune stimulating effects of these plants has been with echinacea, berberine (the active ingredient in goldenseal), burdock root, and pau d'arco (*Tecoma curialis*). The relative amounts of each botanical in the formula are not given, so it is difficult to know how strong the immune stimulating activity of the formula really is.

The Energy Formula™ is advertised to diminish *fatigue* and contains American, Korean, Siberian, and Tienchi ginsengs, kola nut, guarana, damiana, and wild ginger root. Both guarana and kola nut contain caffeine, and various over-the-counter products that contain these herbs have been found to contain very high amounts of caffeine. Because this is a liquid formula, the amount of caffeine in the product would be hard to regulate and difficult to label. If high amounts of caffeine are what is producing the "needed boost throughout the day," green tea or another inexpensive source of caffeine may provide an economical alternative.

Hepatico™

Hepatico™ is a botanical compound that was first used in Russia. It is a combination of three common plants (plaintain, nettle, and immortelle) in a base of three other plants (turmeric, milk thistle, and dandelion root). Each capsule contains 250 mg of a combination of the first three plants in 250 mg of a combination of the base herbs.

The manufacturer does not provide information about the individual action of the first three plants. However, none of them individually is commonly known to have any action on the liver or gall bladder. The base botanicals are known to have effects on the liver and *bile* ducts, but the doses (unknown amounts, but less than 250 mg of each per capsule) are low. The amount of Hepatico™ used in an unpublished study discussed below was one to two capsules three times daily. This means the amounts of the botanicals involved in the study were below the amounts commonly used in published research that has examined the individual action of turmeric, milk thistle, and dandelion root.

The information available from the manufacturer includes a study done in Canada with 23 patients who had either *hepatitis B* or C, or both. The majority were *chronic hepatitis C* patients. Study participants were given one or two capsules of Hepatico™ three times daily (depending on the patient's weight) for a period of 20-40 days. At the end of the study period, four of 23 participants had normalization of their *ALT* levels, and three of 23 participants had normalization of their *AST* levels. Participants who experienced normalization of their *liver enzymes* had varying histories of hepatitis C infection from 2-24 years duration. There is no information about their individual disease progression. A second group of ten hepatitis C patients took Hepatico™ for the first month of a 7-month trial. Two had normalization of their ALT levels. The investigators reported the participants in this study had relief from digestive *symptoms* and insomnia, but they did not document when or for how long this occurred. The study gave incomplete information about the patients' medical conditions. The only other liver function test conducted was for GGT levels, which did not change significantly during treatment. *Liver biopsy* results were not available.

The Internet site for Hepatico™ lists reports from specific institutions and health care providers in Russia who report alleviation of the symptoms of severe cirrhosis, chronic hepatitis B and C, gallbladder disease, and chronic colitis. The studies were done with people who took one capsule three times daily over a period of three to four weeks. The only Russian medical study was on the toxicity of this product when tested in animals. It was found to be nontoxic in doses much higher than the recommended dose.

It is unknown whether the claims for this product could be reproduced in *clinical trials* conducted in the United States. According to the study done in Canada (unpublished), improvement (normalization of ALT levels) occurred in only a small minority of patients.

Hepato-C™

Hepato-C™ is a botanical combination of 15 powdered Chinese herbs contained in capsules. It is advertised as a formula that, "along with lifestyle changes, may minimize the viral effects of hepatitis C." The manufacturer publicizes a trial of 11 hepatitis C patients on Hepato-C™ for nine months. Information on *viral load* levels and liver enzymes in these 11 people is inadequate to allow evaluation of the effects of the product. Follow-up viral counts were unavailable for seven of the 11 study participants. Ten people in the study were taking other substances (vitamins and other herbs) and receiving acupuncture treatments during the study. Liver enzyme levels were normal in five people at the end of the study period, but all of these people were taking other herbs and vitamins that were not specified. Three of these people had been on *interferon* or interferon plus *ribavirin* prior to taking Hepato-C™. According to product literature (May 2000), a few private practice and university-based health care providers have agreed to conduct clinical studies with this product.

IP-6™

Abul Kalam M. Shamsuddin MD, PhD patented IP-6™ (inositol and myo-inositol hexaphosphate). His research demonstrated the immune enhancing and anticancer actions of IP-6™, a combination formula found to be effective against cancer cells in the test tube. Myo-inositol hexaphosphate is a B vitamin combined with phytic acid, a naturally occurring substance found in certain plant fibers (grains such as rice are particularly high in phytic acid). IP-6™ is the subject of many published studies on cancer in animals and cultured cell lines, but this author found only one study on the use of IP-6™ in liver disease.[5] A study in rats that included IP-6 in their diet appeared to prevent the accumulation of fat in the liver that would otherwise have occurred because of a high sugar diet. Whether this finding has any relationship to hepatitis is questionable because different factors are responsible for liver damage in chronic hepatitis C. There is no evidence to date that IP-6™ has any direct effect on chronic viral hepatitis.

LIV.52

LIV.52 is a traditional Indian Ayurvedic medicine currently marketed under several names including LiverCare™ (see below). LIV.52 contains the herbs capers (*Capparis spinosa*), wild chicory (*Cichorium intybus*), black nightshade (*Solanum nigrum*), arjuna (*Terminalia arjuna*), yarrow (*Achillea millefolium*), Negro coffee (*Cassia occidentalis*), and tamarish (*Tamarix gallica*). All of these plants are recognized in the writings of traditional Indian herbal medicine as treatments for liver problems. The combination of these medicinal plants has been widely used and researched in India for over 30 years.

Because LIV.52 has been extensively tested in animals and has been used clinically for a long time, its lack of toxicity has been proven. There has been concern about the levels of the *toxic* metal lead found in Ayurvedic preparations. However, an independent laboratory analysis has shown that the level of lead in LIV.52 is low, and the compound is considered safe.

LIV.52 appears to be beneficial in treating liver disease and may play a role as an antioxidant herbal preparation in supporting the liver function of people with chronic hepatitis C. However, there is no clinical evidence (that is, no human studies have been done) that LIV.52 has an antiviral effect on the hepatitis C virus (HCV), or that it can prevent or treat cirrhosis.

LiverCare™

LiverCare™ is one of the currently marketed brands of LIV.52. Although the LiverCare™ manufacturer's Internet site states that there are over 168 clinical papers published on the use of

LIV.52, only 50 clinical and experimental (animal) studies were found by this author in a search of the medical literature.

The animal studies reviewed showed clear evidence that LIV.52 has an antioxidant-like effect on the liver. It prevented damage from chemical toxins in animals, and from alcohol in both animals and humans. However, only three studies appeared to have been done in people with hepatitis, and none of these involved people with chronic hepatitis C.[6, 7]

One clinical study evaluated 24 people with chronic active hepatitis B who were taking LIV.52.[8] A significant number of patients in this study had *jaundice, ascites,* and cirrhosis, all of which are signs of liver damage resulting from long-term infection. After treatment with LIV.52, 58% of the study participants had significant decreases in their liver enzymes. The researchers considered this an improvement in symptoms. However, we cannot assume that LIV.52 would have the same effect in people with chronic hepatitis C. First, HCV is a very different virus from the hepatitis B virus. Western medications that are effective in treating chronic hepatitis B do not work with chronic hepatitis C. Second, lower viral loads and/or improved biopsy results need to be seen to prove with chronic hepatitis C. Decreases in liver enzymes alone are not enough to prove efficacy. The authors cite an older published study that showed long-term improvement in people with chronic hepatitis who took LIV.52 for nine months. However, this study was unavailable for review.

A separate study examined the effects of LIV.52 on 188 patients with alcoholic cirrhosis. Study participants took LIV.52 for two years. Among patients with the worst cirrhosis, those taking LIV.52 had a higher death rate than those not taking the supplement (23 deaths versus 11 deaths). It is unclear if LIV.52 was related to this observed increase in death rate. An increased death rate was not seen in study participants with less severe cirrhosis.[9]

There is no mention of a recommended dosage on the LiverCare™ Internet site. The standard dosage suggested by Ayurvedic practitioners is two tablets twice daily with meals. However, each individual's dosage should be adjusted by a qualified Ayurvedic practitioner.

Liverite™

Liverite™ is a *nutritional supplement* containing B complex vitamins, phospholipids, cysteine, and bovine liver hydrolysate (cow liver that has been broken down by *enzymes*). There are many references in the European and Japanese medical literature about studies that examined the effects of these preparations on liver cells. However, human studies have failed to show any clear benefit in hepatitis.[10, 11]

Liverite™ contains an unlisted amount of *phosphatidylcholine*, a type of fat found naturally in certain foods. There are approximately 20 years of medical research on the effects of phosphatidylcholine on the liver. Phosphatidylcholine has been shown to have a protective effect on liver tissue in alcoholics and people who are exposed to *toxins*, large doses of liver damaging pharmaceuticals, and viruses.[12] Most studies used a combination of intravenous preparations of phosphatidylcholine and oral doses of 450-700 mg. Other studies used only oral doses of 1,350-2,350 mg per day for alcoholic liver damage or hepatitis. Studies of chronic hepatitis B patients taking phosphatidylcholine and steroid therapy showed improved liver biopsy results. *Acute hepatitis* B resolved more quickly in those taking 1,350 mg phosphatidylcholine daily compared to those not taking the supplement. Phosphatidylcholine has also been studied in people with severe liver disease. In these studies, phosphatidylcholine used both intravenously and orally produced a reversal of *fibrosis* or scarring of the liver, and a return to normal liver function tests.[13] Whether Liverite™ is the best dose or source (practically or economically) of phosphatidylcholine is unclear.

Microhydrin™

Microhydrin™ is a liquid suspension of minerals (silica, potassium carbonate, and magnesium sulfate) and safflower oil in a base of purified water. The manufacturer claims this product lowers the surface tension and raises the pH of water (makes it more alkaline), and increases the absorption of nutrients from drinking water. The researcher who developed Microhydrin™, Dr. Patrick Flanagan, claims its effect comes from the fact that the product carries extra hydrogen atoms and, "acts as a powerful antioxidant." He has published studies with athletes showing the product has the effect of lowering lactic acid levels after heavy exercise. The manufacturer publicizes this product as part of a regimen to improve nutritional status and hepatitis C. Individuals with hepatitis C have given personal testimonials supporting this claim. At this time, there is no evidence from human, animal, or cell studies that indicates Microhydrin™ has any direct effect on hepatitis C.

Mannatech™

Mannatech™ is a proprietary (secret) formula distributed and discovered by Terry Pulse, MD and Reg McDaniel, MD while they were working with AIDS patients. Mannatech™ is distributed by a multilevel marketing firm. It is based on a group of complex sugars called acemannan derived from the aloe vera plant. These sugars are known to have immune stimulating and antiviral properties.[14, 15] The manufacturers also use a product called arabinogalactan, a type of fiber that has been demonstrated to have an immune stimulating effect in humans.[16]

In a study published in the "Proceedings of the Fisher Institute for Medical Research" (a publication that lists research using the Mannatech™ products), a group of eight chronic hepatitis C patients received "glyconutritional powder and an antioxidant supplement."[17] The patients in the study had declined *interferon therapy* or had experienced interferon treatment failure before entering the study. Participants were given the "glyconutritional powder and an antioxidant supplement" twice a day for six months. After six months on this protocol, ALT levels normalized in three out of eight patients, and four reported improvements in energy level. Liver biopsy was done on all eight patients at the beginning of the study, but no information is given about follow-up biopsy results. Viral loads were not available.

Although this small pilot study is interesting because there is reason to think that the ingredients in this proprietary formula may be useful, a much larger and more detailed study would need to be done to determine if these plant nutrients have any antiviral or immune stimulating effect in hepatitis C.

MGN3™

MGN3™ is a molecule called an arabinoxylane that is extracted from rice bran. It has been used in cancer studies and in small trials that showed it has the ability to enhance the immune response of cancer patients, and to decrease the side effects of *chemotherapy* in studies with rats.[18, 19] There is clear evidence from papers published by Mamdooh Ghoenum, PhD and others that this compound increases blood levels of natural killer cells (a special type of immune cell). It also increases levels of gamma-interferon and another substance called tumor necrosis factor. Although the boost in immunity may be useful in cancer therapies, hepatitis C is a different condition. In chronic viral infection, the immune system already makes too much tumor necrosis factor, which may be a large part of the problem in hepatitis C. To date, any direct effects of MGN3 on hepatitis C are unproven.

MTH-68/B Vaccine

The Newcastle disease virus is found in chickens. It can be up to 100% fatal in fowl, but does not have any effect on humans. Dr. Laszlo Csatary developed a *vaccine* made from this virus, MTH-68/H. This vaccine has been used to treat a specific type of human brain cancer called glioblastoma.[20] Recently, Dr. Csatary and his associates have been conducting studies with another virus vaccine in people with hepatitis B and C. The vaccine uses an attenuated (weakened) form of the bursal disease virus and is called MTH-68/B. A recent study on MTH-68/B involved two groups of acute hepatitis patients, 43 with hepatitis B and 41 with hepatitis C. Half were treated with conventional treatment. The other half were given injections of the vaccine. Of those HCV patients on conventional treatment, 26% went on to develop chronic active (symptomatic) hepatitis. Of those given the vaccine, only 9% went on to develop chronic active hepatitis C. Of those who recovered, 79% on conventional treatment *relapsed* while only 32% of those who received the vaccine relapsed.[21] In another study, MTH-68/B was given to three patients with end-*stage* hepatitis B and C. All three patients experienced significant improvement that could only be attributed to the vaccine.[22] Since the research with the live virus vaccine (MTH-68/H) in cancer patients has proven to be free of toxicity, the attenuated virus vaccine (MTH-68/B) used in hepatitis research is also likely to be free from side effects. At this time in the United States, the vaccine is only available in a research setting, although it is available in other countries.

Phlogenzyme™

Phlogenzyme™ is an oral enzyme therapy manufactured in Germany. It contains proteolytic (*protein* digesting) enzymes and a vitamin from the flavinoid family called rutosid. A trial with hepatitis C patients in Egypt compared Phlogenzyme™ to alpha-interferon and ribavirin.[23, 24, 25] Patients in the study were divided into four groups: 20 took ribavirin, 20 took interferon, 20 took Phlogenzyme™, and 20 took a liver support protocol that consisted of vitamins and antioxidants. After four months, the researchers compared the results of the four groups. Phlogenzyme™ was more effective than interferon or ribavirin at lowering liver enzymes (ALT, AST, and GGT). It was also associated with a 50% reduction in symptoms including appetite loss, weight loss, fever, itching, fever, fatigue, jaundice, and spider nevi (small broken blood vessels in the skin). Interferon and ribavirin were associated with smaller reductions in symptoms. The liver support *protocol* was considered ineffective for both symptom reduction and liver enzyme reduction. Tolerance of Phlogenzyme™ was rated as "good" in 14 patients, whereas tolerance of interferon and ribavirin were rated as "good" by only one and four patients, respectively.

This study clearly demonstrates Phlogenzyme™ has an anti-inflammatory effect on the liver. However, with no information about viral loads, the antiviral activity of this product is unknown. It is also unclear how long patients were followed after the four-month treatment period. We do not know how many (if any) of those in the Phlogenzyme™ group relapsed after 6-12 months. Mucos Pharma is the German pharmaceutical company that produces this product. They are reportedly planning larger clinical trials that will follow patients for longer periods. These studies will give us more information about how to most effectively use this natural compound in the treatment of hepatitis C.

Thymic Protein A

Thymic Protein A was formulated by immunologist and research scientist Terry Beardsley, PhD. He currently holds the U.S. patent on this protein and is involved in research evaluating its use in immune disorders.

Thymic Protein A is chemically identical to a protein produced by the human thymus gland. It was originally derived from the thymus tissue of calves, but is now produced with the technology of cell cloning (reproducing cells in the laboratory). It has been shown to be absorbed orally, a problem with other thymus proteins. It increase the body's production of *CD4 cells* (T-helper cells) and natural killer cells, the immune system's virus-killing cells.[26]

One study evaluated the effect of thymic protein A on people with chronic fatigue syndrome (Epstein-Barr disease). Participants were treated with 12 mcg (micrograms) of thymic protein A daily for 60 days. Treatment resulted in significant Epstein-Barr viral load reductions of 50% or greater in 67% of patients.[27]

Thymic protein A has not been studied in hepatitis C. However, the use of another thymic protein, thymosin alpha-1, has been the subject of hepatitis C studies. In one study, people with HCV were treated with a combination of thymosin alpha-1 plus interferon or interferon alone for 26 weeks. A higher proportion of patients treated with the combined therapy cleared virus and had a normalization of ALT compared to patients treated with interferon alone.[28] Post-treatment liver biopsy results were better in the combined therapy group than in the interferon group. In the follow-up period, the biochemical response rate dropped to 14% and 8% in the combined therapy and interferon groups, respectively.

Thymosin alpha-1 is a 28 *amino acid* protein fragment and is much smaller than the 500 amino acid thymic protein A. Therefore, thymic protein A may work differently than the thymosin alpha-1. In general, a larger protein fragment (thymic protein A) would be expected to have a greater effect than a smaller protein fragment (thymosin alpha-1). Thymic protein A has been tested in mice, cats, and humans and has been found to enhance immune response to viral infections. To date, there are no published studies that have evaluated the effects of thymic protein A on hepatitis C infection. Thymic protein A is sold over-the-counter under the brand name of ProBoost™.

Ultraviolet Blood Irradiation

Ultraviolet blood irradiation (UBI) is not a product but rather a technique that was popular in the United States during the early 1930's as a treatment for poliovirus. UBI involves removing blood from the body and exposing it to ultraviolet light. After the discovery of the Salk vaccine for the prevention of polio and the advent of antibiotics in the 1950's, the use of UBI all but disappeared. Recently, there has been a renewed interest in this technique. It has been now been reapproved by the Food and Drug Administration for the treatment of a specific type of cancer called cutaneous T-cell lymphoma.[29] This type of UBI is called photophoresis. It is currently being investigated in clinical trials for the treatment of autoimmune diseases such as arthritis. The UBI process is time-consuming (each treatment takes about five hours) and expensive. A 1959 published study described the use of this process to treat acute *hepatitis A* and B, but there have been no published studies on its use to treat hepatitis C.[30] This process can destroy white blood cells if it is not done properly. Therefore, it should only be performed in a medical setting by a licensed doctor who specializes in this procedure. UBI is available outside of the United States for the treatment of chronic hepatitis.

REASONS FOR USING OVER-THE-COUNTER PRODUCTS AND WHO MAY BENEFIT

People decide to pursue *complementary and alternative medicine (CAM)* treatments for a variety of reasons. You may have decided to decline western therapy at this time. On the other hand, you may have experienced a treatment failure. Or perhaps your doctor has advised you to follow a 'watchful waiting' course (you are monitored for disease progression but are not being treated). The reason for your interest in CAM therapy is not nearly as important as making sure whatever you decide to do is <u>safe</u>. It is extremely important to seek safe, clinically tested CAM treatments.

As you look into your options, realize that any treatment should have proof that it is effective at improving liver function and/or quality of life in people with hepatitis C. A product that has not undergone safety studies in animals or humans may not be a wise choice. Many botanicals (both western and traditional Chinese) have been shown to be harmful to the liver. Your first concern should always be to do no additional harm to your liver.

If you are on treatment and are having side effects from your medications, there are ways to reduce these symptoms. A licensed CAM provider can help you use botanical medicines, acupuncture, and supplements that are specific for the side effects you are experiencing. Their guidance can also help insure that whatever CAM therapies you use do not interfere with your treatment's antiviral, and/or immune enhancing activities. Unfortunately, none of the products mentioned in this chapter have been shown to reduce side effects from interferon-based therapy.

Anecdotal Story of Treatment Success Using Over-The-Counter Products

Gloria is a 49-year-old woman who is coinfected with *HIV* and hepatitis C. She had been using alternative medicine along with her HIV antiviral medicines for the previous eight years. She was doing well but her HIV viral load was starting to climb. She and her doctor were in the process of deciding whether to change her medications. Gloria had diarrhea and fatigue, side effects of her medications. She managed these side effects with herbs and acupuncture. Some days she felt fine, other days she did not want to get out of bed. Then Gloria was diagnosed with hepatitis C. Her doctor was hesitant to give her western treatment for HCV because her CD4 count had dropped below 200 and her HIV viral load was rising. Her liver biopsy showed moderate *inflammation* and no cirrhosis. Gloria decided to add another alternative therapy to her protocol.

After doing some research and talking to her doctor, she looked at a study on Phlogenzyme™. She e-mailed the German pharmaceutical company that produces the product. She found that it was safe for her to take with HIV, and that it is available in the United States. She worked with her acupuncturist to obtain it.

REASONS FOR NOT USING OVER-THE-COUNTER PRODUCTS

Essentially, it is not your personal situation but the product that is in question here. If the manufacturer or provider cannot provide a reference to a published study documenting a positive effect in hepatitis C, you are taking a chance that it may not be safe and/or may have no beneficial effects. Before you take anything, we urge you to consider checking with a licensed CAM provider who treats people with chronic hepatitis C. Many botanicals (both western and traditional Chinese) have been shown to be harmful to the liver. It is best to have someone who is trained in complementary and alternative medicine oversee your alternative treatments. He or she can work with your primary care doctor or gastroenterologist/ hepatologist. You can check with the American Association of Naturopathic Physicians (AANP), the American College for Advancement in Medicine (ACAM), or the American Holistic Medical Association (AHMA) for help in finding a qualified CAM practitioner. (See the *Resource Directory* for contact information.)

Over-the-counter products marketed to people with hepatitis C can be very expensive, especially when taken for months or years. Very few (if any) of these products are covered by health insurance policies.

You also need to be aware that there are no regulations that govern the manufacture of these products. Therefore, it is often very difficult to know if you are actually getting what is listed on the product label. Further, there is no assurance that you will get the same product from one bottle to the next. It is sometimes challenging to find reputable distributors for these products.

Anecdotal Story of Treatment Failure Using Over-the-Counter Products

Rodney was diagnosed with hepatitis C after a period of alcoholism and intravenous drug use six years earlier. Rodney had been in recovery since that time and had become very active in substance abuse treatment. He worked at a local treatment facility. Rodney's liver enzymes were very elevated and his liver biopsy showed evidence of cirrhosis. He was always tired and this was starting to affect his ability to work. His doctor said that he was a good candidate for treatment because he had HCV *genotype* 2, his HCV viral load was only moderately elevated, and he was otherwise in good health. Rodney had limited money and he relied on his health insurance to pay for his treatment. His employer was very supportive of Rodney getting treatment. He agreed to allow Rodney to work part-time and take medical leave if he needed to during treatment. However, Rodney was afraid of getting treatment because he had friends who had become severely anemic during treatment, or who had become *depressed* and did not responded to Prozac© or other antidepressants.

He began to look at alternatives and sought out some that were advertised on the Internet for people with hepatitis C. He found a special kind of water that was supposed to cure hepatitis C and some herbal/vitamin combinations that were only available through multilevel marketing distributors. When Rodney looked at the cost of a month's worth of these products, he realized he would not be able to afford them. After talking to his doctor and finding out he could go off treatment if he got too sick or if he became depressed and did not respond to antidepressants, Rodney decided to use western treatment.

SUMMARY

There are many over-the-counter products that are marketed specifically to people who have hepatitis C. While many of these products may provide benefit to the user, there are very few documented studies on the effectiveness of these products. Reliable advice on which products are or are not appropriate for you to take may be difficult to find. Most western health care professionals know very little about these products, and are generally skeptical about their possible benefits.

It is very important that you learn everything you can about over-the-counter products. Your first priority should be to insure that a product will do no additional harm to your liver. If you are considering using one of these products, you may want to consult with a qualified CAM practitioner before you make a decision. Remember, it is very important to discuss your use of any of these products with all of your health care providers. This will help insure your safety and maximize the possibility of benefit from all your treatments.

YOU AND YOUR HEALTHCARE

Mark White, Peggy McCarthy, Jo An Loren

INTRODUCTION

It is challenging to be an effective health care consumer. The system can sometimes be quite confusing. As a person with *chronic hepatitis C*, you will be meeting new people, learning new terminology, and perhaps living by new rules. Learning about the various medical disciplines and becoming familiar with the new medical terms you will be hearing may help you become a more confident and comfortable health care consumer.

People newly diagnosed with *hepatitis C* are often amazed at how much others with the illness know about it. You may marvel at the easy way they talk with their health care providers and others. Believe it or not, after a surprisingly short period, you will probably be doing the same thing!

This chapter covers the following topics.

- choosing your health care provider(s)
- building a relationship with your health care providers
- maintaining your medical records
- disability and Social Security issues
- health insurance issues
- compassionate use drug programs

CHOOSING YOUR HEALTH CARE PROVIDERS

You are a health care consumer, and you have the right to choose your health care providers. These people will be helping you make decisions that may greatly affect your life. Therefore, it is very important for you to feel confident about the quality of care you receive from your health care providers. Confidence in your doctors comes from knowing they are well informed about hepatitis C, and are both skilled and experienced in their profession. Your comfort with your providers is also strongly influenced by their attitudes toward you as a patient.

There are some sample lists of questions in *Appendix VI: You and Your Health Care*. These question were developed to help you choose health care providers who meet your needs, and to effectively communicate with them.

Choosing your health care providers is the first step in taking care of your health care needs. Deciding on the roles you want your providers to play in your health care is the next step.

Deciding the Roles Your Health Care Providers Will Play

Most health care professionals in the United States are either western or *complementary and alternative (CAM)* providers. Western doctors are either allopaths (MDs) or osteopaths (DOs). CAM providers are trained in one or more health care disciplines such as traditional Chinese medicine (TCM), acupuncture, chiropractic medicine, Ayurvedic medicine, naturopathic medicine, massage therapy, et cetera. We strongly urge everyone with hepatitis C to have a western doctor on your health care team. You need a western doctor because only these health care providers are able to order some of tests necessary to monitor your disease progression.

Your health care goals will largely determine your choices of health care providers. The chapters in Part Two of this manual describe the various western and CAM treatment options available to people with hepatitis C. Your personality, feelings about having hepatitis C, and your health care beliefs and goals will determine which medical disciplines are best suited to meet your needs.

The members of your health care team and their roles are entirely up to you. You will need to select one health care professional to be your primary care provider. This person will help you coordinate your health care plans and will monitor your overall health. You can choose either a western doctor or a CAM practitioner to be your primary care provider. You may choose to see only western medical professionals. You many choose to have western doctor as your primary provider and consult with one or more CAM practitioners. Alternatively, you may choose a CAM professional as your primary provider, and consult with a western doctor to monitor your disease progression.

Regardless of whom you choose as your primary care provider, if you receive care from more than one health care professional, it is <u>very</u> important to keep all of them informed about everything you are doing and **all** of the products you are taking. This is important to insure that treatments prescribed by one health care provider do not change the effects of treatments prescribed by another provider.

Getting Referrals

Finding a western health care provider to either manage or consult on your health care often begins with a referral. You will want a referral to a doctor who is knowledgeable about hepatitis C. The referral will probably come from another western health care provider such as your primary care doctor. When you ask for a referral, keep in mind that some health care providers are uncomfortable saying anything less than complimentary about a professional colleague. You may have to read between the lines. If someone seems uncomfortable, vague, or unenthusiastic about another provider, this may suggest an unspoken concern. A provider who refers all of his or her patients to one provider without considering the circumstances might also raise a concern. As hepatitis C is a complicated disease, we suggest you ask for a referral to someone who specializes in treating hepatitis C. Friends, colleagues, and other people with hepatitis C can also provide referrals based on their own experiences.

You may be referred to a gastroenterologist, an infectious disease specialist, or a hepatologist. Infectious disease specialists treat people with viral, bacterial, and other diseases caused by an infectious agent. Gastroenterologists specialize in diseases of the gastrointestinal system, which includes the liver. Hepatologists are gastroenterologists who treat only people with liver disease.

Whether you choose a CAM provider or a western provider to manage your care, keep in mind that your insurance coverage may limit your choices. This is particularly important if your insurance coverage is through a health maintenance organization (HMO) or a preferred provider organization (PPO). HMOs usually require a referral from your primary care doctor before you are able to see a specialist. Many PPOs also have this requirement. HMOs and PPOs have a list of health care providers who are members of the organization. Usually, you must choose a provider from this member list. Before you see a specialist or a CAM provider, check with your insurance company to see what services are covered under your policy. Coverage for CAM services vary greatly from one insurance carrier to another. Checking about coverage ahead of time will prevent you from being in the unhappy situation of getting unexpected medical bills.

Checking a Provider's Credentials

We urge you to take the time to find out about a health care provider's credentials and experience. It is important to work with providers who are skilled and experienced in the management of hepatitis C.

Many public libraries have guides such as the *American Medical Directory*, *The Directory of Medical Specialists*, and *Top Providers of America*, which can be good sources of information if you are looking for an allopathic doctor (an MD). There are many other resources available on the Internet for allopathic, osteopathic, naturopathic, and other CAM providers. See the *Resource Directory* in this manual for the Internet addresses of these sites. If you do not have your own computer, you may be able to use a friend's computer, or ask him or her to do some research for you. Most libraries have computers available for public use. There are also many businesses such as copy centers that have public use computers available for a small fee. Usually, you pay according to the amount of time you use the computer. Many public gathering places such as coffee shops and cafe's also offer Internet access to their customers.

If you are a veteran, see *Chapter 17: Military Veterans and Hepatitis C* for specific information about the Veterans Administration and your health care.

THE PROVIDER/PATIENT RELATIONSHIP

Your health care provider(s) will be making recommendations about health care decisions that may have lasting effects on your life. How you relate to these professionals is an important factor in achieving successful treatment and ongoing care. When talking with a potential health care provider for the first time, ask yourself if you are comfortable with the way this person treats you. If you intend to use one or more alternative therapies in your treatment plan, you will want to ask any western doctor you interview if he or she will work supportively with you to incorporate these choices into your overall treatment plan. Remember, you are hiring health care providers to work with you, not the other way around.

After you have interviewed someone you are considering as a potential health care provider, asking yourself some questions may help you decide if this is someone you want working with you.

- Was I comfortable with him/her?
- Did he/she take enough time to answer my questions?
- Did he/she treat my questions with respect?
- Did he/she answer my questions willingly and completely?
- Did we agree on issues about which I have strong opinions?
- Does he/she have a thorough understanding of hepatitis C?
- Did he/she adequately explain things to me?

An important consideration in assembling your health care team is deciding on the kind of provider/patient relationship that will work best for you. Answering the following questions may help you figure out what type of relationship best suits your personality.

- Do you want to have a significant role in reviewing information and making decisions? Or do you want your health care provider to tell you what to do and what treatments you should receive?
- Do you want a health care provider who uses only standard western treatments? Or do you want a provider who practices *integrated* medicine and is more likely to suggest experimental or CAM approaches?
- Do you want your provider to provide only facts? Or do you want your health care provider's opinions about what you should do?
- What personality traits are important for your provider to have?

Some people want their provider/patient relationship to be an equal partnership. There are certainly advantages to this type of relationship. You may feel you have lost some control over your life as a result of having hepatitis C. Participating in your health care may help you feel you've regained some of that control. While this type of relationship suits some people, it is not right for everyone. You may find the stresses of everyday living with hepatitis C are challenging enough without adding the additional stress of making all of your own health care decisions. In this case, allowing your health care providers to make decisions about your care removes an unwanted burden. Not having to think about the illness and/or its treatment may give you some much needed peace of mind. Only you know what kind of provider/patient relationship is best for you.

Communicating Effectively with Your Health Care Providers

You and your health care providers must communicate effectively for you to get the best care. All information you provide your health care providers about yourself is important. There is no right approach to treatment. Knowing your ideas and feelings will help your health care provider determine which treatment *protocol* will best match your needs. If you are unable to talk openly and honestly with your health care providers, try to identify what is interfering and work to change it. If the problem persists, you may want to consider seeing a different provider.

Be sure to tell all your health care providers what information you want kept confidential and what information they are free to discuss with your family and friends.

Tips for Talking with Your Providers

Most health care providers will speak with you privately in an examining room. However, it may be more comfortable for you to talk with them about important issues in an office or other private room. If you prefer to have your meeting in an office rather than an exam room, be sure to let the office staff know this when you make your appointment.

As a health care consumer, you have a right to have all of your questions about your health care answered to your satisfaction. You might have to ask questions more than once, but keep asking them until they are answered. If your health care provider or a nurse cannot answer your questions, ask for a referral to someone who can.

Here are a few tips that can make your interactions with your health care providers easier.

- If your health care provider seems distracted or less friendly on one day than another, do not take it personally. It probably has nothing to do with you. Your health care provider is human, too, with different moods, energy levels, and personal concerns. Health care providers often have to protect themselves from becoming emotionally drained so they can provide equal care to all of their patients. Treat your health care provider with the same consideration and respect with which you expect to be treated.

- If you are upset with your health care provider, try not to ask angry questions or make angry statements. Instead, express your angry feelings to someone you trust, a family member, friend, or a member of your support group. When you talk with your health care provider, try to phrase your comments and questions clearly but without a lot of emotional intensity. This will prevent an upsetting situation, and will help you get your needs met in a positive way.

- If you are aware of any extra efforts your health care provider has made for you, express your appreciation. Tell your health care provider if there are things about his or her style of working with you that are particularly helpful. A simple expression of gratitude can go a long way toward establishing a productive provider/patient relationship.

- If your provider does not have time to answer all of your questions during a regularly scheduled appointment, make an appointment just for that purpose. Be sure to say how much time you will need and that you will need your health care provider's undivided attention.

- Ask your health care provider about what kinds of things you should call about, and when it is best to call. This should help you come to an agreement about telephone contact that will work for both of you.

- If you make a telephone call to your health care provider, state your need, ask if your provider can take the call, and say how long you think the call will take. If your health care provider cannot take your call, ask when you should call back or when he or she can call you.

Talking About Sensitive Issues with Your Providers

Even if you respect your health care provider's skill and knowledge, you may not feel comfortable talking with him or her about how hepatitis C affects you emotionally. If this is the case, you may want to speak with a social worker or get a referral to a mental health professional.

There may be other issues you find difficult to discuss with your health care providers such as sexual concerns. Though it may be difficult to bring up sensitive issues, try to keep in mind your health care provider is used to discussing sensitive matters. It is always better to discuss your concerns rather than worry about them. You may find it is easier to talk with a nurse about an issue you may not feel comfortable discussing with your doctor. However, if the discussion affects your care, be aware that the nurse will need to share your discussion with your doctor.

If you have advanced disease and feel strongly about issues such as pain management, the initial interview may be a good time to discuss these issues. Coming to an understanding about issues that are important to you at the start of your relationship can prevent the need to change health care providers down the road.

Handling Communication Difficulties with Your Health Care Providers

If you are not satisfied with the care you are receiving, or if you are uncomfortable with the relationship you share with your health care provider, ask to talk with him or her in person about your concerns. Prepare for the meeting by writing down your questions and concerns ahead of time. Be specific about what you are dissatisfied with, and what changes you would like to see. Following these guidelines may help you specify your concerns and communicate them effectively.

- Describe the specific behaviors that bother you and how they make you feel. Try not to use negative words to describe your health care provider, or his or her attitude.
- Describe specific incidents that you have found troublesome as accurately as possible.
- Admit any part you may have played in the problem.

If you either cannot or do not want to meet in person, present your concerns in a letter. This approach can be useful because it gives your provider time to think about your concerns before getting back to you. Ask for your health care provider's ideas about ways to resolve the problem.

If you are generally satisfied with your health care provider, but have concerns about a particular decision or recommendation he or she has made, you may want to get a second opinion about that particular issue. Your health care provider can give you the names of other providers who can provide a second opinion. Under some managed care plans, you may have to pay for a second opinion. However, you may be able to appeal this decision.

It is important to try to work through any difficulties you might have with your health care provider. However, if it appears that it is just not a good match, you may want to consider finding a different health care provider. This is your right as a patient. Your health care provider should be willing to give you a referral to another health care provider if you request it. You can also get referrals from other health care providers or other people with hepatitis C. You may need to get approval from your insurance carrier before changing care providers. Though it can be somewhat stressful, keep in mind that changing health care providers does not mean there is anything wrong with either you or your health care provider.

Your Role in Treatment: Gathering Information

You can take an active role in your health care by educating yourself about hepatitis C. Your health care providers may have patient education materials available about your medications or supplements, their side effects, and how to manage them. Since product manufacturers often provide these materials, you might ask your health care provider to direct you to additional sources of information. Patient advocacy organizations and hepatitis C support groups can be invaluable sources of information about the disease and its treatment. See the *Resource Directory* at the back of this manual for a list of hepatitis C *advocacy* and support organizations.

If you are comfortable reading technical information, you may want to read medical journal articles about hepatitis C. However, be aware that these journals are intended for health care professionals, so they can be very challenging reading. If you are interested, ask a member of your health care team for recommendations about appropriate journals and/or articles. A hospital librarian or the reference librarian at your local public library can help you locate specific journals or articles.

The Internet is another good resource for information about hepatitis C. Any search engine can lead you to a number of resources. However, keep in mind the Internet is unregulated. Anyone can post just about anything on the Internet regardless of its accuracy. Sites that are reviewed by a medical advisory board are generally more reliable sources of information than sites with no such oversight.

Getting Information from Your Health Care Providers

Gathering information takes time and effort. However, it is important to get answers to your questions. If you have questions for your health care provider, organize and write them down ahead of time. Your time with your health care provider is often limited. Being organized will help you get as many of your questions answered as possible in the time available. Identify the two or three most urgent questions. You may even want to give your list of questions to your provider before your appointment so he or she is prepared to answer them. Ask your provider to read all of your questions, not just those you have marked as most urgent. He or she may see questions on your list that are more important than you realize. Be sure to speak up if you do not understand the answer to a question. If you cannot get all of your questions answered in one appointment, you may want to schedule a follow-up appointment just for that purpose.

Nurses are often good sources of information about treatment and care. They are usually easy to approach, and most nurses will go out of their way to make sure you get the information you need as quickly as possible.

Pharmacists can answer questions about your medications, and are often easily accessible. Be sure to tell your pharmacist about all of the medications and supplements you are taking. The pharmacist can advise you about possible side effects, and potential interactions between drugs and/or supplements. However, it is very important that each of your health care providers knows all the drugs and/or supplements you are taking to be certain the various treatments are compatible with one another, and that there is no risk of harm.

The more you know about hepatitis C, the less confused and anxious you are likely to be. Understanding the reasons for particular treatment options, and taking part in the decisions about what options are right for you may help you sort through your priorities.

MAINTAINING YOUR MEDICAL RECORDS

We suggest you keep your own set of medical and insurance records. Managing your treatment records and filing insurance claims can take a lot of time and energy, though doing so may help you regain a sense of control over your situation. You may need to turn this responsibility over to someone else if you are not feeling well. Family members and friends often feel helplessness when a loved one is sick. The opportunity to help you may come as a welcome relief to this sense of helplessness. A social worker or a community service organization may also be able to help. Some private companies check bills, file claims, track deductibles, and advocate for their clients.

You can create your own medical record file. Start by contacting the medical records departments of any hospitals or clinics where you have received care. Requests for copies of your records usually need to be in writing. Be sure to ask for copies of everything in your file. If possible, get copies of all treatment records and tests including x-rays, biopsies, and other lab reports. These documents will provide you with an easily accessible historical record of your hepatitis C experience. It is also a good way to keep track of the medications and supplements you are currently taking or have taken in the past.

Keeping a diary of your reactions to medications and supplements may help you differentiate those that seem to be helpful from those that do not. Your provider will have a reference for making treatment recommendations, and you will have a record of your reactions to specific drugs and/or supplements.

HEALTH CARE COVERAGE

At times, it may seem that your relationship with your insurance carrier is almost as important as your relationship with your health care provider. You may need to call for authorization to see a specialist. You may need to get permission to have certain tests done. You may need to ask questions about billing procedures and what charges you will have to pay. You may even need to voice a complaint. If you can, establish a relationship with one person in customer service who is familiar with you and your situation. These workers are often called case managers. The more familiar your case manager is with your situation, the easier it will be to get the information you need. He or she may even be willing to advocate for you, if necessary. If you cannot get the help you need or if you are not satisfied with a decision your case manager makes, do not be afraid to ask to talk to someone with greater authority.

Keeping Accurate Records of Medical Costs

It is important to keep records of all of your medical care costs. Ask for a receipt each time you go to an appointment. Before leaving the office, review the receipt to make sure everything is correct. Keep track of all insurance claims and expenses, including such things as mileage to and from medical appointments. You may be able to deduct a portion of your medical expenses from your federal and state tax debt. The Internal Revenue Service can help you to determine which expenses are deductible from your federal tax debt.

When you receive a statement from your insurance company, review it to make sure it is accurate. Call the insurance company immediately if you find a mistake. Ask to have the error corrected, and to be sent a corrected statement. Review the new statement to make sure that all changes have been made and the total is accurate.

When a health care provider submits a claim, the insurance company responds by sending a check for the covered amount. You will receive a statement showing the request for payment, and the amount of reimbursement to the provider. If the amount is not covered entirely, the carrier will instruct you to pay the health care provider whatever amount is remaining. Normally, your health care provider will also send you an invoice for any remainder that is due. As many people with hepatitis C know, medical bills can pile up very quickly. If you are unable to pay the full amount you owe on a bill, call your health care provider and ask to set up a payment plan. Most health care providers are aware of the financial burden of health care and are usually willing to work out a reasonable payment schedule.

Filing Insurance Claims

Most hospitals and many medical offices will file claims to your insurance company for you. However, be sure to file claims for all medical treatments you receive that were not filed by the provider. People often do not get the most from their medical insurance because they either do not know what is covered or are overwhelmed by the paperwork. If you are filing claims yourself and are not sure if something is covered, file the claim anyway. Even if the cost is not reimbursed, it might be applied to your deductible. There is no harm in trying.

There are a number of reasons why your insurance company may not cover treatments or services your health care provider considers necessary. The insurance company may not be up-to-date on the latest treatments. They may not share your health care provider's views on which treatments are standard and which are experimental. Some insurance companies try to keep costs down by covering only older, less expensive treatments. Carriers often refuse to pay for treatments that have not been approved by the Food and Drug Administration (FDA). If a claim is denied, do not panic. Denied claims can be appealed.

Appealing Denied Insurance Claims

If you decide to appeal a denied claim, contact the insurance company to find out about the appeal process. If possible, find out who made the decision to deny your claim and talk with him or her to find out why the claim was denied. If that person does not answer your questions satisfactorily, ask to speak to someone with more authority. If you believe your claim has been unfairly denied, go to the top of the organization if necessary. Your state insurance commissioner's office may be of assistance.

If a claim is denied because the treatment is not considered standard care, a letter from your provider explaining that your treatment is consistent with standard practice may help. Copies of articles from respected medical journals that support the treatment may also help.

If your health care provider's fee is challenged for being above what is customary, check with other local providers to find out if their fees for that procedure are similar to what you were charged. If you need assistance, someone involved in billing at your health care provider's office should be able to help.

Document any conversations you have with a representative of your insurance company in a brief letter to that person. Summarize the conversation and any arrangement or decision that was made.

Submit all requests in writing. Keep copies of all written correspondence you have with your insurance company, billing agencies, hospitals, and doctor's offices. When you speak to a representative of one of these organizations by telephone, make a note of the date and time, who you spoke with, and what you discussed. Consider keeping a notebook by the telephone for taking notes during telephone conversations.

Changing Insurance Plans

If you plan to change jobs, be aware that you may not be able to enroll in your new employer's medical insurance plan for a period of time. Also be aware that some insurance policies have what is known as a pre-existing condition clause. This clause states the insurance carrier will not cover expenses for a previously diagnosed medical condition. This clause may be in effect for a defined period, or it may permanently exclude coverage for such a condition. These clauses are most frequently encountered in policies issued by relatively small companies.

It is very important to find out the details about health insurance coverage before making a decision to change employment. Some people decide to consider a less satisfying or lower paying job in order to get the kind of health insurance they need.

Getting Health Care Without Health Insurance

Many people do not have health insurance. Once you have been diagnosed with hepatitis C, getting health insurance may be difficult. However, there are always options to get the health care you need. For example, many states have a high-risk insurance pool that is set up to provide insurance for citizens who would otherwise be denied health insurance. Many of these pools provide competitive rates and services.

Medicaid is another option. Medicaid provides health insurance for people with low incomes, the disabled, and certain groups of children. Services are provided through your state under federal guidelines. Benefits vary widely from state to state. To apply for Medicaid, contact your state's department of social services.

Patient advocacy organizations, support groups, and social workers are all good sources of information about these and other options for obtaining health care in a difficult situation.

COMPASSIONATE USE PROGRAMS FOR PRESCRIPTION DRUGS

A number of pharmaceutical companies have compassionate use programs. These programs are also known as patient assistance programs. These programs provide drug treatments for individuals with low incomes who do not have medical insurance, and would not otherwise have access to these treatments. To qualify for one of these programs, you will probably need to provide basic information about yourself, and your health care provider's name and contact information. Some programs will only work directly with your health care provider, or a representative such as a social worker or case manager. You will probably be interviewed to verify that you qualify for the program. Most programs request proof of your income level. Review for final approval varies, but many programs make a decision within a matter of days.

For compassionate use programs contact information, see the *Resource Directory* at the back of this manual under "Pharmaceutical Companies".

DISABILITY STATUS UNDER SOCIAL SECURITY

Hepatitis C affects everyone differently. How much the illness affects your daily life depends on the status of your liver, your age, overall health, and a number of other variables. Some people with advanced disease and/or severe *symptoms* find they are unable to work. If you are unable to work because of your hepatitis C, you may want to consider applying for disability benefits from the Social Security Administration (SSA).

Gaining approval for social security disability benefits can be challenging. SSA denies the majority of first time claims. However, an initial denial should not keep you from pursuing this option. If you have been denied, you must appeal the denial within 60 days. You can build a strong case for your appeal by paying close attention to the information and documentation SSA requires. Be sure to follow all instructions carefully. Be honest, accurate, and brief when completing the required forms. You will need detailed medical records that document your symptoms and limitations. You will also need the support of a doctor, psychiatrist, and/or psychologist if you hope to win your case. SSA requires proof that your diagnosis causes your limitations. There must also be medical proof that your limitations are significant and severe enough to prevent you from working full-time on a sustained basis.

If you want to win your SSA disability claim, it is important to receive continuous and consistent medical care. This will allow you to provide SSA and a judge with current and complete medical records that support your doctors' opinions. You can choose to use any CAM therapies you believe are beneficial. However, be aware that SSA and judges are most persuaded by western doctors, and how you respond or fail to respond to mainstream treatment.

You should apply for disability benefits as soon as you and/or your doctors believe your hepatitis C will prevent you from working for at least one year. Waiting to file may cost you benefits that cannot be recovered. Many people recommend consulting with and/or hiring a disability lawyer as soon as possible after you have filed your claim. A lawyer can explain the process and lay the proper foundation for your case. If you decide to hire a disability lawyer, find one who is familiar with SSA rules and regulations. You should have an agreement with your attorney that you will only owe fees if you win your case and receive benefits. For more information, see the *Resource Directory* at the back of the manual.

SUMMARY

Dealing with the health care system can sometimes leave you scratching your head and wondering what you are supposed to do next. You will meet new people, hear and use new language, and very often, live by new rules. Information is probably the most important tool you have for making your way through the maze and getting the best care you can — the care you deserve. Gathering information will put increased demands on your time and energy, but you may be surprised at your own strength and stamina.

There is much you can do to advocate for your own rights and needs. Be assertive about your needs with your current health care providers and when choosing new providers. Look for treatment facilities that meet your needs. Ask about new treatments and clinical trials. Analyze your insurance coverage and other financial concerns.

Remember, there are always options.

Chapter Seventeen

MILITARY VETERANS AND HEPATITIS C

Terry Baker

INTRODUCTION

America's veterans have been plagued with many health issues since the founding of this country. *Hepatitis* has long been associated with U.S. military service. Military training and combat present many opportunities for transmission of viral hepatitis through blood-to-blood contact. Field bleeding, surgery, transfusions, and exposure to blood by military medics and surgeons all constitute high risks. During World War I, thousands of American GI's were stricken with *hepatitis A*. To this day, service men and women still become ill with hepatitis A, B, and C (formerly known as non-A, non-B hepatitis).

Since the identification of the *hepatitis C* virus (HCV) in 1989, physicians and Veterans Administration (VA) officials have seen large numbers of infection among veterans. Veterans appear to have unusually high rates of hepatitis C. While the prevalence of hepatitis C in the general population is approximately 1.8%, various studies in VA facilities have shown hepatitis C virus (HCV) prevalence rates between 10-20% among veterans.[1]

Veterans of foreign combat appear to be at the highest risk for infectious hepatitis. All major engagements of the last 60 years, World War II, the Korean War, and the Vietnam War, were associated with high rates of infectious hepatitis. Viral hepatitis was viewed as a single disease in the early years, and most treatment and documentation of it were for the acute forms of the disease.

VETERANS AND THE HEPATITIS C TIMELINE

1941-1953   Many World War II and Korean War veterans were diagnosed with non-A, non-B hepatitis. Non-A, non-B hepatitis was the diagnosis for unexplained infections that damaged the liver.

1967-1969   Field hospitals performed 364,900 blood transfusions on American personnel in Vietnam. Soldiers, medics, and nurses were exposed to blood while caring for the wounded.[2]

1989   Researchers identified the hepatitis C virus, 48 years after the start of World War II.

1992   Researchers developed an accurate blood test for hepatitis C.[3]

1998   The number of hepatitis C cases at U.S. Department of Veterans Affairs facilities rose to 22,000 in 1998, up from 6,600 in 1991.[1,4]

1999   The VA established two HCV research and education centers and issued HCV treatment guidelines.

VA leaders argued that investing in early treatment would save public dollars by reducing future hospital stays and liver transplants.

AMVETS, Disabled Veterans of America, Paralyzed Veterans of America, and Veterans of Foreign Wars criticized the Clinton Administration's year 2000 budget proposal stating that funding for veterans' health care was $3 million below needed allocations.

Legislation was introduced to ensure wider coverage for hepatitis C treatment through VA facilities.

Veterans Aimed Toward Awareness (VATA) launched a nationwide campaign to alert U.S. veterans they may be at risk for hepatitis C.

A national survey about hepatitis C was conducted with 504 veterans.

Veterans' Hepatitis C Survey

Bruskin-Goldring Research conducted a national survey commissioned by VATA of 504 veterans in 1999. Ages of those surveyed ranged from 40-60, with a mean age of 49. Following are some of the highlights from that survey.

- 74.8% were "not very" or "not at all" concerned about their risk for HCV
- 60.1% had not been tested for HCV
- 58.3% were "not very" or "not at all" likely to be tested for HCV
- 67.5% were "not very" or "not at all" familiar with the disease
- 63.3% recognized flu-like symptoms, and 57.7% recognized yellow skin as possible symptoms of liver disease
- 1.6% knew that hepatitis C often has no symptoms
- 9% initially acknowledged they might be at risk for hepatitis C
- 45% acknowledged they might be at risk after being informed of risk factors
- 65.1% stated their greatest fear about HCV is the possibility of infecting a loved one
- 62.9% stated their next greatest fear was the possibility of having a serious illness or dying from a serious illness

These findings clearly indicate there is a need for HCV education. Veterans must be informed of their risk for hepatitis C, and about the seriousness of the disease.

THE INCIDENCE OF HEPATITIS C AMONG AMERICA'S MILITARY VETERANS

Veterans' *advocates* have grown increasingly concerned in recent years about the incidence of hepatitis C among military veterans. Several studies have suggested veterans may be at higher risk than the general public. According to testimony given before the U.S. Senate Committee on Appropriations, Subcommittee on Veterans' Affairs, 69,000 veterans in VA facilities have tested HCV positive since 1999.[5] Studies at the VA Medical Centers (VAMC) in Washington D.C. and San Francisco found the prevalence of HCV positive inpatients was 20% and 10%, respectively.[1] One of these studies also found 52% of patients requiring liver transplant were HCV positive.[1]

In 1998, a national tracking system analyzed the findings from 95,000 hepatitis C screening tests performed in the VA system.[4] Of those who tested positive:

- 64% were Vietnam veterans
- 18.5% were post-Vietnam veterans

- 4.5% were Korean era veterans
- 4.2% were post-Korean era veterans, and
- 9.1% were Veterans from other periods of service.

Veterans of the Vietnam War: The Largest Military Population Most At Risk

Of the 8.1 million surviving veterans of the Vietnam War, 3.2 million had active duty in Asia between 1964 and 1973.[6] It is conservatively estimated that 10% of these Asian theater veterans are now infected with HCV.[1]

Modes of Transmission of HCV in the Asian Theater of the Vietnam War

There are a number of HCV risk factors for veterans who were in Asia during the Vietnam War, many related to the high prevalence of HCV in southeast Asian countries. It is estimated that 5-8% of the Vietnamese population is infected with HCV.[7]

Transfusions

Transfusion of blood or blood products before 1992 is a known risk factor for HCV infection. Prior to 1992, there were no accurate HCV screening tests to ensure the safety of the blood supply with respect to HCV.[3] Three hundred thousand Americans were wounded and 153,329 were hospitalized during the Vietnam War. Between March 1967 and June 1969, 364,900 Americans in Vietnam received blood transfusions.[2] It is estimated that a minimum of 10% of those transfused received HCV infected blood.[8]

Medical Contact

Surgeons, nurses, medics, helicopter crews, and others involved in the evacuation and treatment of the wounded from Vietnam were also placed at risk for HCV infection because of their blood exposure. An estimated 41.1% of all soldiers deployed to Vietnam, approximately 2.1 million veterans, were involved in combat. Many soldiers assisted the more than 300,000 wounded. Medical personnel on hospital ships were also placed at risk via their exposure to wounded soldiers from the Vietnam theater.[9]

Tattoos

Unclean needles that pierce the skin can transmit HCV. While transmission of HCV by tattooing has not been fully documented in the U.S., it has been documented elsewhere.[10] An estimated 34% of active-duty military personnel have tattoos (personal communication, Capt. John Mateczun, Principal Director, Clinical Affairs, Office of Health Affairs, Department of Defense). Many of these tattoos were and continue to be acquired in countries where sanitation is often substandard.

Sexual Contact

Although sexual transmission of HCV occurs, it is believed to be relatively uncommon. Nevertheless, a portion of those infected with HCV during the Vietnam War were probably infected through sexual contact with Vietnamese nationals.

Recreational Drug Use

Sharing drug paraphernalia is currently the most common cause of newly acquired HCV infections. This was also a risk factor during the Vietnam War. A study from the Centers for

Disease Control and Prevention on the health status of Vietnam veterans found 3% had used "hard drugs," including amphetamines, barbiturates, cocaine, heroin, psychedelics, phencyclidine and methaqualone.[11]

VA MONITORING OF HCV-INFECTED VETERANS

The Department of Veterans Affairs has noted a decided increase in the number of HCV cases diagnosed over the past several years. There were 6,600 HCV cases reported in the VA system in 1991. By 1994, this number had increased to 18,854. Over the next four years, the annual number of newly identified cases increased steadily to 20,203 in 1995, 21,424 in 1996, 24,850 in 1997, and 29,799 in 1998. Since March 1999, over 69,000 additional cases have been identified. VA officials expect this number to continue to increase substantially.[12]

Testing of veterans outside the VA medical system has confirmed the high HCV prevalence in this population. A 1998 screening program that tested 200 apparently healthy leaders of the Vietnam Veterans of America found 9% of those tested were infected with HCV.[13] A more recent screening at a Vietnam Veterans' stand down found 36% of those screened tested positive for HCV.[14] Although these numbers are preliminary, they all point to the fact that veterans have consistently high rates of HCV infection of at least 10%, more than five times the prevalence rate in the general population.

In June 1998, the VA issued new HCV screening guidelines for veterans entering VA facilities who have one or more of ten specified risk factors. The VA has also established two Centers of Excellence located at the VA medical centers in Miami and San Francisco. These centers coordinate treatment and research efforts, and develop educational programs for patients and their families. Health care providers who specialize in HCV and patient counselors are also located at these centers. These centers established the current guidelines for VA clinicians who treat patients with hepatitis C.

The VA expects the new screening guidelines will dramatically increase the number of VA patients identified with hepatitis C. The demand for HCV related services is expected to rise proportionately. The screening guidelines indicate that any veteran who requests HCV testing should be tested regardless of his or her risk factors.

In December 1999, the VA adopted treatment guidelines for HCV infection. The guidelines recommend that eligible veterans be given the very best medical care, including the most recently approved treatment. Of course, only veterans who are income eligible or service connected for HCV can receive treatment through a VA medical center. Despite the treatment guidelines, veterans report problems obtaining care due to constraints put on HCV health care at the Veterans Integrated Service Network (VISN) level.

The one fact on which we can all probably agree is that hepatitis C among military veterans is an overwhelming problem for the Veterans Administration.

THE NEED FOR A SERVICE CONNECTION TO HCV TO RECEIVE TREATMENT THROUGH A VA FACILITY

As a result of the reorganization of the VAMC system, all veterans have been put into one of seven categories according to his or her medical priority. Currently all veterans, regardless of their category, receive medical treatment when they come to a VAMC. However, unless they are 100% service connected, a copayment is required for all services and medicines.

It is critically important for veterans with HCV to be granted presumptive service connection to the disease so they can be treated. However, veterans infected with HCV during their military service are generally unable to establish the necessary service connection. A lack of knowledge about hepatitis C and how it is contracted, a historic lack of a reliable screening test, and the prolonged, often asymptomatic course of disease progression all conspire to make it extremely difficult to prove that infection was acquired during military service. Without a service connection to HCV, most veterans are unable to meet the standard of proof necessary to show that they contracted HCV during their military service. As the VA's budget continues to shrink, we fear that veterans without a service connected injury (including veterans with HCV) will be turned away from VAMCs.

Currently, Vietnam veterans are the military group most significantly affected by hepatitis C. Many veterans who contracted HCV in Vietnam 25-30 years ago are only now exhibiting symptoms of liver disease. When they were first infected, HCV had not been distinguished from other forms of hepatitis. In 85% of the cases, there would have been no acute symptoms at the time of infection.

Detecting HCV infection at the time of discharge was also impossible. Many of today's HCV infected veterans were discharged from the military before tests for hepatitis C existed. Even today, when there are reliable tests for hepatitis C, the military does not conduct HCV testing as part of the discharge physical.

HCV infected veterans who were treated for *acute hepatitis* during their military service and who now appear before the Board of Veterans' Appeals (BVA) to establish service connection are most often denied because they cannot prove their current HCV infection is related to their prior acute hepatitis. The Board often rejects a claim for service connection because the veteran's medical record does not show the presence of HCV at the time of discharge. In fact, in the review of all 1,599 cases of chronic hepatitis brought before the BVA between 1994 and 1996, only 37 resulted in approval of a service-related disability rating for hepatitis.[15]

Making a service connection to HCV will enable veterans to be tested for hepatitis C, and those who are positive and desire treatment to obtain treatment through the VA system. It will also enable veterans who progress to advanced liver disease to get adequate treatment through the VA.

Establishing A Service Connection to Hepatitis C

To establish a successful claim for military service connected disability from hepatitis C, you must meet the following requirements.

1. You must show that you currently have hepatitis C. The VA is obligated to test you for hepatitis C, but it is suggested that you also get a diagnosis from a private doctor.

2. You must show that hepatitis C was caused by or aggravated by military service. Because hepatitis C is blood-borne, you must show that while you were in the military you had:

- a blood transfusion
- hemodialysis
- blood-to-blood contact
- jet injector inoculations (shots), and/or
- shared a razor, tooth brush, or any other item that could carry infected blood.

Successful claims often include a private physician's (often a gastroenterologist or hepatologist) letter indicating that, in his or her opinion, your hepatitis C is a direct result of your military service.

You should be aware that activities that show "willful misconduct" could disqualify you from compensation. These activities include body piercing, tattoos, and/or use of injected recreational drugs, snorted cocaine, and other drug use.

If you are a veteran diagnosed with hepatitis C, the first thing you should do is to find a qualified Veterans Service Officer to assist you in filing a claim for a service connection to hepatitis C. Most Service Officers work for a county or state veteran's service. From the Veterans Aimed Toward Awareness's internet site at http://www.vetsaware.org, you can link to the Vietnam Veterans of America site. From there, go to "Benefits" and then to "Service Representatives" to select a representative from your state. Service representatives know the laws, rules of filing, and the paperwork you will need to complete for a claim.

SUMMARY

Veterans' advocates have made it a priority to see that service men and women are tested for hepatitis C. We are working to ensure that treatment is affordable, and that information will be available for those who need it. It is my heartfelt commitment to work to see these goals accomplished.

HCV/HIV COINFECTION

Section 1

OVERVIEW OF COINFECTION

Misha Cohen, OMD, LAc

INTRODUCTION

Due to similar routes of transmission, an increasing number of people with either the *human immunodeficiency virus (HIV)* or the *hepatitis C* virus (HCV) are becoming infected with the other virus. People with both HIV and HCV are said to be coinfected. Because of the widespread use of highly active antiretroviral therapy (HAART) in developed countries, the survival rate for people with HIV has greatly improved in recent years. Increasingly, people who are coinfected with HIV and HCV are dying from HCV *not* HIV.

HCV appears to progress much more rapidly in people with HIV than it does in people without HIV. Coinfected people have at least double the risk of developing severe liver damage compared to people without HIV. There is also evidence that suggests HCV liver disease progression is faster among people with HIV than it is in people who do not have HIV.[1]

INCIDENCE OF HCV INFECTION, HIV INFECTION, AND HCV/HIV COINFECTION

HCV infection is the most common, chronic, blood-borne infection in the United States.[2] An estimated 170-240 million people worldwide are infected with HCV. As of 2002, the estimated number of people living with HIV/AIDS is 40 million. All people with HIV/AIDS are believed to be at great risk for opportunistic infections, including HCV. Up to 40% of those infected with HIV are believed to be already coinfected with HCV. There is every reason to believe that the coinfection rate will only increase over the next decade.[3]

Researchers at the University of Cincinnati College of Medicine conducted a retrospective study of a diverse sample of the United States population in two *clinical trials* on AIDS. They found HCV infection occurs in all groups of HIVpositive people at an average rate of 35.6%. People between the ages of 40 and 49 who are HIV positive are at very high risk, with more than 50% having active HCV infection. One hundred percent of those in the study who had a *CD4* (an immune cell killed by HIV) count below 100 were coinfected with HCV.[4] Another separate study found approximately 30% of HIV positive people coming out of prison are also infected with HCV.[5]

More than 95% of hemophiliacs who received blood products during the 1970's and 1980's show evidence of viral infection with HCV.[6] The incidence rate of those infected with HIV who are also adult hemophiliacs is between 60-85%.[7]

For those with a history of intravenous (IV) drug use, the coinfection rate is between 60-81%.[8] A 1998 study conducted in a large U.S. urban HIV clinic found 81% of HIVpositive IV drug users were also infected with HCV.[9] A 1998 multi-center observational study conducted in Brazil examined the coinfection rate among IV drug users participating in a needle exchange program. Over 42% were coinfected, slightly over 10% had HCV only, slightly over 9% had HIV only, and 40% did not have HIV or HCV.[10]

INCREASED RISKS FOR THOSE WHO ARE COINFECTED

People coinfected with HCV and HIV are at increased risk for a number of conditions that can lead to more rapid disease progression.

Immune System Changes with Coinfection

Twenty percent of those living with HIV who later contract HCV cannot develop *antibodies* to HCV because HIV has devastated their immune systems. These infected people will most likely go on to develop *chronic hepatitis* C with all its potential harmful consequences. Even if you are one of the 80% of HIV positive people who *do* produce antibodies and your *immune system* can mount an immune defense against HCV, you are still almost twice as likely to sustain severe liver damage as someone infected with HCV alone.

The immune system generally responds to viral infection with two types of responses, a cellular response and a humoral response. A cellular response involves special white blood cells called a *T-cells*. Different kinds of T-cells have different actions that help the body attack virus and moderate the immune system. A humoral response is an antibody response. Another group of white blood cells, B-cells, produce antibodies. Antibodies tag viruses and other *microorganisms* as invaders, thereby alerting the rest of the immune system.

Most people with chronic HCV have elevated *viral loads* (chronic viremia). HCV infection is associated with a broad-spectrum white cell (immune) response to HCV *antigens* (proteins unique to HCV). However, chronically infected patients lack an HCV-specific T-cell response. Further, the antibodies produced in response to HCV infection do not lead to HCV *clearance*. Researchers speculate that this inability of the antibodies to produce viral clearance is the reason people coinfected with HIV have an increased risk of hepatitis C progression to *cirrhosis* and *liver cancer*. In one study, HCV infection was associated with an increase in T-suppressor cell (*CD8* cell) activation. T-suppressor cells lower the immune response. Researchers also found the HCV viral load was inversely related to the level of T-helper cells (CD4 cells). In other words, the lower the level of T-helper cells, the higher the HCV viral load.[11]

In another study, researchers examined how HCV affects the course of HIV disease. They found coinfected patients appeared to have a decreased ability to increase their T-helper cell (CD4 cell) counts after they achieved an undetectable HIV viral load compared to people infected with HIV alone.[12]

A 1999 report stated the survival time in HIV is "normal" in coinfected patients on HAART who have a CD4 count greater than 2,000.[13] However, the progression of hepatitis C is greater in coinfected people with lower CD4 counts. Overall, coinfected people have a faster rate of hepatitis C disease progression than do people infected with HCV alone. It takes less time to develop cirrhosis, liver *decompensation*, and/or liver cancer (*hepatocellular carcinoma*).

Research suggests that HCV undergoes an increased number of *mutations* when the CD4 count is less than 200 compared to when the count is greater than 200. The increased number of mutations may be associated with more virulent (agressive) forms of the virus.[13]

Inability of Liver to Detoxify Antiviral Drugs

People who are coinfected and are taking HIV combination therapy that includes *protease inhibitors* and other *antivirals* may be at increased risk of harmful side effects from the HIV medication. This is because a damaged liver cannot properly process and detoxify many HIV medications. It appears that in some cases, the use of HIV medications can accelerate the progression of an existing HCV infection.[14]

It is common for those who are coinfected with HIV and HCV to have a jump in their *liver enzyme* levels after starting an HIV antiviral drug combination. The most *toxic* HIV antiviral medications for coinfected patients appear to be the protease inhibitors ritonavir and indinavir. However, other antivirals such as nelfinavir and those in a group of drugs called *nucleoside reverse transcriptase inhibitors* (NRTIs; for example, ddI, ddC and AZT) have also been found to produce elevated liver enzymes and/or life-threatening episodes of liver *toxicity*.[15, 16, 17]

Studies of people taking HAART found coinfected people were almost three times as likely to experience liver toxicity as people infected with HIV only.[18] HCV and HAART medications both have the ability to damage the mitochondria of the liver cells (*hepatocytes*). This effect is even more powerful when HCV and HAART drugs are present together. This is thought to be the cause of the increased liver toxicity seen in coinfected patients on HAART.[17] Mitochondria are the powerhouses of cells. They provide the energy needed for cells to function properly. When mitochondria are damaged, liver cells do not have the energy to function normally and liver damage occurs. Because of the increased risk for liver toxicity, all coinfected people on HIV antiviral therapy should have regularly scheduled blood tests to assess liver function for the duration of their drug treatment.

Although it appears that all people with chronic hepatitis C have an increased amount of *free radical* damage in their liver mitochondria, this damage is greatest in people with HCV *genotype* 1b.[19] Studies of people with HCV genotype 1b who were not HIV positive showed this damage occurs along with a loss of *glutathione*, an important *antioxidant* (a substance that limits free radical damage).[19] The loss of this important nutrient and the liver damage that follows may be the result of increased levels of free radicals in liver tissue. These free radicals may accelerate disease progression, and may also be partly responsible for the resistance to treatment that most people with HCV genotype 1b experience.[20] These studies show that the loss of glutathione, resistance to treatment, and accelerated disease progression are more significant for those who are coinfected *and* have HCV genotype 1b.[20] See *Chapter 14: Nutritional Supplementation* for more information on free radical damage and antioxidants.

A major problem in treating coinfection is that certain HIV medications themselves (for example, NRTIs, AZT, ddI, and ddC) cause mitochondrial damage. This toxic effect appears to be increased if *ribavirin* is taken along with these antiviral agents.[21, 22, 23] This is one reason treatment for coinfected people is usually undertaken one virus at a time. Either HIV or HCV is treated to avoid the risk of the toxicity that can occur when medications for both viruses are taken together.

Treating coinfection is a new and complex area of medicine. There are no specific guidelines about how to do it. Decisions about treatment need to be made in close communication with a knowledgeable health care provider.

Fibrosis and Cirrhosis from Alcohol Consumption

Alcohol intake increases the risk of *fibrosis*, cirrhosis, and severe liver disease. Alcohol is especially harmful to coinfected people who are taking antiviral medications.[24]

Increased Liver Enzymes (AST and ALT)

Doctors have noticed over the years that treatment for HIV commonly leads to increases in liver enzymes such as *ALT* and *AST*. These increases were previously attributed to the *hepatotoxicity* of the drugs used to treat HIV. However, it now appears that hepatitis viruses are cofactors in the development of increased liver enzymes after starting HAART for HIV. Among HIV positive people on HAART, it has been shown that liver enzyme levels increase faster in those who are coinfected with HCV or hepatitis B virus (HBV) compared to those who are not coinfected.[24]

Accelerated Progression of Liver Fibrosis

HCV disease progression is faster in people who are coinfected than in people who have only HCV. HCV appears to be able to replicate faster in coinfected people because the immune system is altered and can no longer produce specific antibodies to HCV. HCV can easily escape the immune system's surveillance, reproduce faster, and possibly mutate more easily in the presence of HIV infection.[25] Generally, coinfected people have higher viral loads of HCV than do those who are infected with HCV only. Coinfected people progress more rapidly to cirrhosis, liver failure, and/or liver cancer. Without treatment, they are more likely to die from liver disease than those without HIV. Studies show the average time to liver cirrhosis is 26 years in coinfected patients, eight years sooner than in HCV infected people who were not coinfected with HIV.[24, 26, 27, 28]

Although studies show that a low CD4 count (less than 200) increases the risk for liver damage and accelerate hepatitis C disease progression, there is no evidence that those with higher CD4 counts are protected against this accelerated disease progression.[29] Some studies have found no relationship between CD4 counts and the rate of hepatitis C progression.[30]

Development of Lipodystrophy

There is evidence that HCV may be related to the development of HIV related *lipodystrophy*. Lipodystrophy is a condition of altered fat metabolism. Fat is lost from the arms and legs and is redistributed to the abdomen, upper back along the spine, and the breasts in women. Blood fats are elevated and lipomas (fat deposits in the skin) are often present. Both HIV antiviral medications and the HIV virus itself have been thought to be the cause of lipodystrophy. However, new research suggests that HCV has the ability to interfere with fat metabolism. It damages the mitochondria of the liver cells, an important site of fat breakdown and storage. Studies show that a large percentage of people with a specific form of lipodystrophy called lipodysatrophy (loss of fat in the arms and legs) also have hepatitis C.[31] The redistribution of fat to the abdomen includes increased fat in the liver. This increase of fat in the liver adds to the damage already caused by HCV. The decreased mass of functioning liver cells decreases the liver's ability to take in and metabolize *glucose*, which can lead to diabetes.

Another *symptom* of lipodystrophy that occurs in those on HIV protease inhibitors is *insulin* resistance. Protease inhibitor insulin resistance occurs more commonly in people who are coinfected than in those infected with HIV alone. Although insulin resistance is associated with an increased risk of heart disease, we do not have proof that taking medications to increase insulin sensitivity will decrease this risk of heart disease.

The exact causes of the lipodystrophy associated with HIV are still being determined. Cofactors that may be involved include therapy with a protease inhibitor, therapy with certain NRTI drugs, injecting recreational drugs such heroin and cocaine, the duration of HIV therapy, age, gender, and *body mass index* (BMI; an indicator of healthy body weight).[32]

Recurrence or Activation of Hepatitis C

There are only a few reports in the medical literature on the effects of HAART among people who are coinfected with hepatitis viruses. However, a new report from Europe implicates HAART in the recurrence or activation of HBV and/or HCV.[33]

Infection with Other Hepatitis Viruses

People infected with HIV and HCV are at increased risk for other forms of hepatitis, especially *hepatitis B* and D. Scientists predict that 1-3% of those already coinfected with HIV and HCV will also become infected with HBV. It is also estimated that those who are infected with HCV and later contract *hepatitis A* have a 40% chance of dying from the acute infection with hepatitis A. These coinfections can create serious medical crises and raise many complicated treatment issues. Everyone with HIV should be tested for HCV and the other hepatitis viruses. Early detection is the best advantage one can have in treating any coinfection.

More Rapid Progression to End-Stage Disease

Researchers from the Centers for Disease Control and Prevention report an increasing percentage of deaths in people with HIV involve at least one form of liver disease such as hepatitis C as a cofactor. Ten percent of people with HIV who died in 1997 had liver disease as a cofactor in their deaths. Most of these cases appear to be associated with viral hepatitis coinfection, HAART, or both. Nearly all of the viral infections would have been due to either HBV or HCV. Researchers believe that protease inhibitor drug therapy is the most likely component of HAART that would have been associated with these deaths, although other components of HAART were not excluded.

RISK REDUCTION

Lifestyle Changes

Reducing your risk of acquiring any other disease or infection is important even if you only have HCV infection, but it is especially important if you are already coinfected. There are things you can do to reduce your risk of additional coinfections. You can practice safe sex. If you cannot stop using IV drugs, you can adopt scrupulously clean injection habits. You can avoid reusing or sharing needles.

People who are coinfected and drink alcohol are at a greatly increased risk of developing severe liver disease, cirrhosis, and/or liver cancer. If you are infected with HCV, but especially if you are coinfected, you should not drink *any* alcohol. If you have difficulty abstaining from alcohol, consider that you might be addicted to alcohol. It would be in your best interest to seek treatment and/or attend group meetings such as Alcoholics Anonymous.

Vaccination

Acute infection with other forms of viral hepatitis is highly dangerous for people coinfected If you are exposed to hepatitis A virus, you can be treated with *immune globulin* for temporary immunity for up to three months. However, you must get the immune globulin as soon as possible, but no later than two weeks following exposure to the virus.

Hepatitis *vaccinations* are generally recommended for those at risk of becoming infected and for children. These vaccines are available free of charge or at low cost at public health clinics in the United States and many other countries.

COINFECTION UPDATE FROM THE XIV INTERNATIONAL AIDS CONFERENCE BARCELONA, SPAIN 2002

It was reported that the most significant hepatitis coinfection issues are the same in all countries. The priority issues are:

- making testing for HCV and HBV readily available
- reducing disease spread of viral hepatitis through education about transmission, and
- preventing disease progression through education about lifestyle changes, and
- making treatment decisions about when to treat for each virus

In areas where HAART and/or hepatitis treatments are not readily available, the priority for western medical treatment lands at the bottom of the list of priorities.

The range of topics reported on in oral and poster sessions included:

- epidemiology of HIV, HBV, and HCV
- risk factors including IV drug use, sexual transmission, and vertical (mother-to-infant) transmission
- prevention of infection
- progression of liver disease in those with coinfection
- risk of fibrosis in coinfection
- harmful side effects of antiretroviral treatment in people coinfected with HCV
- hepatotoxicity with the use of HAART, and
- integrating hepatitis C into HIV/AIDS programs.

Some of the key issues that dominated the coinfection reports at this conference are discussed below.

• More rapid progression to liver fibrosis and cirrhosis in HIV/HCV coinfected patients

New reports added to previous knowledge with results from large studies from Spain[34], the United States[35], the United Kingdom[36], and Germany.[37] Each study confirmed earlier indications that there is more rapid progression to fibrosis and cirrhosis in those coinfected with HCV and HIV than in those infected with HCV alone. There were also indications from some of the studies that the more rapid progression to fibrosis was in those with higher HCV viral loads and lower CD4 (T-helper cell) counts.

• Increased sexual transmission of HIV and HBV, but not HCV in non-injecting drug users

New IDUs (injection drug users) are at substantial risk of sexually transmitted HIV. In particular, female IDUs and new IDUs who share syringes are more likely to engage in unprotected sex, and to have high-risk sex networks. Especially among new female IDUs, sex risk and syringe sharing both need to be targeted to prevent HIV, HBV, and HCV transmission among new IDUs.[38] NIUs (non-injecting drug users) who engage in unsafe sex and have high-risk sex networks are at risk of becoming infected with HBV and HIV. However, HCV seroconversion was not associated with sex risk.[39]

- **Pharmaceutical treatments for hepatitis have moderate effects**

There was little new information about coinfection treatment. Combination therapy with pegylated *interferon* plus ribavirin has about the same range of efficacy in HIV/HCV coinfected people as in those with HCV alone.

- **Pharmaceutical treatments for HIV may increase HCV emergence and liver toxicity in coinfected people**

Abstracts from several countries including Cote d'Ivoire[40], Italy[41], Canada[42], and Australia[43] suggested HIV positive people might suffer increased liver toxicity and HCV emergence from HIV antiretroviral medications.

- **Harm reduction strategies reduce transmission and need to be used more widely**

Reports from Thailand, Argentina[44], the United States, Canada[45], Romania, Pakistan[46], Indonesia[47], China, Brazil[48], Spain[49], and France indicated both the success of and need for harm reduction strategies to prevent transmission of HIV, HBV, and HCV. These strategies included needle exchange programs, encouraging drug users to switch to non-injection drug practices, and use of condoms. One interesting report stated U.S. military personnel who have become HIV positive since 1994 have an extremely low rate of HCV coinfection compared to other HIV infected populations. Researchers attributed the low rate of HIV infection among soldiers to be due to the 'no drug use' policy in the U.S. military that requires soldiers to undergo periodic, random drug screenings.[50] On a different note, there was also a call for the United States prison system, the second largest in the world, to adopt harm reduction strategies such as needle exchange, methadone maintenance, and condom and dental dam distribution to prevent the growing epidemic of HIV, HCV, and HBV within prisons.[51]

- **Barriers to treatment for coinfection must be overcome for treatment availability and success**

Several studies showed that mental health and psychiatric problems were prevalent among people with coinfection. However, there was a relative lack of treatment for both HIV and HCV in these populations.[52, 53] Current drug addiction was also found to be a treatment barrier.[54, 55] Pilot programs showed that it is important to review treatment options on a case-by-case basis rather than not offering treatment based on mental illness or current drug addiction.[56]

Conference Summary

The International AIDS Conference 2002 confirmed much of what health care providers and researchers have previously theorized about hepatitis/HIV coinfection. New studies are helping us better understand risk factors, epidemiology, harm reduction, and the serious consequences of coinfection.

We can draw the following conclusions from the conference.

- Coinfection with HCV and HIV is a growing problem. People coinfected with viral hepatitis and HIV are at increased risk for rapid disease progression, especially advanced liver disease.
- HIV drug therapy may increase emergence of HCV when given to people with coinfection.
- Risk reduction is especially important for people with either hepatitis and/or HIV infection to avoid coinfection. Harm reduction strategies need to be more widely implemented to reduce disease transmission and severity.
- Health care providers need to improve and create more inclusive treatment for coinfected patients who also have psychiatric illness and/or addiction.

UPDATE FROM THE HEPATITIS C CONSENSUS DEVELOPMENT CONFERENCE NATIONAL INSTITUTES OF HEALTH, 2002

HIV/HCV Coinfection and the NIH Consensus Statement

Given the severity of liver disease experienced by people coinfected with HIV and HCV, and the high mortality rate associated with coinfection, it was disappointing to have reconfirmed during this conference that we still have very little knowledge about coinfection. In the 38-page Preliminary Draft Consensus document, there were only thirteen references to HIV. The main section of the document that related to HCV/HIV coinfection reads as follows.

HIV Coinfection: All HIV infected persons should be screened for HCV. Patients with chronic hepatitis C and concurrent HIV infection may have an accelerated course of HCV disease. Therefore, although there are no HCV therapies specifically approved for patients coinfected with HIV, these patients should be considered for treatment. Thus far, studies have enrolled only patients with stable HIV infection and well-compensated liver disease. In coinfected persons, an SVR[1] can be achieved with HCV treatment. Preliminary data suggest better responses to pegylated interferon with ribavirin than to standard interferon with ribavirin. Although treatment of HCV has not jeopardized control of the HIV infection, additional data are needed.

SVR = Sustained Viral Response

To view the complete Preliminary Draft Consensus Statement on Hepatitis C, go to: http://consensus.nih.gov/cons/116/116cdc_intro.htm.

SUMMARY

Up to 40% of all HIV positive people are also chronically infected with HCV. People coinfected with HCV and HIV are at increased risk for rapid disease progression, especially advanced liver disease and its complications.

Risk reduction is especially important for people with HCV/HIV coinfection. Vaccination against hepatitis A virus and HBV is particularly important. Making lifestyle choices such as practicing safe sex, using clean needles, and abstaining from alcohol can enhance health and improve quality of life.

HCV/HIV COINFECTION

Section 2:

WESTERN TREATMENT OPTIONS

Misha Cohen, OMD, LAc

INTRODUCTION

Treatment decisions are particularly challenging for those who are coinfected with the *human immunodeficiency virus (HIV)* and the hepatitis C virus (HCV). It must be decided whether to treat both infections simultaneously or to treat them individually. The repercussions of treating both diseases simultaneously must be taken into consideration. If the infections are treated individually, it must be decided which infection to treat first. For people infected with both HCV and HIV, the benefits of therapy for *hepatitis C* have not been demonstrated conclusively.

The concerns about treating both infections at the same time center on the risk of *hepatotoxicity*, and possible interactions between *ribavirin* and certain *nucleoside reverse transcriptase inhibitor* (NRTI) *antivirals*. The interactions between *interferon-based therapy* for hepatitis C and other HIV antiviral drugs (*nucleoside* analogs, non-nucleoside reverse transcriptase inhibitors, and *protease inhibitors*) are not yet known.

For a person coinfected with HCV and HIV, western treatment for hepatitis C is often begun before antiviral treatment for HIV. However, treatment for HIV is sometimes stopped so that treatment for hepatitis C can be given. This approach has two advantages. It addresses the immediate threat of rapidly progressive liver disease, and it may restore liver health. A liver that has been partially or completely restored to normal function is better able to process the antiviral drugs when HIV treatment is initiated or resumed.

On the other hand, some doctors advocate treating HIV infection first. Although this allows HCV *viral loads* to rise, doctors who use this approach believe there is sufficient time in the progression of hepatitis C to tend to the liver disease after HIV viral loads have been reduced. For the person faced with this dilemma, the choices are challenging. If you are dealing with coinfection, it is very important to consult with all the health care providers involved in your care.

There has been little research on the use of western treatment in people coinfected with HCV and HIV. A small observational study followed the course of 20 coinfected patients simultaneously treated with highly active antiretroviral therapy (HAART) for HIV and interferon-based therapy for *chronic hepatitis* C. The study showed that treatment of HCV *genotype* 1 is difficult, as it is in people with HCV alone.[1] In the United States and Europe, HCV genotype 1 occurs more often in coinfected people than in those infected with only HCV. It appears people who are coinfected and have HCV genotype 1b are at increased risk for liver damage compared to those who have another HCV genotype.[2]

One large study called APRICOT began in 2000 and is ongoing.[3] The study is examining the potential benefits of adding interferon plus ribavirin therapy for HCV to HAART for HIV in coinfected people. This study will assess the risks and benefits of treating both viruses at once. However, it will be several years before the results of this study are known.

SIDE EFFECTS OF HAART AND HCV THERAPY

At the 2002 International Conference on AIDS in Barcelona, researchers reported several cases of lactic acidosis that occurred as a complication of nucleoside analog therapy among coinfected people undergoing interferon therapy.[4] This rare but serious condition is related to mitochondrial *toxicity*. *Symptoms* include *fatigue*, shortness of breath, weakness, and numbness. Researchers from the APRICOT study reported that out of more than 750 patients, eight developed lactic acidosis.[5] Study participants are coinfected and are being treated for both infections simultaneously. HCV treatment is *pegylated interferon* or standard interferon, plus ribavirin. Most of the people who developed lactic acidosis had been on stable HIV therapy including d4T or ddI. Lactic acidosis developed when ribavirin was added to the treatment regimen. One person died during treatment. Although the rates of lactic acidosis in this study were not significantly higher than rates seen in people taking d4T or ddI without concurrent HCV therapy, there remains a concern that ribavirin could heighten the risk of mitochondrial toxicity.

One of the most concerning side effects of HAART is increased blood *lipid* levels, which can lead to heart disease. Interestingly, a study of HCV/HIV coinfected people taking HAART found they were significantly less likely to have high cholesterol levels than those with HIV alone who were taking HAART.[6] In this study, coinfection was associated with lower levels of both total cholesterol and low-density *lipoprotein* (the fat most closely associated with cardiovascular disease risk). Researchers have suggested this finding may be due to the way HCV binds to lipoproteins.[7]

HAART improves *immune system* function. However, it apparently does not help fight HCV. A recent study found HCV viral loads did not decrease after 12 or more months on HAART.[8] It seems increased numbers of *CD4 cells* are not associated with an increased ability to fight HCV infection. However, another study found HAART leads to improved survival in coinfected patients just as it does with HIV alone.[9]

Liver Transplantation

Until recently, HIV infection has been considered a *contraindication* to liver transplant based on the poor *prognosis* of those infected. However, since the introduction of HAART, the prognosis for HIV infected people has improved significantly. Although the numbers are still relatively low, coinfected people are now undergoing liver transplantation. Researchers are currently studying the long-term outcome of this treatment in people coinfected with HIV and HCV.

Issues Associated with Western Treatment for HCV

There are a number of side effects associated with the various western drug therapies for HCV. These include flu-like syndromes, headache, fatigue, fever, loss of appetite, nausea, vomiting, hair loss, and *depression*. Low white blood cell and *platelet* counts are also possible due to bone marrow suppression. Ribavirin may cause sudden, severe *anemia*. It can also cause birth defects. Ribavirin is currently unavailable for use in pregnant women because of this risk.

Interferon plus ribavirin therapy is currently the recommended western biomedical treatment for most people with chronic hepatitis C. If you are interested in western treatment for coinfection, you should talk with your western doctor about your eligibility for treatment.

SUMMARY

Western treatment for HCV is available to people who are coinfected with HIV. However, the effectiveness of this treatment is still being studied. *Clinical trials* are currently underway to determine the effectiveness of using multiple western medications to treat HCV/HIV coinfection. Western treatment for HCV may be appropriate for some people. However, for many, choosing no western treatment remains a viable option.[10]

HCV/HIV COINFECTION

Section 3:

ALTERNATIVE EASTERN TREATMENT OPTIONS

Misha Cohen, OMD, LAc

TRADITIONAL CHINESE MEDICINE FOR HCV/HIV COINFECTION

Many people with hepatitis C virus (HCV) and/or the *human immunodeficiency virus (HIV)* are turning to traditional Chinese medicine (TCM) for treatment. TCM has a rich history in the treatment of *chronic hepatitis. Hepatitis B* and *C* infections are prevalent throughout China, accounting for the increased risk of *hepatocellular carcinoma* in the Chinese population. The Chinese medical system has been dedicated to solving these problems for many years. The Chinese are working to eliminate sources of hepatitis, and to develop treatments for chronic viral hepatitis using both TCM and western medicine.

At the International Symposium on Viral Hepatitis and AIDS held in Beijing, China in April 1991, more than 100 papers on viral hepatitis were presented. Several of these papers documented the positive results of studies involving Chinese herbal medicine. Studies on the use of herbal antivirals, and blood cooling and circulating herbs for liver damage repair were presented. These studies corroborated hundreds of years of treatment experience with Chinese herbs for the symptoms of hepatitis.[1, 2, 3]

A 1995 literature review revealed there are at least 55 herbal formulas that can be used to treat hepatitis. Some recent herbal studies from China and Australia showed positive results in hepatitis C using herbal formulas similar to those widely used in the United States.[5, 6, 7]

In the United States, TCM is a popular *complementary and alternative medicine (CAM)* therapy among patients with chronic liver disease. Anecdotal reports from one of the largest western medicine *hepatology* practices in San Francisco suggest that at least 20-30% of patients report use of TCM herbs for hepatitis.[8] The rate of use of TCM therapies by HIV positive people is believed to be around 40%.[9] The actual use of TCM may be underestimated because patients often choose not to divulge the use of CAM therapies to their western health care providers.

TCM uses nutrition, acupuncture, heat therapies (such as moxibustion), exercise, massage, meditation, and herbal medicine to treat people infected with HCV. *Protocols* have been developed that have successfully helped people infected with HIV and HCV decrease *symptoms*, normalize or lower *liver enzymes*, and slow the progression of liver disease. A 1995 pilot study conducted among people coinfected with HIV and viral hepatitis (B and C) at San Francisco's Quan Yin Healing Arts Center indicated acupuncture alone may have an effect in lowering and/or normalizing liver enzymes.[10]

Chinese Medicine Philosophy

The primary goal of TCM is to create wholeness and harmony within a person thereby allowing the mind, body, and spirit to heal themselves.

Chinese philosophy states there are two opposing principles of life, *yin* and *yang*. Imbalances between *yin* and *yang* within a person can manifest as illness because the body is considered a microcosm of the world.

TCM defines the physiological components of illness using the concepts of *qi* (vital energy), *xue* (blood), *jin-ye* (body fluids), *jing* (essence), *shen* (spirit), and organ systems. Organ systems are domains within the body that govern particular body tissues, emotional states, and activities.

TCM theory states the key to health is the internal ability of the body to remain strong. According to this theory, people are born with a certain amount of original *qi* (pronounced "chee"). The *qi* is easily depleted as energy is used by the body and not replaced. It is not easy to increase the original *qi*. A person must work hard during life just to retain it. Exercise such as tai chi and *qi gong*, healthy eating, and good sleeping habits are highly recommended for maintaining the original *qi*. If a person consistently lacks sleep, does not have a healthy diet, abuses drugs or alcohol, and/or has excessive or unsafe sex, he or she becomes *qi* deficient. When weakened and *qi* deficient, a person is more susceptible to infection by harmful external elements.

Traditional Chinese Medicine Diagnoses for HCV/HIV

According to TCM literature, people in China have experienced the various syndromes associated with both HIV and HCV infection for over 2000 years. This is because TCM diagnoses are based on symptoms, not on detection of *antibodies* to a specific virus. TCM treatments for these syndromes have been used over the past millennia and are generally considered safe and effective for all patients. However, TCM recognizes that each person has a unique constitution and pattern of disease that exists in conjunction with the age-old syndromes. TCM contends that the best form of treatment is to modify, alter, or supplement the base therapies to create an individualized treatment that meets each patient's unique characteristics and needs.

Chinese medical theory states that HIV and viral hepatitis are not singular diseases, but are combinations of *stages* and syndromes. The diagnosis and staging of HIV and HCV are accomplished using tongue diagnosis, pulse diagnosis, and questioning to determine if the patient's initial western diagnosis is consistent with TCM theory.

According to TCM, the initial organ systems affected by HIV are the spleen and stomach, although all organ systems are involved. The spleen and stomach organ systems influence digestion and appetite, the lymph system, and muscle mass.

In both HIV and HCV infections, toxic heat enters the body. Manifestations of an invasion of heat include feelings of warmth, sweating, agitation, hot sensations, and itching skin. Examination may reveal a fast pulse and a red tongue. Small red spots on the tongue are a likely finding in nearly all cases of chronic infection. A review of over 5,000 tongue slides from HIV infected subjects on a Chinese herbal treatment protocol revealed that small red spots were present in nearly every person, ranging from very obvious to barely noticeable.

The organ systems primarily disturbed in hepatitis are the liver and spleen organ systems. These disturbed organ systems affect digestion and energy. According to TCM, acute viral hepatitis is generally associated with excess damp heat or damp cold conditions. While a few people acutely infected with HCV may have or notice symptoms, this is rare. The TCM stage at which one is diagnosed with hepatitis C is usually either the chronic stage of *qi* stagnation, or the stage of *qi* and *yin* deficiency. Advanced chronic disease includes development of the patterns of *xue* stagnation and *xue* deficiency. All HCV infection is associated with toxic heat or the *li qi* (the pestilence/epidemic factor).

Traditional Chinese Medicine Therapy for HCV/HIV

In western medicine, extremely harmful external elements include severe bacterial or viral infections such as HIV and HCV. However, those terms are inappropriate in TCM. Instead, it is said Chinese medicine,

> "…recognizes the existence of Pestilences called *li qi* or *yi qi*. These are diseases that are not caused by the climatic factors of Heat, Cold, Wind, Dampness, or Summer Heat dryness, but by external infectious agents … that are severely *toxic* because they strike directly at the interior of the body." [11]

In the case of HIV and/or HCV, the particular pestilence is identified as toxic heat. Toxic heat is considered by TCM to be both an epidemic factor (something that is seen in a number of patients) and its own individual, treatable syndrome. However, HIV and HCV are not identical invasions of toxic heat. They are each characterized by a different set of syndromes, both involving toxic heat.

The various modalities of TCM therapy include diet, massage, heat therapies, exercise, meditation, and acupuncture. Heat therapies include the use of moxibustion. Moxibustion is the burning of the herb mugwort over certain areas of the body to stimulate or warm these areas. Exercise therapy ranges from martial arts to more subtle forms of movement such as tai chi and qi gong. Acupuncture is perhaps the most well-known form of TCM in the United States. It is the art of inserting fine, sterile, metal filiform needles into acupuncture points on the body in order to control the flow of energy. Acupuncture therapy can include electrostimulation and/or hand stimulation. This form of therapy is most appreciated for its ability to relieve pain. However, acupuncture is also able to help change body energy patterns, which promotes the body's ability to heal itself of organic syndromes and symptoms. In these treatments, TCM often does not distinguish energetic effects from physiologic effects.

The different modalities of TCM have different aims. Some focus on balancing the body's energy, while others focus on building the physical body and adding substances to both balance and change the body materially. For example, the Enhance® herbal preparation that is widely used in HIV and HCV contains herbs to tonify the spleen *qi*, and build *xue*. *Qi* tonification increases the amount of energy in the body that is available for certain functions. *Qi* tonic herbs often have the specific effect of increasing digestion and food absorption. This increases the quality of the blood (*xue*).

Acupuncture is associated with balancing the body's energy levels, while herbal substances are more like drugs or foods in that they have specific organic effects. Breathing exercises are known to strengthen *qi*. One meaning of the Chinese word *qi* is air. By learning how to breathe correctly, more oxygen becomes available to enter the bloodstream.

Specific Chinese therapies are discussed below.

Chinese Herbal Medicine

TCM treatment for HCV/HIV coinfection depends on the stage of the disease and the syndromes involved. Herbal medications in conjunction with rest and dietary recommendations can treat the symptoms of *acute hepatitis* fairly rapidly. Chronic hepatitis C is more difficult to treat. Research and experience both from China and from TCM clinics in the United States suggest that a one-year course of TCM therapy is the minimum needed to alter the progression of hepatitis C. In our clinics, TCM therapy for chronic hepatitis C usually includes combinations of herbal preparations, which are often specifically designed for the disturbed organ system patterns. For example, the combination of Enhance® and Clear Heat® herbal formulas were developed for the treatment of HIV and other chronic viral disease. These formulas were tested in an herbal study at San Francisco General Hospital. Hepatoplex One®, Hepatoplex Two®, and other herbal formulas have been designed specifically for the treatment of chronic hepatitis and related problems.

A few Chinese medicine practitioners in the U.S. have developed specific treatments for HCV and HIV infections. Two such practitioners are Dr. Subhuti Dharmananda of Portland, Oregon and Dr. Qing-Cai Zhang of New York, New York. (See *Chapter 12: Modern and Traditional Chinese Medicine* for additional information on Dr. Zhang's protocol.) My own experience treating people with HIV and/or HCV led me to develop the following herbal formulas. These formulas can be recommended and prescribed by licensed TCM practitioners who have been trained through the Quan Yin Healing Arts Center's Hepatitis C Professional Training Program.

For acute hepatitis C:
    Coptis Purge Fire®
    Clear Heat®
    Hepatoplex One®
    Ecliptex®

For chronic hepatitis C, choose from:
    Hepatoplex One®
    Hepatoplex Two®
    Ecliptex®

For immune disorders, choose from:
    Cordyseng®
    Enhance®
    Tremella American Ginseng®

For toxic heat related to chronic viral inflammation:
    Clear Heat®

Other recommended herbal formulas:
    Licorice 25®
    Ginger Tabs®
    Milk Thistle 80®

Hepatoplex One® is given for acute and chronic hepatitis symptoms. It may be used when liver enzymes are elevated. It can be used with Clear Heat® to increase the Clear Heat® toxin effect. It is designed to regulate the *qi*, vitalize *xue*, clear heat, and clean *toxin*.

While there are herbs to help protect the digestion in Hepatoplex One®, this formula should usually be used in conjunction with formulas that protect the spleen and stomach, as there are a number of herbs that are cooling or cold and vitalize *xue*. For example, to increase the effects of tonifying *qi* and *yin*, this formula can be taken with Cordyseng®. If there is spleen dampness and deficiency with loose stools, add Shen Ling®. If there is liver invading spleen, a common scenario in chronic hepatitis patients, you may add Shu Gan®.

To protect the *yin* in liver disease and specifically in chronic hepatitis, you may use Ecliptex®. For immunodeficiency disorders, you may add Enhance® or Tremella American Ginseng®.

For *xue* stagnation including liver *fibrosis, cirrhosis*, and decreased blood circulation, add Hepatoplex Two®.

For *qi* stagnation with *xue* deficiency, add Woman's Balance®.

For *xue* deficiency and *xue* stagnation, or to protect the bone marrow during interferon/ribavirin treatment, *chemotherapy,* or radiation, add Marrow Plus®.

In chronic hepatitis, you may also add the individual formulations Licorice 25® and olive leaf extracts.

For digestive problems, you may add Ginger Tabs® or Quiet Digestion®.

Milk Thistle 80® is used for all forms of liver inflammation and chronic hepatitis.

For gallstones or gallbladder inflammation, add GB6®.

Hepatoplex Two® is designed to vitalize *xue*. When used in chronic hepatitis, it should be used in conjunction with other herbal formulas. Its special uses are for liver fibrosis and cirrhosis, and to decrease an enlarged liver. It may also have an effect on splenomegaly. As Hepatoplex Two® is a formula designed to vitalize *xue*, it should increase circulation of the blood and improve *microcirculation* in the capillaries.

Cordyseng® is used as an adjunct to other herbal formulas to increase the function of *qi* tonification and increase energy. The formula tonifies both *yin* and *yang*. It primarily strengthens the spleen, stomach, kidney, and lung, and helps digestion. It is especially good for the chronic *fatigue* found in chronic hepatitis and AIDS.

An example of how these herbal formulations are combined is presented below.

> A person presents with HIV and hepatitis C with stage III fibrosis, grade II *inflammation*. The patient is fatigued. The tongue and pulse configuration match the Chinese diagnoses of toxic heat, *qi* and *xue* stagnation, and possible *qi* and *xue* deficiency. The recommended herbal *protocol* for this patient would be:
> - Cordyseng® or Enhance®
> - Hepatoplex One®, and
> - Hepatoplex Two®.

Acupuncture

TCM uses acupuncture extensively in the treatment of chronic hepatitis. Though some of the herbal theories already discussed may apply to acupuncture, the primary goal of acupuncture treatment is to readjust the body's *qi* in order to enable the body to heal itself. Therefore, acupuncture treatment can be used to treat both specific symptoms, and a general epidemic pattern. After a TCM diagnosis is given for a patient infected with HIV and HCV, an acupuncture treatment plan is developed by considering the epidemic nature of the disease, the individual presenting complaints, and any underlying constitutional TCM patterns of illness. On a symptomatic level, acupuncture treatments for HIV and HCV infections address digestive functions, appetite, energy level, stress, anxiety, depression, pain associated with organic illness, and skin complications. Acupuncture has also been used to lower elevated liver enzymes as part of a chronic hepatitis protocol using special acupuncture points.

Moxibustion

An important part of TCM treatment in HCV/HIV coinfection is the use of moxibustion. Moxibustion is the burning of the herb mugwort (called moxa in Chinese) over certain points or areas of the body. Moxa is rolled into a cigar-like stick or used loose over protected skin to create warmth and tonification. In Chinese studies, moxa has been shown to increase digestive function, white blood cell and *platelet* counts, and may have an effect on the transformation of *T-cells* (one type of immune cell). Moxibustion is often used for pain syndromes and areas that appear or feel cold on the body. It is often prescribed for home use in treating both HIV and HCV infections.

Qi Gong

Qi gong meditation and exercise is a common practice in China. It is growing in popularity in the United States among people who have HIV and other life-threatening illnesses such as cancer. There are many studies from China, Japan, Germany, and the United States that show the positive effects of qi gong on immune function. Quan Yin Healing Arts Center and many other locations around the United States offer medical qi gong classes specifically designed for people infected with HIV and HCV.

Dietary Therapy

A healthy diet is considered a key part of maintaining original *qi* and harmony in the body. Most TCM practitioners recommend that their HIV infected clients eat a cooked, warm diet. Other recommendations are based on the specific organ pattern diagnosis. For example, those suffering from chronic diarrhea may be advised to eat white rice (not brown rice) daily, especially in the form of an easy to make rice porridge called *congee* or *jook*.

COMBINING EASTERN AND WESTERN THERAPIES

If you decide to use a combination of eastern and western therapies, you must discuss all of your treatment approaches with both your eastern and western practitioners. The use of some herbal therapies in conjunction with *interferon therapy* may be inappropriate. However, Chinese medicine can be highly effective for the management of side effects from drug therapy. TCM may also be used as an alternative to western drug therapy in some cases.

A list of herbs and drugs that are considered liver toxic can be found in *Appendix VII: HCV/HIV Coinfection*.

SUMMARY

Many people with HIV and HCV coinfection are turning to TCM for primary treatment, or to complement other forms of treatment. TCM uses a number of therapies for the treatment of coinfection such as acupuncture, moxibustion, Chinese herbs, qi gong exercise, and dietary therapy. While these therapies have not undergone clinical trials in the west, many of these therapies have been used for centuries in China for hepatitis and other conditions. Modern Chinese research on herbs and other modalities is used in the development of current Chinese medicine treatments for HCV/HIV coinfection.

It is important to discuss all treatment approaches with both your eastern and western practitioners in order to ensure the safety of and to gain the greatest benefit from all of your treatment modalities.

For recommended reading on traditional Chinese medicine, please see the *Resource Directory*.

HCV/HIV COINFECTION

Section 4:

NATUROPATHIC TREATMENT OPTIONS

Lyn Patrick, ND

INTRODUCTION

This section is a discussion of the naturopathic treatment options available for people who are coinfected with the hepatitis C virus (HCV) and the *human immunodeficiency virus (HIV)*. See *Chapter 13: Naturopathic Medicine* for more information about the naturopathic approach to treating viral *hepatitis*. See *Chapter 14: Nutritional Supplementation* for additional details on the *nutritional supplements* mentioned in this section.

ANTIOXIDANTS

An important similarity between *chronic hepatitis C* and HIV/AIDS is that both infections appear to progress more rapidly in situations of increased *oxidative stress*. Oxidative stress refers to state in which there is an overabundance of molecules called *free radicals*. Free radicals can damage cells and are involved in the processes of *inflammation* and scarring. Increased oxidative stress is evidenced by low levels of the active form of *glutathione* in the *lymphocytes* and blood of people who have HIV and/or HCV. Lack of glutathione can lead to immune suppression, decline of *immune system* function, and an increase in HIV *replication*.[1] While glutathione levels are low in those infected with HCV or HIV alone, they are lowest in those who are coinfected.[2]

Glutathione is produced by the liver. Low levels of glutathione are associated with more active liver disease on *liver biopsy*, and increased levels of the *liver enzyme ALT*.[2] Researchers have suggested that low glutathione is a factor in resistance to treatment that is seen with both *interferon treatment* for HCV and *antiviral* therapy for HIV.

Several studies have been done in both HCV and HIV to look at the role of *antioxidants* in raising glutathione levels. These studies show the use of antioxidants such as N-acetyl cysteine and vitamin C has a positive effect on glutathione levels in the blood and white blood cells of those infected with HIV. Antioxidants have also been shown to significantly lower HIV *viral load*.[3]

N-Acetyl Cysteine

Not all studies of N-acetyl cysteine (NAC) in HIV/AIDS and chronic hepatitis C have shown significant effects. However, the studies that showed no effect were small and lasted only a few weeks. In the major studies that showed NAC has a glutathione elevating effect in people with HIV, this effect was seen only after eight weeks of therapy.[4] A small study found HCV positive, HIV negative patients who were given 600 mg of NAC three times a day for four weeks experienced a normalization of ALT levels. These normalized ALT levels may relate to increased glutathione levels.[5] There are several drugs called cysteine pro-drugs that are currently in *clinical trials*. These drugs increase glutathione levels in people who are HIV infected. They may be useful in coinfection, but we need more information about them before that determination can be made.[6] NAC has been shown to be safe in doses of 1,500-2,000 mg per day. Researchers in this field suggest this dose is sufficient to affect glutathione levels in people who are HIV infected (personal communication, Lenore Herzenberg, Stanford University).

Alpha-Lipoic Acid

Alpha-lipoic acid (ALA) is an antioxidant that exists in small quantities in the food we eat. It has been shown to increase glutathione levels in those with HIV when given at doses of 450 mg per day. This dosage is considered moderate and has been shown to be safe. This dosage was also effective at significantly raising the level of *CD4 cells* (a type of immune cell) after 14 days in the same study patients.[7]

ALA has positive antioxidant effects in mitochondrial *toxicity*, a common problem in coinfected people. In addition, ALA has been shown to prevent damage that results from free radical production in both the nervous system and the liver.[8] Oxidation or production of free radicals occurs in the white blood cells and liver of coinfected persons. This can lead to neuropathy (nerve damage) and liver damage. Although there have been no large scale studies on the effects of ALA in coinfected individuals, it has been proven to be safe at dosages of up to1,200 mg daily in those who are HIV positive.[9]

ALA may be useful in decreasing the risk of kidney stones, a side effect of the *protease inhibitor* indinavir, an antiviral drug used to treat HIV infection.[10]

SAMe

S-adenosylmethionine (SAMe) is a *protein* made in the liver. It is also available as a nutritional supplement. SAMe has been found to be an effective treatment for certain types of *depression*. SAMe is also used to treat liver disease. SAMe has been shown to be effective in raising glutathione levels in the liver cells of those with *cirrhosis,* and in the nervous systems of HIV positive patients.[11, 12] Dosages of 1,200 mg daily raised liver glutathione levels in people with liver diseases. This dose has been used in other conditions, and has been shown to be safe and free of side effects.

Vitamin E

Vitamin E deficiency is common in HIV infection.[13, 14] While vitamin E has not been shown to raise glutathione levels, it does play an important role as an antioxidant in coinfection. Increased intake may be related to slower HIV disease progression. A study of HIV positive men who were followed for over six years showed a decreased risk of disease progression to AIDS in those who took vitamin E.[15]

At a moderate dose of 200-400 IU per day, vitamin E has also been shown to protect against the bone marrow toxicity that is a well-established side effect of the HIV drug zidovudine (AZT).[16, 17]

As an antioxidant, vitamin E has been shown to protect cell membranes from *lipid* peroxidation, a specific type of free radical damage. This is one of the reasons why vitamin E is particularly helpful in preventing liver damage. As explained in *Chapter 14: Nutritional Supplementation*, vitamin E has been found to interrupt the biochemical pathways that lead to liver *fibrosis*. However, this does **not** mean that vitamin E can completely stop the damage caused by HCV, or that it is okay to continue drinking alcohol if you take vitamin E. The research *does* indicate that vitamin E is protective against liver fibrosis and plays a role in preventing the free radical activity that can lead to HIV replication. Vitamin E is nontoxic in doses up to 2,000 IU per day, unless there are blood clotting problems. In this case, vitamin E should only be used with guidance from a doctor. The most beneficial forms of vitamin E are d-alpha tocopherol, d-alpha tocopherol succinate, and mixed tocopherols.

Selenium

Selenium is probably one of the most important nutrients for people who are HIV positive. One research study of HIV infected people showed that those with the lowest levels of selenium had a 10-fold greater risk of dying from the disease than those with normal levels of selenium. This risk was independent of the CD4 count at the time of the study (often an important marker of HIV prognosis), the use of antiviral treatment, and the levels of other important nutrients.[18] Studies have found that selenium levels in people with coinfection are even lower than in those with HIV only, even in people without *symptoms*.[19] Selenium has been shown to raise blood levels of the active form of glutathione in people who are HIV positive.[20]

Clinical trials involving HIV/AIDS patients have shown that taking 400 mcg of selenium per day resulted in significant increases in blood selenium levels, improved appetite, better digestion, and fewer recurrent infections.[21]

AMINO ACIDS

L-glutamine

L-glutamine is an *amino acid* found in large quantities in muscle, intestine, and immune cells. L-glutamine and the amino acid cysteine are both required for the body to make glutathione.

L-glutamine is particularly important in people with HIV. L-glutamine is one of the nutrients the body loses because of HIV infection. This loss is compounded by the body's demand for additional L-glutamine resulting from the rapid turnover of immune cells and the stress of infections (including coinfection with HCV and other viruses). This added demand usually results in an L-glutamine deficiency. Glutamine deficiency appears to be one of the causes of wasting (weight loss and muscle loss) that occurs in people with AIDS.[22]

L-glutamine is a main source of fuel for the cells in the intestines. An L-glutamine deficiency can lead to problems absorbing nutrients from the intestine. About 20% of people with AIDS have abnormal intestinal absorption. This problem has been treated successfully with L-glutamine.[23] Giving supplemental L-glutamine to people with HIV-related wasting has been shown to be beneficial in regaining lost muscle and lean body mass (body weight that is not fat). In one study, the daily doses of L-glutamine supplementation ranged from 8-40 grams. The patients who gained the most lean body mass took daily doses of 40 grams per day (divided into four equal doses of 10 grams) for a period of 12 weeks.[23, 24, 25] See *Chapter 14: Nutritional Supplementation* for more information.

L-Carnitine

L-carnitine is an amino acid that is particularly important for muscle and immune cells. L-carnitine appears to be another nutrient that can become deficient in certain groups of HIV infected individuals. One study found carnitine deficiencies in 72% of a group of AIDS patients on AZT.[26] HIV positive patients are at risk for L-carnitine deficiency as a result of malabsorption, kidney problems, specific antibiotic and antiviral medications, and lipoatrophy (weight loss that is mostly fat tissue).[27, 28]

There are preliminary studies that show chronic hepatitis C patients have a deficiency of acylcarnitine, a specific form of L-carnitine.[29] It is not fully understood why this deficiency occurs, but we know that HCV damages the mitochondria (the powerhouses of cells) of the liver. We also know that mitochondrial function uses acylcarnitine. Therefore, by causing mitochondrial damage, HCV may cause a need for more L-carnitine in people with chronic hepatitis C. More studies are needed to clarify this issue.

Studies in HIV patients have shown that L-carnitine has a positive effect on the immune system, normalizes high *triglycerides* (blood fats), reduces muscle wasting that results from taking AZT, and improves symptoms of neuropathy (nerve damage) that result from taking any of the NRTI class of antiviral medications.[30, 31, 32, 33, 34] Carnitine and acetyl-L-carnitine (a specific form used to treat mitochondrial toxicity) are used in Europe to treat the peripheral neuropathy that often occurs in HIV patients as a side effect of some antiviral drugs. Dosages of 3-6 grams per day of L-carnitine are used to treat elevated blood fats and muscle wasting in people with HIV. Carnitine is available both as a prescription drug and over-the-counter as a nutritional supplement.

SUMMARY

The biological effects of HIV and HCV on antioxidants in the body make it necessary to restore these nutrients with nutritional supplements. Research has shown that taking N-acetyl cysteine, alpha lipoic acid, SAMe, vitamin E, selenium, L-glutamine, and L-carnitine is safe when the appropriate doses are used. These supplements can also be used safely in combination with western therapies and/or traditional Chinese medicine. A health care provider who is trained in *clinical* nutrition and the treatment of coinfection should be consulted for optimal benefit from an antioxidant *protocol*. It is important to discuss your nutritional supplementation with all of your health care providers to make sure your protocol is safe and effective.

Chapter Nineteen

MY JOURNEY, MY CHOICES

Randy Dietrich

INTRODUCTION

This is the story of my journey with *hepatitis C*, and of my choices. My motivation for sharing my story with you is to try to help both you and myself. When I was first diagnosed with hepatitis C, I wanted to know about the experiences of other people with hepatitis C. I thought that hearing about others' experiences would help me make my own decisions. I still believe that. But there was very little information available. I am sharing my story with you as one man's contribution toward trying to help us **all** find our way in this journey. I am a true believer in the power of teamwork, and in the motto of the Hepatitis C Caring Ambassador Program, "Working together, we can make far more significant advances than could be achieved by anyone working alone." We are all in this together. Just as hearing others' experiences motivates me, it is my sincere hope that sharing my story will help motivate you, too.

As you read my story, it is important to understand that everything I have decided to do or not do reflects what I believe is right for me. Based on your own personal circumstances and your intuition, you must decide what is right for you. I want to stress that the most definitive medical test to determine disease progression is a *liver biopsy*, but the results are not always conclusive. I have had two liver biopsies, one at the time of my diagnosis and another two and a half years later. Unfortunately, there was no conclusive information from my second biopsy to determine whether my liver disease has progressed or not.

I should mention that I do not know how I got the hepatitis C virus. And since I do not know how I got the virus, I also do not know when I got the virus. This makes it very difficult to determine the progression of my liver damage. For the most part, I am symptom free. I occasionally experience tightness or slight pains in the liver area. On rare occasions, I have night sweats and indigestion. Fortunately, I was diagnosed prior to developing any significant *symptoms*.

One important question you need to ask yourself before you decide on any given treatment or treatments for your hepatitis C is, "What are my goals?" Is it important to you to clear the virus, or are you comfortable living with the virus so long as you are able to feel healthy and well? These can be difficult questions to answer, but it will be important as you make your decisions about various treatments. My treatment goals are:

1.   to have good health for as long as possible, and
2.   to get rid of the hepatitis C virus.

For me, it is important that I do not sacrifice the first goal in order to achieve the second goal. Ideally, I hope to one day achieve <u>both</u> goals.

If clearing the virus is important to you, I want to share with you the fact that I have done a lot of research about various treatments for hepatitis C. Although I have heard anecdotal stories about people who have cleared the virus without *interferon-based therapy*, I have never seen any proof. If you or someone you know has cleared the hepatitis C virus without interferon-based therapy, I, personally, would very much like to hear from you! However, to date, the only therapy I am aware of that has been proven to clear the virus in some patients is interferon-based therapy. But, I encourage you to do your own research, too.

Based on my experience with hepatitis C, my advice to you as you go through your journey is:

- Get as much information as possible.
- Talk to and use the services of as many health care professionals as possible, from as many different disciplines as possible.
- Use your support network; develop one if you need to.
- Make choices that work best for you.
- Focus on your overall health, not just on hepatitis C.
- Make the best of your hepatitis C situation. Enjoy and learn from your journey.

THE BEGINNING OF MY JOURNEY: MY DIAGNOSIS

My story began in January of 1999 when I had a routine physical. Because my blood tests showed high liver enzymes (*ALT* 88, *AST* 82), a hepatitis check was done. The test came back positive for hepatitis C. My doctor had me come in for more specific blood tests. He also told me it would be a good idea if I did not drink alcohol while we waited for the results of the new tests. He said if the results were positive, then we would talk about what they meant. I did not think much of it. I assumed hepatitis was a short-term problem. I did not stop drinking alcohol, though I did reduce the amount I drank.

In the meantime, my mother was having a heart valve replaced. My sister and I traveled to Cleveland to be with her and help her make decisions. While we were waiting for my mother to come out of recovery after the surgery, my sister and I went to the hospital library and got on the Internet to do some research on hepatitis C.

I was in shock! I could not believe my eyes! Every article I pulled up talked about how more people were going to die from hepatitis C than from AIDS, and that it was the leading cause of liver transplants, and how nobody was talking about this silent epidemic. There were numerous articles about treatment for hepatitis C and how terrible the side effects were. The successes were very limited. I could not find any articles that said there was a cure, but many that said there was not a cure. My sister and I were stunned. We just could not believe that an energetic 42-year-old man who was feeling good could be suffering from a deadly disease. We printed a number of the articles so we could take them back to our hotel rooms to read.

The next morning, from my hotel room, I called my doctor's office. They read me the results. Not only was I positive for hepatitis C, but I also had a *viral load* of 799,000. I was alone in my hotel room when I got the news. I just sat on the bed and cried. Questions were running wildly through my head. How much time did I have? What were my odds of beating this thing? How had I contracted it?

I was about to be named president of my company, Republic Financial Corporation. I thought to myself, not now! I did not need this in my life, especially not now when I was getting ready to take on a new job. One of my favorite sayings that I have learned on my journey is, "How do you make God laugh? Tell him your plans!" This was definitely not in my plans.

After about 20 minutes of crying, I got up off the bed, and the thought hit me: So what? You thought your whole life was going to be easy? Did you really think you were never going to have to deal with any major problems? I had always encouraged others with serious health challenges to become experts on their disease, and to fight it. I had given out copies of Bernie Siegel's book <u>Love, Medicine and Miracles</u>, to friends who were fighting cancer. It quickly became apparent to me that I had 'talked the talk,' but now I was going to have to 'walk the walk.'

My sister came to my room, and we cried together for a while. Then we started to pore through the articles we had printed looking for names of people I could call. My first phone call was to Hep C Connection, a national organization for people affected by hepatitis C. I spoke to a very helpful gentleman there. As we spoke, I quickly realized that many others were in the same situation as me. I was walked through a series of questions that helped me begin to understand my disease. I learned some basic information such as the meaning of viral load, and that my level was not necessarily high. I learned my *ALT* and *AST* levels were above normal, but not off the chart. Still, I did not have a very good understanding about what this disease might mean to me. What was my prognosis? How fast or slow would the liver damage occur? Was I likely to need a liver transplant?

One of the scariest thoughts for me at that point was whether I had infected my wife or any of my three children. Everyone was tested immediately and thankfully, all the tests were negative.

Following my mother's successful surgery, I returned home. After we put the kids to bed, I sat down with my wife and told her about my diagnosis. I explained the limited information I had gathered. We cried together, and then vowed that we would fight this together, although we had no idea how to go about doing that.

My wife and I were leaving in two days for a 12-day trip to Australia. I wanted to take this opportunity to learn more about hepatitis C, so I called Hep C Connection to get recommendations about useful reading material. I purchased five books on hepatitis C, and got more articles off the Internet. I had plenty of reading for my trip! I read every book and article I took with me. After a while, I started to get a better picture of the disease.

It seemed that for most people, hepatitis C is not a death sentence! Simple terms that used to send fear through me were now starting to make sense. For example, I learned the term *"chronic hepatitis C"* simply meant the virus persists in the liver. It did not necessarily mean that I would have all the symptoms of the disease, that my liver would become cirrhotic, or that I would need a liver transplant. Based on my understanding of the material, it quickly became clear that alcohol was definitely out, and I should avoid fried foods, coffee, red meat, and many of my other favorite foods.

On my way home from Australia, I drew a diagram similar to the one on the following page:

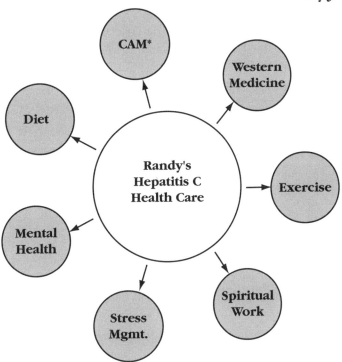

*Complementary and Alternative Medicine

I looked at the diagram and played a little game. I would cover up one of the circles on the diagram and ask myself, "Can I ignore this aspect of my health care?" Playing this game, I realized each category of care was important to maintaining my health. It became obvious to me that I needed to investigate <u>all</u> the various disciplines to figure out what I needed to do.

After the initial shock of my diagnosis wore off, I met with the then president of my company, Jim Possehl. We had a lengthy discussion. I told Jim about my liver biopsy and that the doctor had recommended I begin interferon-based therapy immediately. He asked me what I was going to do. I told him I thought I needed to do some research before making that decision, a <u>lot</u> of research. We discussed the possibility of having my secretary help me with the research. Then we talked about perhaps hiring a medical secretary to assist me in this task. We even considered hiring a medical doctor to help me investigate my options. But as we talked, we both realized that any one person we could hire would be biased by his or her own training and experience. Together, we concluded that a team approach was needed.

At my company, Republic Financial Corporation, we make decisions by bringing together in the same room all of the different business disciplines such as sales, legal, operations, financial, and management. Each discipline challenges the others. We call this process, "teamstorming." We believe the people representing the different disciplines have different experiences and insights into any given problem. If we all challenge each other to be creative enough to come up with a solution that works for <u>all </u>of the different points of view, then it is probably a better decision than any single individual would have come up with on his or her own.

As in business, there is a wide variety of health care disciplines. However, in medicine, it is often very difficult to get people from the various health care disciplines into the same room, let alone for them to seek and agree on a common solution. Part of the problem is that many of the individuals in a particular medical discipline have little or no knowledge about what the other disciplines do. This lack of knowledge can lead to an uninformed prejudice that other disciplines have little medical value.

At the end of our discussion, Jim and I agreed that I would postpone becoming the new president of the company until I had a better feel for what this disease meant to me, and what my long-term prospects were. We also agreed that I would take a three to five month sabbatical from the company so that I could assemble a team of health care professionals to brainstorm possible common solutions for people affected by chronic hepatitis C. I took the next four and a half months off.

This was the founding of the Hepatitis C Caring Ambassadors Program started by my company and me. For myself, I wanted to be able to participate in a teamstorming session in which representatives from each of the various medical disciplines would present his or her ideas of how I should either clear the virus or live with it. I wanted to see all of their theories tested against and challenged by health care professionals from other disciplines. I believe decisions become much easier when a person has information. I wanted as much information as possible before deciding what my own treatment choices would be.

My sabbatical was to last however long it would take to get the Hepatitis C Caring Ambassadors organization started, and for me to come up with a good plan for how to approach my own hepatitis C infection.

MY EXPERIENCES WITH VARIOUS TREATMENTS FOR HEPATITIS C

I want to share with you my experiences with various treatments for hepatitis C that I have encountered along my journey. Of course, these are my experiences and yours may be different. I share these experiences with you in the hope that by openly sharing my experiences, I may be able to help others who are still considering various treatment options For each treatment discipline, I will tell you about both what I liked and what I did not like about my experiences. Personal anecdotes of specific experiences I have had with the various health care disciplines are offset in italics.

Before I begin to tell you about my experiences, I would like to tell you about my belief in what I call "the 95/5 rule." According to this rule, 95% of people are good people who do their very best to live life in a positive way. The remaining 5% are the people who do not do that. Often times, although the vast majority of people are good, we find ourselves spending inordinate amounts of time thinking and talking about the actions of those few people who are not making an honest effort. I believe this same rule applies to health care professionals, too. The vast majority of people in the healing professions are caring people who work very hard trying to do their best for their patients. Only a small minority fall short of this level of commitment. Although, there are great differences of opinion about how best to help people with hepatitis C (based on an individual's training and background), in my experience, the vast majority of health care practitioners are genuinely trying to do their best to alleviate the suffering associated with chronic hepatitis C. To the extent that I have had negative experiences, I ask that you view these as one man's experiences. My experiences should not be misinterpreted to be representative of the potential contributions of any given health care discipline.

Western Medicine (Allopathic Medicine)

What I Liked

Western medicine has been and continues to be a very important part of my treatment choices. First, it was through western medicine that I was initially diagnosed with hepatitis C. I consider having the diagnosis to be the most important information a person with hepatitis C can receive. Had I not been diagnosed, I would still be drinking alcohol. As stated earlier in this manual, stopping drinking is the one of the most important things you can do for your hepatitis C.

In addition to providing my initial diagnosis, western medicine has also given me information about the damage the hepatitis C virus (HCV) has caused in my liver. My first liver biopsy done shortly after my diagnosis pointed out to me not only how much damage my liver had sustained, but also helped me understand how much time I had to try different treatment options.

I also use western medicine for monthly blood tests to determine my *liver enzyme* levels and my viral load. In my opinion, western medicine does the best job of gathering data regarding disease progression, how a person is affected by the disease, the length of time between various stages, etc. All of this information was and continues to be very important to me as I make decisions regarding my treatment.

I would like to share with you my ALT, AST, and viral load test results over time. I am sharing this information because people do not generally share their medical data. I hope that by sharing my medical information, other people will feel less afraid to do the same.

The tests shown in the graphs below were performed at different laboratories. It is important to be aware of the fact that each testing laboratory has its own range of normal values for each test. A laboratory's normal value range means that the majority of people in good health tested by that laboratory have values within this range. Another fact to be aware of is that a laboratory may periodically change their normal ranges. Therefore, in order to know whether your test results are normal or abnormal, you have to know the testing laboratory's normal ranges for those tests at the time you were tested. I have found it is easiest for me to get a copy of the laboratory report. These reports have the normal ranges listed for each test, making it easier to interpret the test results.

The ALT and AST graphs below show how far above or below the upper limit of the normal range each test result was. This means the blue and red bars above zero represent test results that were higher than the upper limit of the normal range. The higher the bar, the further out of the normal range that test result was. The green bars below zero represent test results that were in the normal range.

The viral load graphs shows actual test results since there is no normal range for HCV in the blood. Any detectable virus is abnormal. There are two graphs because two different testing methods were used.

ALT: Number of Units Above or Below
the Upper Limit of Normal

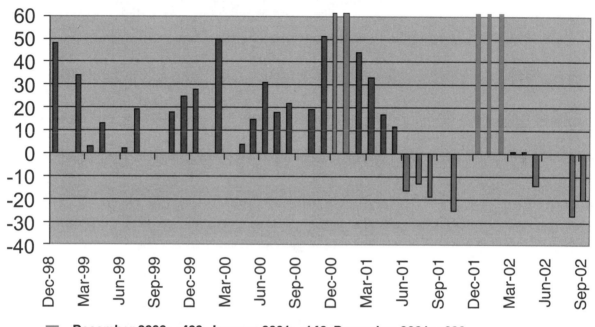

December 2000: +486, January 2001: +146, December 2001: +629
January 2002: +169, February 2002: +89

AST: Units Above Upper Limit of Normal

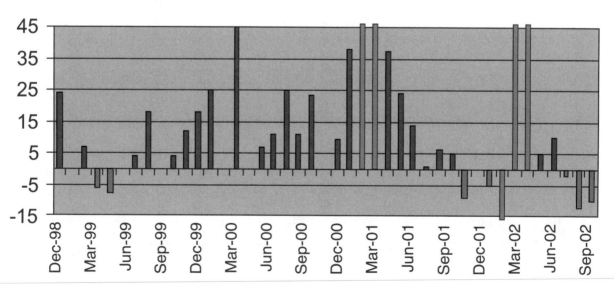

December 2000: +332, January 2001: +96, December 2001: +563
January 2002: +100, February 2002: +65

Hepatitis C Viral Load by PCR:
March '98 - October '01

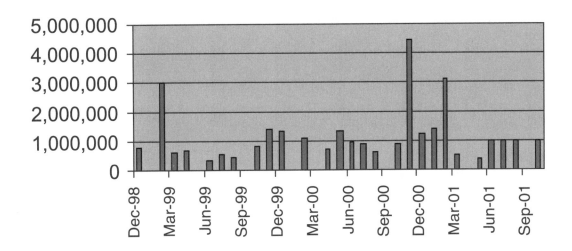

Hepatitis C Viral Load by Heptimax:
December '01 - September '02

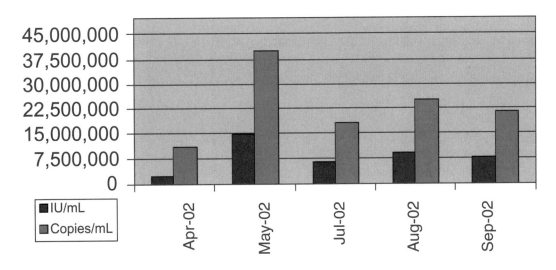

IMPORTANT NOTE: Viral load testing performed using different testing methods give different results. Notice how much higher the viral loads are once my laboratory changed from a PCR test to their own high sensitivity test called the Hepitamax™. At first, I was very worried, but after discussing it with my doctor, I realized that the difference was the testing method, not something happening with my hepatitis C. For more information about viral load testng, see *Chapter 5: Laboratory Tests and Procedures.*

My treatment approach is an integrated approach, and my primary care doctor is an allopathic doctor (an MD) who practices integrated medicine. He has not only been very supportive of my treatment choices, but actively works with me to find alternative treatment options. He is open to alternative treatment options and dedicated to determining the effectiveness of various treatments. We are interested in determining the effect of various treatments on: 1) reducing and/or eliminating liver *inflammation*, and 2) clearing the virus. We agree that in the end, we want treatments that will not only make me feel better, but that can also be **shown** to be effective through improvements in my test results. I have chosen a treatment approach that integrates western, Chinese, homeopathic, and naturopathic medicine and various forms of bodywork, all of which are supported and encouraged by my primary care doctor.

What I Didn't Like

I get my ALT, AST, and viral load levels tested every month. Unfortunately, I have come to find out these tests do not mean much. The ALT and AST levels are indicators of liver cell damage, but do not tell you anything about liver cell repair or replacement. As such, these tests do not tell me if my liver is getting better or worse. My viral load levels have varied from 295,000 to 3,030,000 with most of the measurements being in the 500,000 to 1,500,000 range. It took me a long time to understand that these differences in viral load are fairly insignificant.

My first liver biopsy was done shortly after I was diagnosed. I recently had another biopsy, two and a half years after the first one. I had great hopes that the second biopsy would be able to tell me definitively if my liver disease had improved or gotten worse since my diagnosis. Unfortunately, I did not get the definitive answer I was seeking.

Three different doctors looked at my liver biopsy slides to look for any changes. One said there was slightly more *fibrosis*, while a second determined the level of fibrosis was unchanged. A third pathologist felt it could not be determined if the fibrosis was worse because of sampling errors. All three did agree that there was less inflammation present in the second biopsy. I was very disappointed that there was no clear consensus on the status of my disease. When speaking with one of the doctors about my frustration over this lack of consensus, he told me, "It's just not that good of a test. It is not that definitive." Although a liver biopsy is the best test we currently have to determine what is happening in the liver, it is **not** the definitive test everyone wishes it could be. One of the major projects of our brainstorming team is to figure out better noninvasive techniques to determine what is going on in the liver. The key to doing this will likely be through western medicine, though insights into how new technology might be used may come from non-western medical practitioners.

Ironically, it was because of the information I obtained through western medical tests that I have decided not to use any of the western medicine treatment alternatives at this point. I reasoned that if my first liver biopsy showed that I had Stage II (out of IV) fibrosis while I was drinking 10-12 glasses of wine or beer per week, I could slow the progression of the disease considerably if I stopped drinking altogether. And, if that was the case, I probably had plenty of time to review my options. It is my opinion that, if you have a strong *immune system*, quit drinking alcohol, and are willing to significantly adjust your diet, progression of liver disease can be significantly slowed. Of course, I do not know this to be true, but it makes sense to me based on all of the data and statistics I have reviewed.

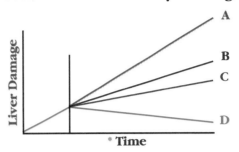

Natural Progression of Hepatitis C in an Individual Patient

Progression of Hepatitis C in a Patient Who Made Lifestyle Changes

*Diagnosed and began lifestyle changes including no alcohol, dietary changes, CAM therapies, stress management, et cetera

As I try to figure out where I am in terms of my disease, I consider the following two graphs.

If I had not been fortunate enough to find out I have hepatitis C, I would be moving somewhere along the line on the graph on the left. But since I was fortunate enough to be diagnosed, I have made a number of lifestyle changes in an effort to slow the progression of the disease as seen in the graph on the right. The only problem is, I do not know how my lifestyle changes have shifted my personal disease progression. Logically, it seems unlikely that I am on line A. But whether I am now on line B, C, or D, no one knows. I had hoped when I had my second liver biopsy that I would finally have enough information to be able to figure out what line I am on now. But since the results were inconclusive, I still do not know. What I do know is that my fibrosis is somewhere between stage II and III, and the inflammation in my liver seems to have decreased. The fact that I do not know how long I have had the virus makes it even harder to try to figure out where I am at in terms of my disease progression.

In short, I do not know whether what I am doing to treat my hepatitis C is helping or not. It is possible that many of the decisions I have made will turn out to be a waste of time and money. Some could actually end up damaging my health. I ask you to read this with the understanding that I have no proof that anything I have done has improved my chronic hepatitis C. On the other hand, I have no proof that anything I have done has made my condition worse either. And with the many lifestyle changes I have made, I feel better and healthier than I have ever felt in my adult life. Further, what is right for me could be totally wrong for you or someone else.

When considering *interferon-based treatment*, I could not get comfortable with the side effects it seemed to produce in so many people. Further, I have found no *clinical* data on the complications and the long-term effects of these treatments. However, in my discussions with people along the way, I have heard a number of anecdotal stories from people who have had other illnesses come up once they started interferon therapy. With no clinical studies, it is impossible to know whether interferon therapy had anything to do with the sudden onset of these illnesses.

For now, I have chosen to hold off on interferon-based therapy. This may be a mistake, but the decision is very clear to me at this time. I have a number of reasons for making my decision. First, my disease appears to be stable at this point, so I feel I have time. By this I mean that I feel no urgent need to begin a therapy about which I am uncertain. Further, interferon-based therapies are rapidly improving. The success rates of clearing the virus are going up; the length of treatment for non-responders is shortening. With these rapid advances, if I ever do decide to take this form of treatment, I will probably receive a much better form of the therapy than I would have gotten had I taken interferon-based treatments when I was first diagnosed in early 1999. In addition, since I have never taken interferon-based treatment, I remain a good candidate for any future therapies that may be developed. This notion has been confirmed by several doctors specializing in HIV and AIDS who have told me they support my decision. I believe this is because many HIV and AIDS patients who took the earlier treatments have experienced viral mutations making current treatments ineffective or less effective than they are in treatment naïve patients. With the power of western medical research and rapid technological advances, I am excited about the future prospects for new and/or improved options.

I have had some negative experiences with western medicine. The first was with the specialist my doctor referred me to following my diagnosis. As I stated earlier, I was leaving for a long trip in two days. I placed a number of calls to the specialist just to discuss my diagnosis and what it meant. I talked to his assistant numerous times, but could not seem to get through to the doctor.

Finally, I got the assistant to agree to have the doctor call me on my cell phone in 15 minutes. There was a mix-up, and instead of calling me on my cell phone, the doctor called my house and spoke with my wife. All he said was that he would see me when I got back from my trip, and not to worry. I now know that this was not bad advice, but at the time, it was devastating not to be able to talk to someone knowledgeable about hepatitis C, what it meant for me, and what my next steps would be.

Even after I returned from my trip, it took me nearly three weeks to schedule an appointment to see the specialist. Once I did get to see him, he told me that my only real option was to use interferon-based therapy. We discussed other alternatives and diet. He said there might be something to milk thistle, but other than that, nothing else had proven scientific benefit. He told me diet did not matter. I questioned him about this since it was in conflict with everything I had read.

At the conclusion of my visit, the specialist agreed to my request for genotype testing, and suggested that I have a liver biopsy as soon as possible to which I agreed.

When I went in for the blood tests for my biopsy, I found out my genotype test had never been ordered. I explained the error to the doctor's assistant and asked her to order the genotype test since it had not been done previously. She told me she could not do that since the doctor was out of town, and he had not ordered it on my chart. I explained that the doctor wanted me to consider interferon-based therapy and that genotype was an important factor. She told me she had 50 people on the interferon-based therapy and had only ordered this test once before.

Since different genotypes not only determine the length of treatment, but also the odds of success, this was critical information to me. I can only guess as to why the doctor did not order this test for all of his patients. My guess is that since he only considered one type of treatment, the odds of success were not all that relevant.

The liver biopsy was described to me as a "routine" procedure. It would take about 15 minutes, I would then rest for another 15 minutes, be checked, wait around the hospital for a little while, and then have my wife take me home. I was advised pain in my shoulder was a potential side effect, and that I should refrain from strong physical activity for about a week.

The procedure itself went smoothly, and the doctor told me I should rest for about 15 minutes at which time they would check for bleeding. I soon began to have sharp pains over my liver area and they were growing more and more intense. It turns out they had hit an artery and I was bleeding internally. I was sent for a CT scan to determine the extent of my internal bleeding. The doctor told me this was 1 in 1,000 occurrence.

My wife and I spent the night at the hospital. It was not until about four or five in the morning that the pain finally subsided enough for me to sleep. I was taking pain medication, but the biggest relief came when I asked for a bag of ice to reduce the swelling. As an aside, I want to mention that my second biopsy went very smoothly. I experienced only temporary sensitivity over the biopsy area that lasted for about a day.

Following my biopsy, the specialist called me on the phone, told me the results, and stated that he wanted me to start on interferon-based therapy immediately. I told him I was still doing research and that I was not sure what I wanted to do. He immediately responded that it was fine to consider some of my "witchcraft remedies," but he wanted to see me in a month, and he wanted to see my plan. I was horrified. I had mainly talked to him about diet and various supplements and to refer to these treatment options as "witchcraft" seemed very inappropriate.

However, this specialist did a very good thing for me. He made me mad enough that I did schedule an appointment with him in thirty days. At that time, I laid out a very detailed plan of how I intended to find information about various treatment options, and how I intended to treat myself in the interim. For this motivation, I am very grateful.

Complementary and Alternative Medicine (CAM)

Overview

What I Liked

When I was first diagnosed with hepatitis C, I mentally grouped all *complementary and alternative medicine (CAM)* treatments together. Now I understand that each CAM discipline is distinct. After studying CAM treatment options, I drew the following chart.

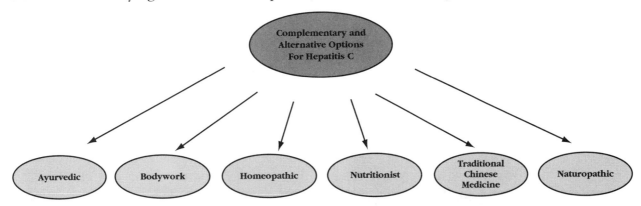

What I like about all of the CAM disciplines is that the underlying goal is to improve my overall health, and that by doing so, I will be better able to live with and fight the virus. I did not know if any of these treatments would be effective against my hepatitis C, but it seemed likely that they could help me feel better and have more energy. It just made common sense to me that, while I was searching for treatment options, doing things that would make me feel better had little downside and lots of upside. The other aspect of each of the CAM disciplines that I appreciated is that they required me to deal with all aspects of my health, not just my disease.

What I Didn't Like

The down side of CAM approaches is that there is little scientific testing or documentation about the effects of the various prescribed treatments. There are few *clinical trials*, and some CAM practitioners do not keep statistics on their patients. This lack of scientific data makes it difficult for many western doctors to believe in or recommend CAM treatments, regardless of how beneficial they may be.

Several times in my search for my treatment options, I would meet a CAM practitioner who had claims of a treatment option with great success, only to have them disappear when I suggested we complete a survey of their patients and medical records to document their success.

Many CAM practitioners judge the effectiveness of a given therapy according to how the person is feeling. Depending on the situation, this may or may not be an accurate way of measuring the progress of the disease. Below is a brief summary of my experiences with my complementary and alternative medicine treatment choices.

Acupuncture

I had always wanted to try acupunture, but never had a reason. My wife had successfully used acupuncture to cure tennis elbow in the past, which told me that there was probably something to it. I had also been fascinated by the fact that the Chinese have a system for body energy channels that map out similarly to anatomical diagrams of the human circulatory system, yet western medicine doesn't acknowledge the Chinese energy system. The Chinese have been practicing acupuncture for thousands of years. But outside of this and the fact that they stuck needles in you, I knew nothing about acupuncture.

I started asking question about whether I should consider acupuncture, and if I did, who should I see. People I spoke with recommended I try acupuncture, and that I should see someone with years of experience which probably meant someone who had received training in China. This lead me to a practitioner at the Chinese School of Medicine in Denver. With the thought that I was going to voluntarily let someone stick needles in my body, I went off to my first treatment.

What I Liked

When I first sat down, the acupunturist asked me a few questions, then felt my pulse. I noticed he wasn't counting. Then he asked me to stick out my tongue and he looked at it. It was clear to me that whatever I was about to experience, acupuncturists used different methods than western doctors to assess a person's health.

I was delightfully surprised. Not only did the treatment **not** hurt, it was extremely relaxing. After the acupuncturist placed needles in various parts of my body, he told me to relax for a while. I fell into a deep sleep, having dreams and images come to my mind. When the treatment was over, I felt as though I'd had a great massage. I decided if acupunture made me this relaxed, it was probably a helpful thing to have as a part of my treatment protocol. I now have monthly accupucture treatments as part of my protocol.

I feel acupuncture treatments effectively help me relax, and are beneficial to my overall health. My recommendation regarding acupuncture treatment for a wide variety of ailments would be, try it and see if you get the results you are seeking.

What I Didn't Like

As with other treatments, I have no western medical tests to prove that acupuncture has been beneficial to my overall health or my chronic hepatitis C.

Ayurvedic Medicine

Ayurvedic medicine originated in India and has been widely publicized in the United States in recent years by Depak Chopra. I had a basic understanding that Ayurvedic medicine involves the mind, body, and spirit, but at the time of my diagnosis, I knew little about how Ayurvedic medicine might be used to treat hepatitis C.

> *Early in my journey of determining my choices, I was attending a National Institutes of Health conference on CAM treatments for liver disease. A gentleman approached me and told me that he had used Ayurvedic medicine as his primary therapy for hepatitis C. He told me that his virus was undetectable for nine months. But after he stopped the treatment, the virus returned. Ayurvedic medicine had my attention! It was also interesting to me that a person with a pitta dosha (which most closely describes my body type) is prone to liver disorders. Pitta doshas are driven individuals.*

What I Liked

I was interested in pursuing Ayurvedic medicine as a possible treatment option for my hepatitis C. I started by trying to find an experienced practitioner who had worked specifically with people who have hepatitis C. I was looking for someone who was available locally so that I would be able to visit on a regular basis. Unfortunately, I was unable to find such a practitioner in the Denver area.

I currently use information from Ayurvedic medicine to help me remind myself that I need to relax and practice moderation. Although I am not specifically using Ayurvedic medicine as one of my treatment options, in general, there seems to be many similarities between an Ayurvedic protocol and my current methods of treatment. Each involves following a restricted diet, working on the mental aspects of the disease, and practicing spiritual activities.

What I Didn't Like

The major drawback to Ayurvedic medicine for me has been the lack of an experienced practitioner in my area. I did meet with an Ayurvedic doctor from India who examined me and walked me through his treatment methods. Unfortunately, he explained that in order to treat me, I would need to be under his care for a few months in India. Given my personal circumstances, going to India for two months is not possible at the present time. Although I have been very impressed with everything I have learned about Ayurvedic medicine, I have not chosen it as a treatment approach because of the limitations I have described. I also have not seen documentation that Ayurvedic medicine results in either decreased liver inflammation or *sustained viral clearance*. This documentation may exist, but I have not seen it.

Body Work

Overview

There are many forms of body work that can help improve the body's immune system and/or reduce stress. I believe the benefits of different forms of body work vary depending on both the practitioner and the individual receiving the treatment. The forms of body work I have chosen to practice are those for which I found experienced practitioners who are also focused on developing themselves as healers. Each one practices some type of spiritual work for their personal benefit. What type of spiritual work they practice is not important to me.

Body work is one of the easiest things to test. Try a particular type of body work. Notice if you feel better, or more relaxed. I will share with you the body work practices I use, but there are many other forms of body work that I have tried or heard about. I would recommend you try different forms of body work to see what is most beneficial for you.

What I Liked

Bowen is a series of manipulations of the soft tissues of the body designed to open up your lymphatic system.

> *Years ago my mother came to Denver to receive Bowen work. My mother was suffereing from Reflex Deficiency Syndrome in both feet. She was walking on crutches, and getting steadily worse. She had been told she would never walk unassisted again. She had tried a number of different treatments before deciding to try Bowen to heal her feet. We will never know for sure what cured my mother, but after two Bowen treatments, she walked across the room. After her third treatment, she was able to walk normally. She was skiing six months later!*

Because of my mother's experience, I tried Bowen work for general health and enjoyed the positive effect on my body. Before being diagnosed with hepatitis C, I received a Bowen treatment every 6-12 months for my general health. After my diagnosis, I decided to make Bowen work a part of my regular treatment protocol. I currently have a Bowen treatment once a month.

I feel better after Bowen treatments. The treatments seem to open up my body and get the energy flowing more freely. The Bowen treatments seem very complementary to my chiropractic and acupuncture treatments as well. I recommend Bowen work to people for a wide variety of ailments.

What I Didn't Like

As with other CAM treatments, I have no medical tests to prove that Bowen treatments have produced any positive benefit. However, my personal experience is that Bowen work has been a beneficial part of my overall treatment protocol.

Chiropractic Medicine

What I Liked

Prior to my hepatitis C diagnosis, I used chiropractic medicine intermittently for occasional back problems. But an experience I had just prior to my diagnosis led to me consider chiropractic therapy as part of my hepatitic C protocol.

> *I hadn't had any back problems for years, so I hadn't been to see my chiropractor for quite some time until just prior to my hepatitis C diagnosis. About one month prior to my diagnosis, my wife mentioned that our chiropractor had moved to a location near our home. I decided I would stop by and get an adjustment.*
>
> *The chiropractor asked me a series of questions about how I was feeling, and told*

me he wanted to see me on a regular basis. He questioned how much water I was drinking and told me that my whole body felt dehydrated. Over the years, I had always been amazed at how he could tell about things going on in my body just by feeling my back. For example, if I drank too much alcohol the night before, he would always make a comment. Or, if work was particularly stressful, he would know.

Despite his past accuracy in diagnosing problem areas for me, I didn't take his comments about my health very seriously. About a week later, my wife came back after a visit to the same chiropractor and told me he was really worried about me, that something was very wrong with my body. Although he didn't know specifically what the problem was, he knew something was wrong. Again, I didn't pay much attention, and did not go back to see him.

When I was diagnosed with hepatitis C three weeks later, he had definitely my attention!

I went to see my chiropractor and we spoke about my hepatitis C treatment options. He told me studies have shown that chiropractic treatments are effective in stimulating the immune system and reducing stress. Because of my belief that anything I can do to help my body fight the virus with my own immune system is a good thing, I decided to add chiropractic treatments to my protocol. I usually have treatments once or twice per week.

Since beginning regular chiropractic treatments, my neck and back adjust much more easily than they did in the past. My posture has also improved. I feel better and attribute a portion of this effect to my chiropractic treatments. When I am particularly stressed, I have immediate relief following an adjustment. If nothing else, I believe this reduction in stress is probably helping my immune system and overall health.

What I Didn't Like

As with other treatments, I have no medical tests to prove that chiropractic care has improved my overall health or my hepatitis C.

Far Infrared Therapy

Far infrared (FIR) energy is one of the many forms of energy emitted by the sun. Far infrared therapy is based on the principle that FIR energy is deeply absorbed by the body. When FIR is applied to an area of the body, that area is warmed and the water molecules begin to vibrate. The combination of warmth and vibration causes increased circulation and clearing of *toxins*. FIR has been used for several years in Japan and various regions in Asia, but it is available on a very limited basis in the United States.

There are many types of FIR therapy devices including blankets, lamps which shine on large areas of the body, and paddles which focus FIR energy on smaller areas of the body. Because of the limited availability of this form of therapy and its relatively new introduction into the United States, I would caution you that it is extremely important that you find a skilled practitioner if you decide to try this form of therapy.

What I Liked

My western doctor suggested I try FIR therapy to improve my immune system, rectify imbalances, and eliminate toxins. He uses a paddle device to deliver the FIR energy to various parts of my body. Those places where I have imbalances become the warmest when exposed to the FIR energy. Sometimes, these areas become painfully hot.

The addition of FIR therapy is a fairly recent change to my treatment protocol, so it is a bit too early to know with any certainty how this addition will affect my liver health and general health. However, both my doctor and I feel this form of therapy is worth further investigation and research.

At this point, I can tell you that I feel better since I began FIR treatments. I think the treatments have helped me, and I also feel more relaxed.

What I Didn't Like

When the FIR machine is applied to various areas of my body, it can get so hot that it hurts. However, the pain only lasts as long as the machine is on my skin.

As I mentioned, I have no proof that FIR therapy has improved my liver or overall health. However, from my limited experience, I believe FIR therapy has had beneficial effects on my health.

Exercise

What I Liked

Many scientific studies over the years have shown that moderate exercise stimulates the immune system, improves the cardiovascular system, strengthens bones and muscles, reduces stress, and improves sleep.

> *Exercise and athletics have always been part of my life. In high school, I played sports, including running track. In the late 80's, I ran two marathons just to see if I could do it. For the last twenty years, I have run two or three times a week, and played basketball once a week. Physical activity has always been and continues to be an enjoyable part of my life.*

After being diagnosed with hepatitis C, I read that exercise was good for maintaining health in people with hepatitis C. My Chinese medicine doctor advised me to do things in moderation, and to give up running and replace it with walking. I knew from my marathon days that too much exercise depletes the immune system and places a tremendous amount of stress on the entire body. Though I agreed with taking a more moderate approach, I decided not to give up running entirely. I reduced my 3-5 mile runs to 2-3 miles, two to three times per week. I have learned to do yoga for deep breathing and stimulating the immune system. Some mornings, instead of running, I jump on a mini-trampoline. I also practice *qi gong* (see my section on Spirituality). And, happily, I still play basketball once a week!

Since I was diagnosed with hepatitis C, my exercise program is more varied and moderate. My approach to exercise now is primarily as a means to increase my energy and keep it flowing. And of course, I want to have fun, too.

I believe exercise keeps me healthy, full of energy, helps reduce stress, and increases my stamina. Whether it is the exercise or the combination of all of things I am doing for my health, I feel like I am in better shape now than I was five years ago.

What I Didn't Like

Although I have no tests to prove that my exercise program has had any direct effects on my liver health, I am certain exercise plays at least some role in my overall feeling of good health.

Homeopathic Medicine

Like everyone else, from time to time, I have had some unusual experiences in my life. My introduction to homeopathic medicine was one of those unusual experiences. I share the following story with you to help you understand that at least for me, the healing powers of homeopathic treatment have been something more than just mind over matter.

I have been using homeopathic remedies since I was 19 years old. It began when my mother's friend, who had just completed homeopathic medical school, was visiting our family. I had sprained my ankle a month earlier, and it had never quite healed. It often ached when I was inactive, and hurt a bit when I played basketball. After my mother's friend helped her with some problem she was having, I jokingly asked him if he could fix a sprained ankle. To my surprise, he said he could.

He had me lay down on the floor, and he tested my strength while I held different tubes of homeopathic remedies. My arm was stronger with two of the remedies than with any of the others. This was pretty weird to a 19-year-old kid who not only did not believe in any of this stuff, but did not want to believe it either. The doctor gave me two tubes homeopathic remedies. I was laughing while I put the remedies under my tongue. As I was driving back to my house with my friends who had witnessed this whole weird examination, we laughed about the whole experience.

About half an hour later, I started to have a strange sensation in my ankle as if the blood was racing through my ankle faster than through the rest of my body. One of my friends joked, "Hey Randy, is your ankle fixed yet?" I was almost embarrassed to admit the feeling I was having in my ankle.

In a couple of days, my ankle was fine with no further aching or pain. Despite the immediate results, I was still a disbeliever and rationalized that my ankle was probably ready to heal anyway.

About three months later, I tore a ligament in the other ankle. This injury was bad. I was on crutches and the ankle was three times its normal size. The doctors wanted to cast my ankle. But my friends who'd had the same injury and had gone with casts had not experienced full recoveries, so I was hesitant to go that route. I tried icing and heating several times every day. But after three weeks, I was still in intense pain with no sign of improvement.

I called the homeopathic doctor who had treated my previous ankle injury. He asked me to send him a few strands of my hair for analysis, and then he would send me some remedies. The day before I received the remedies, I had an appointment with a western doctor who could not believe my ankle was still swollen after five weeks. He strongly urged me to consider a cast, and I was. But I thought first, I would give the homeopathic doctor a chance to work his "magic."

The next day I received the homeopathic remedies, two substances to ingest and one to rub on my ankle. I could not believe the results! The swelling in my ankle started to go down by the next morning. Within a week, the injured ankle was only slightly larger than the other one. More importantly, I was walking again.

My ankle healed with no significant problems. I still play basketball to this day, and I have no problems with my ankles.

What I Liked

Following these experiences, I was no longer skeptical about homeopathic medicine. My personal experience over the years has been that in some situations, homeopathic medicine does nothing to help a condition, but at other times, it works wonders clearing things immediately or in half the normal time for me.

Regarding homeopathy for the treatment of my hepatitis C, three individuals prescribe homeopathic and similar forms of energetic medicine for me. Both my medical intuitive and my BioScan practitioner have to approve a given remedy before I take it. I take specific remedies until my medical intuitive and BioScan practitioner agree that I no longer need it.

I feel good, and continue to feel healthier over time. But given the various protocols I use, it is difficult to determine whether this is in any way attributable to the homeopathic remedies. In the end, it is just my opinion that homeopathy is benefiting my overall health, and therefore adding to my body's ability to live with and fight the virus.

What I Didn't Like

I have been given many homeopathic supplements that were called, "hepatitis C remedies." These remedies may be helping my body live with the virus. However, taking these remedies has not had any significant effect on my viral load, ALT, or AST levels. As with other CAM treatments, I have no proof that homeopathic treatments are helping me. But it is my opinion that homeopathy does contribute to my overall health.

Naturopathic Medicine

Naturopathic medicine uses the healing power of nature. Naturopaths treat the whole person, trying to support and promote the natural healing powers of the body. Many different therapies are used by naturopaths including such things as herbs, supplements, homeopathic remedies, nutritional therapy, and various forms of body work. Some who are licensed acupuncturists also incorporate acupuncture into their treatment regimens.

Given the lack of testing of CAM products, I had to figure out a way to determine which of the numerous herbs, supplements, and remedies would be right for me. I came up with a two-pronged approach. I decided to consult with two CAM practitioners. One consultant is a naturopathic doctor who is also a medical intuitive. The other practitioner is trained in chiropractic medicine, but devotes most of his practice to a technology called a BioScan. The BioScan instrument is an FDA registered biofeedback device that measures the energy flow through the body's energy channels (acupuncture *meridians*) to identify imbalances. This technology is based on the Chinese medical theory that improper energy flow through the body can lead to imbalances, which if left untreated, can cause disease.

As I came across a product or supplement I was considering, I took it to each practitioner independently to see if he or she recommended the product for me. Every month or two, I took a large bag of supplements to each practitioner. To be honest, in the beginning I was very skeptical. However, over time I found that both practitioners agreed about 90% of the time about which products I did or did not need.

What I Liked

My exposure to naturopathic medicine started shortly after my diagnosis with hepatitis C. Although I could not find any information that naturopathic medicine could cure hepatitis C, I received recommendations from others who have hepatitis C. They told me they felt better after being under the care of a naturopath and taking the various vitamins, supplements, and homeopathic remedies. Based on these recommendations and my basic theory that everything I can do to make my body healthier to either live with or fight the virus is helpful, I decided to give it a try.

The first naturopath I met with took the time to explain naturopathic medicine to me. He asked me a series of questions about my life and my general health. He then prescribed various supplements and had me go through a detoxification diet to clean out my system. He also suggested that I meet with a nutritionist to discuss my diet following the intense detoxification diet. The nutritionist basically agreed with the diet I had already been following (see my Nutrition and Diet section).

Shortly after starting on my naturopathic program, an acquaintance suggested I go to see a naturopathic practitioner who is also a medical intuitive. So with a significant amount of skepticism, I went off to see this woman.

When I got to the office, I was instructed to go in and lay down on the examination table in another room. The practitioner walked into the room and asked me how many bowel movements I have. I had just come off the detoxification diet and was a little constipated. I told her this information, thinking she probably started every visit like this. About half way through the visit, she asked me to write down some things that were making me very angry. I explained that I am a very calm person and did not really have anything to be angry about. This woman, whom I had spoken no more than 15 words to, proceeded to describe my personality very accurately - what I am like, how I think, how I bury my feelings. I felt naked. She definitely had my attention.

The next time I saw this practitioner, my bowel movements had become regular again. When she walked into the room, before I had said anything, she stated, "Well I'm glad we cleaned that problem up."

I was placed on a yeast-free diet to clean up my system. Since that time, I have consulted with this naturopathic doctor regularly.

The protocol that I follow, a combination of diet, herbs, homeopathic remedies, and supplements is generally a naturopathic approach. I continue to use the input of my medical intuitive and my BioScan practitioner to determine what products I need at any given point in time. The supplements I use most frequently are:

Supplement	**Frequency**
Vitamin C	Always*
Bee propolis	Always*
Greens (wheat grass or barley greens)	Always*
Chinese herbs (various)	Most of the time**
Flax seed oil	Most of the time**
Homeopathic remedies	Most of the time**
Multiple vitamin (iron-free)	Most of the time**
Milk thistle	Occasionally
Vitamin E	Occasionally
Thymus	As needed

* See Spirituality section
** Remedies and herbs used varies over time; I rarely take more than one of these supplements at a time

I have always subscribed to the theories that "less is more" and "moderation is the key." I tend to take less of a product than might be recommended because I do not want to put too much into my body if it is not needed. This may be a mistake, but my theory has been that since my diet is so strict, it does not take much of a supplement to balance my system. This theory of mine has been supported by my experience. When my medical intuitive and my BioScan practitioner recommend I take a certain supplement, I have found that I generally need to take only small amounts before the imbalance is corrected and I am taken off the supplement.

To be clear, I am not advocating that you take lesser amounts of the medicines or supplements than your health care providers recommend for you. I am simply trying to point out that more is not always better, especially when it comes to treating liver diseases. Sometimes, out of frustration and/or fear, people with hepatitis C begin taking large amounts of a number of different supplements. Because the liver processes virtually every medicine and supplement we put into our bodies, overloading the body with large amounts of medicines and supplements may end up doing much more harm to the liver than good. I would urge you to check with your health care provider(s) before beginning any new supplement or medicine to determine first if you need the supplement, and if you do, what the appropriate dosage is for you.

Although I have no medical tests to prove that my naturopathic treatment has improved my liver or overall health, I know that I feel better. And from time to time, my naturopath and my BioScan practitioner have independently detected that I have a particular condition. For example, following a trip to Mexico, my liver enzymes suddenly went up to over five times the normal level. Both my naturopath and my BioScan practitioner independently stated that I had picked up a parasite in Mexico. After a short treatment period, both independently concluded that the parasites were gone, and my liver enzymes came back down to their previous levels. I have experienced many similar situations where both CAM practitioners stated I had a certain condition, and after a period of time, they both independently stated that the condition had cleared up. This is hard to correlate with western medicine because we do not have tests that adequately show all the subtle changes that are going on in the body.

What I Didn't Like

I feel it is important to add a note of caution here about some of the many products marketed to people with hepatitis C. I have taken many of these products to my naturopath and my BioScan practitioner. Both agree that many of these products will provide an initial boost of energy, but that the products should not be taken long-term. If taken long-term, many of these products have the potential to eventually begin to start taking energy from the body. This experience of an initial boost of energy followed by a subsequent feeling of decreasing energy is fairly common among people who have taken some of these products.

It is important to remember that manufacturers cannot patent an herb. Frequently, combinations of herbs and other supplements are packaged together to create a product that can be marketed as something unique. I encourage people considering natural products to investigate the products. Try to find out if the products actually do what they claim to do.

Nutrition and Diet

When I was first diagnosed, much of the information I was able to find on the role of diet in the treatment of hepatitis C was contradictory. I was unable to find any scientifically controlled studies that evaluated the role of diet in the treatment of hepatitis C. However, many books and other sources of information stressed the importance of good nutrition in managing hepatitis C.

As I looked to other diseases and how diet affects them, I found that the general trend was toward the consensus that diet *is* important.

After considering the various opinions, I decided that modifying my diet and nutrition was very important because even if it did not help my hepatitis C, I would still be healthier overall. In addition, since the liver is involved in processing everything we eat or drink, it makes sense to me that the less taxing the diet is on the liver, the more energy it will have to stay healthy and regenerate.

A recent study out of Australia showed there is a relationship between body weight and fibrosis among people with chronic hepatitis C. The study found that the more overweight you are, the more likely you are to have *steatosis* or fat deposits in the liver cells. Further, the amount of fat in the liver was related to the amount of fibrosis seen on liver biopsy.[1] This study reinforces the notion that nutrition and weight management are important factors to consider for people with chronic hepatitis C. I am looking forward to more studies on the relationship between diet and hepatitis C disease progression.

What I Liked

There is no doubt that my diet now is much healthier than it was before my diagnosis with hepatitis C. And since in a very literal way, we are what we eat, I believe my new diet has improved my overall health.

About one month after my diagnosis, I met a woman who had recovered from pancreatic cancer seven years earlier. Her doctors had told her she was going to die and had stopped treating her. She started using diet as the major form of treatment for her disease. And today, she is a healthy, active person. No one knows what cured this woman of her pancreatic cancer, but she certainly feels that diet was a major part of her healing process.

My new acquaintance worked in a natural foods store. She spent about two hours walking my wife and me around the store, teaching us about foods and reading labels. She told us about her theories regarding which foods were good for me and which ones to avoid. As we walked around the store, I was horrified. I wanted to keep my "normal" diet; I did not want to change. But we talked further, and I saw this woman's great life energy and realized changing my diet had little downside and lots of upside. About an hour into our two-hour walk around the store, I finally decided. Why not? Many foods are an acquired taste. I realized I could acquire tastes for different kinds of foods that might be healthier for me.

The example I use to help people understand this is milk. When I first changed from whole milk to 2% milk, I did not like the taste. Eventually, I switched to 1% milk, and at first, I did not like that change either. But now if I went back to drinking whole milk, I would hate it. It is far too rich and creamy for me. Our taste buds adjust. Now that I use rice milk instead of cow's milk on my cereal in the morning, I like the taste of rice milk and have adjusted my taste buds such that I wouldn't want to go back to cow's milk.

My current diet is a combination of what my natural foods acquaintance outlined for me with slight modifications based on advice from my naturopath and other health care providers.

My general dietary guidelines are:

- No alcohol
- No sugar
- No fried foods
- No coffee or colas
- No cow's milk or dairy products
- No food with preservatives or chemicals
- No red meat
- No shellfish
- Eat organic products whenever possible

I try to eat things that are as fresh as possible, organically grown, and without chemicals or antibiotics. When you first hear this, you might wonder what you can eat. There are plenty of choices! It is just a matter of getting your taste buds to adjust.

One of the main aspects of my diet is that I juice raw vegetables. Three to five mornings per week, I have a 24-ounce drink of vegetables prepared with a Vitamix™ juicer. The juicer is a modified blender in which the vegetables are ground up with all their pulp into a juice. I use a variety of vegetables, but limit vegetables high in sugar such as carrots. This is my way of eating raw vegetables on a regular basis.

Following are the specifics of my diet since January 1999:

FOODS I EAT

Fish	• Mainly deep water fish such as salmon, tuna, sea bass, and halibut
Poultry	• Chicken and turkey – preferably free-range, not smoked, and without the skin
Dairy Products	• Sheep and goat milk yogurts and cheeses • Rice cheeses
Fresh Vegetables	• Salad greens, carrots, spinach, cucumbers, broccoli, etc. • Juice fresh vegetables every morning, including wheat grass, using a Vitamix® juicer
Starchy Vegetables	• Potatoes, sweet potatoes, yams, pumpkin, acorn and butternut squash
Fresh Fruits (in moderation)	• Citrus fruits, kiwi, melons, apples, pears, peaches
Legumes	• Lentils, split peas, black-eyed peas, pinto beans, lima beans, kidney beans
Rice and grains (limit white flour and wheat products)	• Pasta, couscous, quinoa, millet, kamut, spelt, aramath • Yeast-free breads, rice cakes, Crispini® crackers, tortillas and tortilla chips (baked)
Condiments	• Nuts and nut butters • Honey, maple syrup, apple butter (very limited) • Grape seed oil mayonnaise, organic salsa, guacamole (made without mayonnaise or vinegar) • Bragg's Liquid Amino® (in place of soy sauce or teriyaki) • Flaxseed oil, virgin olive oil • Rice Dream or almond milk for cereal
Beverages	• Eight glasses of bottled water daily (at least 64 ounces) • Unsweetened juices, filtered water • Herbal teas, including milk thistle and dandelion root, ginger, licorice, green and raja's cup

FOODS I DO NOT EAT

Shellfish	• Lobster, shrimp, clams, mussels, etc.
Red Meats	• Beef, veal, and pork
Cow Dairy Products	• Milk, cheeses, margarine, yogurt, cottage cheese, ice cream, etc.
Specific Condiments	• Ketchup, mustard, mayonnaise, soy sauce, Tabasco®, teriyaki, barbecue sauce (except organic made with apple cider vinegar) • Vinegar (except apple cider vinegar) • Pickles
Sweeteners	• Sugar • Artificial sweeteners such as Sweet-N-Low® and NutraSweet®
Specific Beverages	• Alcohol, including all beer, wine, hard liquor or anything fermented • Caffeinated or decaffeinated coffee or soft drinks • Guarana, chai, and other teas with caffeine
Other Food Rules	• No fried foods • No chocolate

I follow my diet fairly strictly because that is what is easiest for me. I have learned over the years that it is easier for me to have lines I do not cross instead of leaving myself gray areas. Some of my health care practitioners have suggested to me that I should feel free to modify my diet from time to time, if I do it in moderation. I agree with them. I strongly believe that anything in excess is potentially harmful, and anything in moderation is probably okay. But it is difficult at times to know what moderation is.

Take alcohol as an example; what is moderation? We know alcohol consumption has a significant effect on the course of hepatitis C. But we do not know the effects of different amounts of alcohol. How much is safe? Is it a sip or maybe a glass of wine? How frequently can one safely drink? The simple truth is, we do not know. Before my diagnosis, I would drink 8-10 glasses of wine or beer per week, and I really enjoyed them. Now, I do not drink **any** alcohol, not even a sip. It is easier for me not to drink at all than to try to maintain my discipline if I open the door a crack. I follow the advice to draw the line and just say no. I believe it is easier if you do not let yourself get started, because once you start, it is hard to figure out where to stop.

For a long time I applied this logic to all areas of my diet. No sugar means no sugar. No cow dairy means no cow dairy, etc. One Chinese medicine practitioner advised me that I should pick one day a week to eat whatever I want. His theory was that since a healthy liver is about flowing with life, I should not be so rigid in my diet. So recently, I have carefully allowed myself to have certain things in very limited amounts.

I have learned to enjoy my diet and make it part of my daily life. I am very fortunate in that my wife is an angel! She makes it so easy to eat well. Every morning she gets up and makes my morning vegetable drink and my lunch. She takes the time to purchase fresh organic vegetables and foods. Without my wife's help, I could never maintain my diet as well as I do.

In his later years, my father often joked, "If I knew I was going to live this long, I would have taken better care of myself." Unfortunately, this is a reality for all of us. The better we take care of ourselves on a daily basis, the less likely we are to have to deal with aches, pains, or more serious ailments as we age. It makes sense to me that what we put into our bodies matters! My recommendation to everyone is to eat as well as you can. If you do, you will probably feel better and be healthier.

What I Didn't Like

People sometime ask me what I miss the most about my previous diet. My reply is simple: it is the convenience. The foods I eat taste fine. But it takes time to prepare the food, and to anticipate my food needs when I am traveling or doing various activities around town. Again, this is where I am very fortunate to have the support of my wife. Her constant care preparing and making foods available make my diet very easy to follow. If I was not so blessed with my wonderful wife, I may have had to make other choices. I am also blessed in that financially I can afford to buy organic foods and high quality fish, chicken, and turkey. I know for many individuals, this is not an option.

I do not know whether my dietary changes will alter the course of my hepatitis C. But I can tell you that I feel healthier and have more energy now than I did when I was eating as I used to.

Spirituality

I have never been a religious man, but I have always believed there is a universal spiritual power. I never spent any real time developing my spiritual side. I had begun to pray just before my diagnosis with hepatitis C, and then, it was only to help someone who was sick. After I was diagnosed with hepatitis C, I found many of the books I read and individual health care practitioners I spoke with talked about developing a spiritual practice.

I made the decision to explore a spiritual practice, but not because I was afraid of dying. Within a month or so of my diagnosis, I understood that I could live with this disease for a long time. So my decision to explore a spiritual practice was borne of a desire to heal. Once I got started, my practice grew and took on a life of its own.

I practice various forms of *qi gong* (a Chinese method of developing one's spirituality). I also practice two forms of yoga, astanga and bikram. Astanga yoga is a rather strenuous form of yoga that is intended to realign and detoxify the physical body. The poses require very focused concentration that bring the mind and body into synch with one another. Bikram yoga is practiced in a heated room to facilitate profuse sweating. The heat is used to bring about deeper stretching, prevent injuries, and reduce stress and tension. Bikram yoga is designed to build strength, flexibility, balance, and mental focus. In addition, I sometimes meditate using either an 'ahh' sound or an 'ohm' sound.

I would recommend any of these activities for anyone looking to improve his/her general health and to develop his/her spirituality. As with other forms of therapy, I recommend that you work with experienced practitioners to gain the greatest benefits from these practices.

What I Liked

Spirituality has opened my eyes to a world I barely acknowledged before. I believe each person has his or her own spiritual journey. I do not think it matters what type of spirituality you practice in your life, as long as it works for you and you feel you are continuing to grow.

I want to share a couple of truly amazing things that have happened to me. To be honest, they are pretty strange. So as I sat down to write these incidents, I hesitated because I realize they may sound quite weird to many of you. The fact is, *I* thought they were very strange when they happened to me. But they did happen to me – a very normal guy, with a very normal job, and a very normal life. In considering whether or not to share my experiences, I realized that in all likelihood, I am not the only person who has had these kinds of strange, even weird, experiences. I am hoping that by sharing my experiences with you, maybe I will help you to understand you are not 'the only one.' And maybe it will help us all understand how much more in tune with life we can be if we pay closer attention to our spirituality.

> *The first experience that really opened my eyes to my spiritual side, and truly shook me up, was a dream. In the dream, someone and I were digging up a man who died of a liver disease. He had been buried in the 1950's. As we reached the part of the grave that held his casket, I noticed there was a piece of paper on top. As I reached for the piece of paper, a ghost came out of the casket, grabbed me by the ankles, carried me across a room, and dumped me on a couch.*
>
> *I turned to the ghost and asked, "Are you mad at me?"*
> *The ghost responded, "No."*
> *"Are you trying to help me?" I asked.*
> *The ghost said, "Yes." Then it said, "Take this."*
> *"What is it?" I asked.*
> *"Bee propolis." the ghost responded.*
>
> *Then I woke up. Immediately I knew this was no ordinary dream. It was so clear and vivid. And I was a little freaked out. I was up in the mountains for the weekend when I had the dream, but I was very curious to research bee propolis on the Internet to see what it was about. I had heard of it, so I knew it existed, but that was about it.*
>
> *When I returned home, I looked up bee propolis on the Internet. The first article explained that bee propolis is a substance bees use to fight off viruses. Now I was really freaked out. But, now I was convinced that this message was not an accident or some kind of weird coincidence.*
>
> *I immediately went to the store and purchased all the different types of bee propolis I could find. I took them to my medical intuitive/naturopath and to my BioScan practitioner. And sure enough, both independently confirmed that I should be taking bee propolis. Other than vitamin C, it is the only substance that is always part of their recommended protocol.*

Ultimately, I think there will be something more to the message than just taking bee propolis, but that part of the journey has yet to become apparent.

So now you ask, "What does this have to do with spirituality?" My answer is that I do not think it is an accident that as I started to practice more spirituality in my life, things like this started happening to me. Many other little things started to happen, too, such as knowing that someone was pregnant or had died without being told. In so many ways, I am much more aware of the world around me.

> *The second significant spiritual event happened during a meditation. Someone told me that if you pray with emotion it has a lot more effect than if you just pray. I was lying on the floor meditating one day when I decided to do it with emotion. Suddenly, my body started shaking all over. Again, I was freaked out. I could stop the shaking by stopping my meditation. But when I started meditating again, the shaking started again.*

> *It was clear to me that this, too, was no accident. I have made this shaking meditation part of my spiritual work. I can now do my shaking meditation by just starting to breathe deeply.*

I believe my spiritual practice is helping me develop into a better person in so many subtle ways. And I also believe that my spiritual practice has improved my health.

What I Didn't Like

I cannot prove that any particular aspects of my health have improved based on my spiritual practice. But I can say that the development of my spiritual practice is the greatest gift I have received from my hepatitis C.

Stress Management and Mental Aspects of the Disease

It is well documented that stress reduces the strength of the immune system. It is my belief that everything I can do to improve my immune system will help me live with and fight HCV. This is an important area of my health care. The two main areas of stress I have to deal with come from my work and from the mental aspects of living with hepatitis C.

I have a very demanding job. I am president of a financial services company, and my business life rarely goes smoothly. On the other hand, I love my job and the company. I really enjoy the challenges of this competitive business. It is a major part of my life and part of what makes me tick. Even when my company gave me five months off to set up the Hepatitis C Caring Ambassadors Program, I still worked very hard. This helped me realize that controlling my work-related stress has much more to do with controlling me than it does with the demands of any particular job.

So how do I balance a demanding job with trying to reduce my stress? Not very well. This is the one area of my health care in which I believe I have done the poorest job. This does not mean I ignore the problem; I am working on it. As time goes on, I am getting better at managing my stress and achieving a sense of balance in my life. I am just not as good at it yet as I would like to be.

My goal is to be able to do both, have a demanding job and be very good at maintaining a balance that allows me to be calm in a stressful environment. I have taken this on as a personal challenge and a great learning experience. I know myself well enough to understand that if I did not have this particular job, I would have another that was equally as challenging. I realize I need to learn to balance my driven personality with learning to be more flowing and balanced.

The other major stressor in my life is dealing with the mental aspects of having hepatitis C. As soon as my doctor said, "You have hepatitis C." I started to be sensitive to every feeling in my body. Every little discomfort or pain I related to having hepatitis C. I realized I not only had the hepatitis C virus to get rid of, but I had a 'mental virus' to get rid of as well.

I have read several books that address the mental aspects of having a disease, and how powerful they can be. One particular book reported that people who thought the terms their doctors used to describe their conditions sounded very serious were more likely to die suddenly in the hospital even though their conditions were relatively harmless. The power of suggestion can be very strong.

The power of suggestion works both ways. The *placebo* effect has been studied extensively. A placebo is a sugar pill that is used in place of a medication to determine if it is the medication or the belief that the medication is helpful that is responsible for any observed improvements. As many as 30% of people with a wide variety of conditions report feeling better when they take placebos. This placebo effect is another example of the power of suggestion.

Having a disease can be used to exert power over others. People often go out of their way to help someone who is ill. Someone with a chronic disease may find that his or her whole life starts revolving around the disease, so that eventually it is hard to relate to that person without also thinking about the disease. This is a very easy trap to fall into.

The challenges for me following my diagnosis were to:

- get rid of the mental virus, and
- not make my life and the people around me dependent on my hepatitis C.

Although these sound simple, they are things that are easy to say, but hard to do.

The areas of our lives that cause us the most stress varies from person to person. I hope in sharing what I have learned about managing my main stressors, you may find some helpful ideas about how to identify and manage your own stressors.

What I Liked

In order to try to manage my stress, I have chosen to make sure I allocate enough time for my spiritual practice, exercise, diet, and visits with my health care providers. I do this by getting up every morning at 6:00 AM, but not getting to work until 9:00 AM. In this way, I take care of myself first before going to work. I may end up working until 7:00 PM, but at least I get myself balanced before I start the day.

I also read a lot of self-help books. Each one has some little lesson about balance, stress management, and being at peace with life that I can apply to my daily life. I believe this is a life-long journey, and I just try to be thankful and appreciate the little steps I have taken. My belief is that someday I will look back and realize I have come a long way.

My approach to dealing with the mental virus has been to try to replace the mental virus with positive thoughts. I search out information about hepatitis C and the real effect it has on people. I also look for success stories from people using all of the various medical disciplines. I have tried to put all these pieces together so that they make sense to me.

What I Didn't Like

I have no proof that my attempts to manage my stress have improved my health, but I believe that my efforts to control the stress in my life have been beneficial. Knowing that stress has a negative impact on the immune system, it make sense that reducing stress can improve immune function which will help me live with and fight the hepatitis C virus.

Traditional Chinese Medicine

Traditional Chinese medicine and/or modern Chinese medicine have been a part of my protocol since I began seeing Chinese medicine doctors in late 1999. I have been examined by three different Chinese medicine practitioners, and have reviewed each of their protocols with my medical intuitive/naturopath and my BioScan practitioner.

What I Liked

Some of the herbs prescribed by Chinese medicine practitioners have been independently confirmed to be important for me to take by my medical intuitive/naturopath and my BioScan practitioner. What particular herbs I need seems to change every 3-4 months. Some of the herbs are prepackaged and some are loose that we boil into a tea. The loose herbs that we boil into a tea are more often picked by my testing methods as more appropriate for me than the processed herbs of the same name.

In talking with others who have tried Chinese medicine to treat their hepatitis C, I have found there are people who have taken Chinese herbs who feel better and have experienced an improvement in their quality of life. This is consistent with the Chinese medicine goal of trying to enhance the body's ability to live with the virus rather than trying to eliminate it. In my experience, there are a number of Chinese herbs that are beneficial in helping the body deal with the virus. I use Chinese herbs from time to time when my medical intuitive/naturopath and my BioScan practitioner agree they are what my body needs.

Chinese medical philosophy states that an imbalance in the liver is associated with anger. I have had many messages that part of my healing process is to deal with anger that I have previously suppressed. Further, I appreciate the Chinese medical model because it deals with all aspects of health. I use acupuncture as a form of body work and qi gong as a form of spiritual practice. My diet is also influenced by Chinese medicine. In short, I use those parts of Chinese medicine that I believe support my healing.

What I Didn't Like

I encountered one Chinese medicine doctor who claimed he had cleared many people of the hepatitis C virus with his protocol. Unfortunately, when we asked to review his medical records and to speak to his patients, we were unable to document that anyone had actually cleared the virus on this practitioner's protocol. This experience points out the importance of doing your own research to try to document the effectiveness of a treatment before beginning a new protocol.

My advice in this area is to find a Chinese medical practitioner who specializes in hepatitis C. Then talk to some of his or her patients to find out if they have experienced the type of benefits you are seeking.

Once again, I do not have any scientific evidence that Chinese medicine is contributing to my liver health or my overall health. But, I believe Chinese medicine has helped me feel better and has improved my general health.

WHAT I'VE LEARNED SO FAR

The Big Picture

The big thing I have learned so far is that hepatitis C is not a death sentence.

Although the natural history of hepatitis C infection is still somewhat unclear, most numbers that I have seen project that after 20 years of chronic infection, approximately 20% of those infected will have *cirrhosis*. After 30 years of chronic infection, the number goes up to about 30%. I look at these numbers and wonder what they mean for an individual with hepatitis C – what do they mean for me? I believe that if you eliminated alcoholics, people with other serious liver conditions, and people with other co-infections, these numbers would go down substantially. This would mean that for an individual who does not have other risk factors, the probability of developing cirrhosis is probably significantly less than the general numbers imply.

I operate with the belief that if people with hepatitis C are willing to make the necessary lifestyle changes and stop drinking alcohol, very few will actually die of their infection. I believe it is possible for the vast majority of people with hepatitis C to die **with** the virus, not **because** of the virus. This is an experience shared by many people with other chronic conditions such as diabetes or high blood pressure. The illness is something that must be dealt with because if it is ignored, it could become very serious. But for the vast majority of people with chronic conditions, their ailment is something manageable. For me, having hepatitis C is something I must manage, but at this point, I do not consider it a threat to my ability to live a long, happy, productive life.

Another related lesson that I have learned along my hepatitis C journey is that there are no concrete answers. Blood tests are an indicator of liver damage and liver function, but they offer little information about disease progression or arrest. Liver biopsies are the best measure we have for disease progression. However, there are factors such as sampling errors and variability in the interpretation of the slides that make this test far from exact. I have had two liver biopsies, one shortly after I was diagnosed and another approximately two years later. I was hoping that a comparison of the two results would give me a definite answer about whether my liver is getting better or worse. But much to my dismay, the results were inconclusive. I was looking for an answer, and did not get one. I now realize there are no concrete answers regarding what exactly is happening with my disease. The closest any of us can get to answers are percentages and probabilities. I can look at the probability that a certain treatment will or will not work for me. But the usefulness of statistics for me as an individual is limited. For an individual, a treatment that aims to get rid of the virus is not 50% effective; it is either 100% effective or 0% effective. A treatment either works or it does not. Since there are no concrete answers for any of us right now, each of us has to learn what we can about our options, make our choices, and wait to see what the outcome will be.

One of my favorite jokes goes like this:

> *A man was caught in a flood. The water was up to his waist when a boat came by. The people in the boat yelled, "Get in." "No," said the man. "I have lived my life as God desires. God will save me. Go help someone else." Soon the water was up to his shoulders and another boat came by. The people in the boat yelled, "Get in." "No." said the man. "I have lived my life as God desires. God will save me. Go help some-*

one else." A while longer, the water was over the man's head, and he could barely keep his head above water when a helicopter came by and dropped down a rope to which the man said, "No, I have lived my life as God desires. God will save me. Go help someone else." A short time later, the man drowned. When he got to heaven, the man was confused and in disbelief, he asked God, "God, I lived my whole life just the way I thought you wanted me to. I had so much faith in you. Why didn't you save me?" To which God replied, "Well, I tried! I sent two boats and a helicopter!"

This is a good analogy of my journey with hepatitis C. I have been sent many boats and helicopters. So many times, I ignored the first boat and the second one. Sometimes, I was stubborn enough that I needed a helicopter to get the message. I have learned to trust the fact that if something is really important for me to do, I will get a lot of messages.

Another big lesson for me in this journey has been to appreciate all the help I get from so many people—all of my health care practitioners, friends, family, even people I just bump into once. I could not begin to list all of the help (the boats and helicopters) I have gotten from so many people.

The health care practitioners I have seen have all been 'boats' for me. Although I may not accept all of their advice, they were all coming from a good place and wanted to help me in their own way. This is a group of people who spend their careers trying to help people feel better and live longer, although each has different methods for trying to achieve the same goal. It would certainly be nice if one of them had 'the answer' for everybody, but unfortunately, that is not the case. That is what makes it tough sometimes, that we each have to decide what choices to make. Each choice has risks and benefits. Each person must decide what is right for him or her.

Western Treatment for Hepatitis C

For me, interferon-based treatments represent two extremes in terms of treatment options. Interferon-based treatments are the best in that they offer the greatest chance for the getting rid of the virus. Yet at the same time, in my mind, they also pose the greatest risk. I wonder about the potential long-term complications of these powerful drugs. Is it possible that this form of treatment can unmask other conditions or lead to the development of long-term complications? At this point, there are no satisfactory answers to these questions. For that reason, I have chosen not to use interferon-based therapy at this time. However, these treatments are improving rapidly. Experience is a great teacher, teaching us what to do and what not to do to make this form of therapy easier and more effective. Further, researchers are learning more every day about viruses and how to effectively treat them. Clearly, the large amounts of money spent on HIV and AIDS research have helped and continue to advance our knowledge about viruses. I fully expect that in two or three years, western therapy for hepatitis C will be significantly better than it is today. Great advances and improvements have already been made; there is every reason to believe the trend will continue.

In summary, I have learned that western medicine is a good treatment option for hepatitis C. Although there are some significant risks associated with current interferon-based therapy, it is an option I believe everyone should consider.

Complementary and Alternative Treatments for Hepatitis C

Based on my experience, I have learned that CAM treatments for hepatitis C are effective at improving overall health, relieving symptoms, and making people feel better. What that means for the long-term prognosis of people with hepatitis C, we do not yet know.

I have yet to find any CAM treatments that show a consistent pattern of significantly reducing liver inflammation and/or viral load. I have also never seen proof of a CAM therapy that resulted in clearing HCV. That is not to say that CAM treatments are not capable of these things. It is possible that we simply have not adequately documented these finding yet. Or, it is possible that, like western treatments, CAM treatments are evolving and have yet to be developed to the level where they can consistently accomplish these things. But as I have noted in my experience with western treatments, significant improvements are also being made with CAM treatments.

One aspect of CAM treatments I have learned about during my hepatitis C journey is that CAM treatments require discipline. With CAM treatments, it is not just about the virus. It is also about changing the conditions that allow the virus to flourish, conditions such as one's general health, diet, exercise, stress, anger, emotions, etc. This is one of the lessons I have had to learn, dealing with all of the personal aspects of this disease rather than just the simple things I would rather deal with. It may be part of my genetic make-up that allows HCV to flourish in my body. But my stress, anger, emotions, and diet also contribute. Though I very much wanted hepatitis C to be something I was a victim of, something I was not responsible for, I have learned over time this is not true. I have accepted responsibility for the things I have done that have allowed this virus to flourish and cause damage in my body. In accepting responsibility, I realized it is within my control to make the necessary changes and adjustments, too. Much as I would like there to be a magic pill without any side effects that would take away my hepatitis C as if it were a common cold, that does not yet exist.

On the positive side, I **do** feel better since I have started taking better care of myself. I feel healthier, I have more energy, and I have the stamina to do things that I could not have done three or four years ago. Even though I have hepatitis C, I have more stamina and energy than most of my friends or business associates my age and younger who do not have a chronic condition. I have found it is not hard, it just requires discipline and a long-term view. I do not think of the changes I have made as short-term changes. The changes I have made are lifestyle changes; this is how I am going to live from now on. There may come a time when I make other choices, but for now, these are my choices. I must admit, I have had to coach myself in order to get comfortable with and feel good about my choices. But the bottom line is that the changes I have made have had a very positive effect on how I feel. Now that I have been following my protocol for a while, I sometimes forget how good I feel. I have to remind myself to be thankful for feeling so good because there are many people without any ailment who don't feel half as good as I do. I am grateful I have the opportunity to take care of myself this way, and that I am able to feel as good as I do.

WHERE I'M GOING FROM HERE

I once asked one of my Chinese medicine practitioners when I would get rid of the hepatitis C virus. He replied, "Have you learned all you need to learn from the virus?" I joked, "I have learned all I **want** to learn from the virus!" Is my role to live with the virus a long time, to get rid of it using western medicine or complementary and alternative medicine, or is my role something I have yet to discover? That is part of the fun and challenge of life – the unknown. I am just trying to take one day at a time and to enjoy my journey.

I have told friends that if I were given a choice of whether or not I would be infected with hepatitis C that I would pick my hepatitis C journey. This may surprise you. But through my journey, I have learned so many lessons, had so many positive experiences I would not have had were it not for this infection. My journey with hepatitis C has taught me so many valuable things about medicine, my overall health, my view of life, and my spiritual development. Because of my infection, I have made many new friends and acquaintances. Of course, I will never know for sure, but I believe I will live a longer and healthier life because I got hepatitis C than I would have if I had not gotten it. But I must also honestly say, even though having hepatitis C has been a gift for me, my goal is still to get rid of the virus without doing significant damage to my body. My goal is not to be known as Randy 'with-hepatitis-C' Dietrich, but just Randy Dietrich.

What are the steps remaining in order for me to get rid of the virus? At this point, I am continuing to look for messages and following the advice that makes the most sense to me. I consider myself to be a very fortunate person in that:

- I work for a great company that gave me time off to research my treatment options and has supported me throughout my journey.
- My financial resources allow me to investigate many different treatment options.
- I have a great family and wonderful friends who provide a strong support system for me.
- I have always been a healthy person and came to this point in my life with a strong immune system.
- I have a naturally strong will that I exert in everything I do. Therefore, it is easy for me to have the discipline to stay on a strict regimen.

All these aspects were very important when I considered which choices were right for me to treat my hepatitis C.

Every form of treatment has its own positives and negatives, its own potential risks and rewards. I intend to stay on my current protocol while I continue to explore other options as they become available. As western therapies improve, I will re-evaluate my choices and decide whether or not this form of therapy is appropriate for me. I will also continue to explore various CAM treatment options. I intend to try to document and understand CAM successes or lack thereof, and make decisions based on what I learn. My long-term treatment goals remain unchanged:

1. to have good health for as long as possible, and
2. to get rid of the hepatitis C virus.

I feel strongly that I want to get rid of the virus, but I am not willing to sacrifice long-term health in order to do so.

I have often remarked to friends that I have three current goals in life:

1. to get rid of the hepatitis C virus
2. to grow my hair back, and
3. to get my step back in basketball.

A friend of mine once responded to my list by asking, "What about your fourth goal?" Confused, I asked, "What's that?" He laughingly replied, "To get rid of your delusions!"

I tell this story to communicate two things. First, it is important to keep your sense of humor. And second, dream big because anything is possible. None of my three goals has happened yet, although I **am** playing better basketball. I think it is very important for all of us with hepatitis C to realize there are all kinds of goals out there, and that we need to focus our lives on more than just hepatitis C. By shifting your focus onto something other than hepatitis C, you reduce some of the stress and fear associated with the illness. This is important because stress and fear can be just as great an impediment to good health and healing as any other aspect of your body.

I am going wherever my hepatitis C journey takes me! I honestly believe that getting hepatitis C has been a true gift for me. It has taught me many valuable lessons, and has opened many doors for me. I do not look at having hepatitis C as something that just happened to me. Rather, it is a journey that I both participate in and make choices about. I try to enjoy every day of my journey. I focus on all of the wonderful opportunities this journey places before me instead viewing hepatitis C as a detriment. I choose to make my hepatitis C as positive an experience as it can be.

As each of you makes your way along your own personal journey, I want to encourage you to share your experiences, both positive and negative, with others. It may seem as though one person's experience is insignificant, but if we **all** begin to share our experiences, we may begin to find some commonalities. We need more data to develop better statistics on how this disease affects individuals on a long-term basis. We may begin to see certain trends that we have not previously been aware of, and will be able to design studies to investigate these trends in a scientific way. Sharing your story can have more immediate personal benefits, too. Often, people with hepatitis C feel alone with their disease. By sharing your story openly, I think you will find that more times than not, you have much more in common with others than you may have thought. Sharing in this way is beneficial for all of us because it helps us come together to a place where we can support and help one another.

I hope that each of you will enjoy your journey, find the positives, and make the experience the best it can be for you and the loved ones in your life.

Good luck with your choices and enjoy your journey!

Chapter Twenty

A LOOK TO THE FUTURE

Lorren Sandt

INTRODUCTION

Hepatitis C is a major public health problem throughout the world, yet it is largely a preventable disease. Prevention requires excellent education programs, rigorous efforts to protect the blood supply, and major intervention programs for at-risk populations such as injection drug users (IDU's).

Despite major advances in the diagnosis and treatment of hepatitis C over the past decade, there is still much more we do not know about the virus than we do know. Research is being conducted on a number of fronts in the race to gain control over the virus. *Advocates* are working diligently to raise public awareness and provide information to the millions infected with the hepatitis C virus (HCV). Health care providers from all disciplines are looking for better ways to treat their patients with hepatitis C.

Where do we go from here?

EDUCATION AND AWARENESS

Despite the fact that hepatitis C is largely a preventable disease, it continues to spread. The need for education and public awareness is critical. Many consider the worldwide HCV prevalence rate to be grossly underestimated. For example, current estimates for the United States do not include infected prisoners, homeless people, injection drug users, and probably many others who do not participate in the mainstream health care system. We may never know the true HCV prevalence rate.

Education, public awareness, and effective, affordable, early testing are essential for disease prevention. When prevention fails, effective treatment is imperative.

The federal government is responsible for educating the public about communicable diseases such as hepatitis C. The Centers for Disease Control and Prevention is the principal agency managing this task. However to date, much of the education and awareness about HCV has actually come from the many grassroots hepatitis C organizations and support groups around the country. Hepatitis C is essentially an 'unfunded epidemic' meaning neither the federal government nor the private sector has earmarked funds for combating this growing public health problem. Funding will not become available until the magnitude and severity of hepatitis C become widely recognized. Both government and private funding are desperately needed to support HCV public awareness campaigns. Many of the grass roots organizations that provide the bulk of hepatitis C education and awareness programs are funded solely by monies from pharmaceutical companies that manufacture drugs used to treat hepatitis C. While this has caused some people to mistrust the information provided , without this funding, public awareness about hepatitis C would be even less than it currently is.

AREAS OF RESEARCH

Almost unbelievable advances in medical research have been made during the past six decades. Each decade seems to bring advances even more rapidly than the one before. Our knowledge increases, and as single pieces of the large puzzle are put in place, a more complete picture is revealed. Computer technology has been an incredible boon to the advancement of medical research especially with respect to viral illnesses. Computer modeling of viral *genomes* has allowed scientists to carefully target and attack specific genetic patterns of viruses.

HCV is not yet thoroughly understood. The process by which it causes an acute or a more problematic chronic infection are still a mystery. Until more answers are available, we must do the best we can with treatments that work for some, but not all, and that can cause significant discomfort while they are being used.

The Eternal Question: Is It The Virus or Is It The Host?

Every day HCV researchers around the world ask the same questions. Is it characteristics of the virus or the host (the infected person) that make this such a terrible disease for so many? How does HCV infect the cell? Why do some people have an acute infection that quickly resolves, while others develop a chronic infection? Why do many people go on to develop *cirrhosis* and/or *liver cancer* as a result of chronic HCV infection? Why do some chronically infected patients have only mild disease with few *symptoms*?

Virologists who are trying to answer these questions generally believe the characteristics of the virus are primarily responsible for all this devastation. However, the immunologists who study the immune response to HCV infection in humans and chimpanzees work from another premise. They believe limitations of the host's *immune system* are primarily responsible for the severe consequences some people experience in response to HCV infection. In the end, most HCV researchers agree that both the virus and the host's immunological capabilities play a role in the natural history of the disease in any given person.

HCV's ability to reproduce itself, a process called *replication*, is staggering. In **one** day in **one** HCV infected person, there may be more copies of the virus produced than there have been humans on Earth since civilization began. Considered another way, a viral particle can replicate roughly 600-900 generations of HCV **each year**. By comparison, it is estimated there have been only 300 generations of humans on Earth **since civilization began**. The numbers are too great to comprehend fully.

Western Medical Research

Western researchers are studying people who spontaneously clear HCV to identify regions of the virus particle that may be involved in triggering a specific, successful immune response. This work is providing potential targets for the development of *vaccines* that may be used to prevent or treat HCV infections.

The federal government funds the majority of clinical and scientific research conducted in the U.S. Areas of HCV research currently being funded through the National Institutes of Health (NIH) include:

- non-invasive liver tests
- development of cost-effective alternatives to *liver biopsy*

- natural history of HCV: why some sustained responders to *interferon-based treatment* still show signs of chronic infection
- humoral and cell-mediated immunity to HCV
- development of a viral cocktail (a mixture of antiviral drugs) for HCV similar to the HAART cocktail used to treat HIV/AIDS
- liver transplants
- decreasing the risk of HCV infection to the transplanted liver in an HCV infected person
- *living donor liver transplantation*

Medical researchers around the world are making great strides in all areas of hepatitis C research. Just six years ago, people treated with interferon-based therapy had only a 12% chance of a sustained response. Today, approximately 50% of people who are treated with *pegylated interferon* plus *ribavirin* achieve a sustained response. The sustained response rates for some patients with specific *genotypes* may be as high as 80%.

Complementary and Alternative Medicine (CAM) Research

The use of *complementary and alternative medicine (CAM)* treatment approaches is common in many countries of the world such as China and India. Its use is becoming increasingly popular in western countries as well. This is particularly true among people with hepatitis C. Frustrated by the inability of western medicine to clear the virus in everyone who is treated, many people have turned to CAM therapies. Much of the upsurge in interest in these therapies has been facilitated by easy access to information via the Internet. However, there are concerns about the use of CAM therapies to treat hepatitis C.

The National Center for Complementary and Alternative Medicine (NCCAM) was established by NIH in 1998. NCCAM's functions are:

- to explore complementary and alternative healing practices in the context of rigorous science
- educating and training CAM researchers, and
- disseminating authoritative information to the public and professionals.

NCCAM's vision is, "to advance research to yield insights and tools derived from CAM to benefit the health and well-being of the public, while enabling an informed public to reject ineffective or unsafe practices."[1]

NCCAM must work to overcome the reluctance of western health care providers to consider CAM treatments for their patients. We need *clinical trials* that establish exactly what herbs and *nutritional supplements* do, and to evaluate their efficacy and safety. NCCAM is conducting research on some herbal therapies and other CAM practices, but they cannot possibly look into all of the thousands of products currently available. According to NCCAM, there has been only limited research on hepatitis C and alternative treatments. [2]

The Amount of Rigorous Research About Hepatitis C

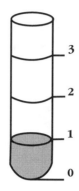

3—Extensive Research: Numerous high quality, scientific studies have been done, including clinical trials and other research published in major peer-reviewed journals. Reliable scientific information is available.

2—Some Research: Some good quality, scientific studies have been published in peer-reviewed journals. Some reliable scientific information is available.

1—Limited Research: A small number of scientific studies have been done, but few have been published in peer-reviewed journals. Some scientific information may be available.

0—No Research: No scientific studies have been done. No scientific information is available.

Note: The above levels of research are based on the amount of published, rigorous clinical research conducted or sponsored by NCCAM, other Institutes and Centers of NIH, and other biomedical research institutions in the United States and internationally.

Manufacturers and other proponents of CAM products must get involved in funding clinical trials that will carefully define the risks and benefits of these products. While it is important that medical research be scientifically sound, many people are questioning the need for randomized, double blind, controlled trials for complementary therapies to establish reliable *clinical* information. Randomized, controlled trials are very costly and time-consuming. While it is true that current research on CAM therapy can be a compromise, it is also true of western research. The best information will come when there is true collaboration between the two worlds.

Until research is conducted on the efficacy and safety of CAM approaches, few western doctors will recommend them. Currently, people interested in using these approaches must rely on their own sources of information. Unfortunately, much of this information is from people who are not knowledgeable. If you are considering CAM products, you should use the same precautions you would use if you were taking prescription medicine. Just because a product is "natural" does not mean it cannot harm you. If you intend to use CAM in your hepatitis C treat approach, gather information from someone who is trained and knowledgeable about CAM therapy, someone you trust.

THE FUTURE OF MEDICINE — AN INTEGRATED APPROACH

Can, should, or must we explore combining CAM and western treatments? Would this provide potentially less expensive and more effective treatments with better quality of life, not only for people in the U.S., but for the rest of the world's population as well?

As we move forward in the 21st century, the general public, CAM practitioners, and western doctors are increasingly accepting the idea of *integrated medicine.* As CAM therapies and interventions are incorporated into western medical education and practice, the exclusionary term "complementary and alternative medicine" will hopefully be replaced with the more inclusive term "integrated medicine."

A number of respected health care institutions, medical schools, and teaching hospitals are setting up or already have integrated medicine clinics. Physicians-in-training are being taught not only about western medical treatments, but also about the many herbs, supplements, and other forms of treatment their patients are using and/or requesting. Respected professionals from all medical disciplines are talking, listening, and working together as colleagues, much like the authors of this manual. We hope that in the not too distant future, integrated medicine will be seen as providing novel insights and tools for whole-body health. Health care providers everywhere will practice this new form of medicine after learning the numerous traditions and disciplines that contribute to the whole art of medicine.

THE ROLE OF THE PATIENT ADVOCACY COMMUNITY

Patient advocates play a major role in many areas of medicine. HCV advocates have been largely responsible for the hepatitis C public awareness and education programs that currently exist. They work in communities and in prisons. They work with the many military veterans who have been infected with HCV through infected blood transfusions for war injuries. They work with police and firefighters, and with injection drug users. They speak before Congress and state legislatures, appear on television, and reach out to other media outlets. They have been responsible for setting up testing sites where people can be screened for HCV free of charge. They are encouraging states to develop their own testing plans to help prevent the continued spread of this disease. They are organizing the development of community-based HCV task forces.

Advocates are clearly a necessary and vital component in the fight against HCV.

Get involved with one or more of your local HCV groups. Volunteer your time if you can. These groups need your help. Just a few hours a week can make a big difference. If there is no HCV group in your area and you would like to start one, give us a call. We would be happy to give you information about how to establish an HCV advocacy group. If you do not have time to volunteer, you can still help by writing your state and local representatives. Tell them you want hepatitis C moved to the top of their agenda.

HCV advocacy organizations provide essential services and a more powerful voice to people diagnosed with this potentially life-threatening illness. They need and deserve everyone's support.

The National Hepatitis C Advocacy Council

The Hepatitis C Caring Ambassadors Program's mission statement addresses the need to motivate the many HCV advocacy organizations to work together. In the summer of 2000, all the HCV advocacy groups were invited to participate in a meeting to determine if a collaborative approach would benefit people with HCV. The meeting resulted in the formation of The National Hepatitis C Advocacy Council.

Since the Council was formed, we have grown to a 24-member, national organization. The Council is a forum for discussing common goals and for strategizing on ways to become a formidable national force to advance the issues of importance to all people affected by hepatitis C. The Council has established ethical guidelines for all participating groups. The Council's guidelines promote a better quality of life for people living with hepatitis C, and stress that all member organizations must act responsibly and provide accurate, unbiased information.

The Council's Mission Statement

The National Hepatitis C Advocacy Council is an association of organizations that creates a unified voice, promotes ethical guidelines, and improves the quality of services for people affected by hepatitis C.

The Council's Ethical Guidelines for Organizations

- Place the needs of people living with hepatitis C and those affected by hepatitis C first.
- Activities should be culturally and linguistically appropriate for the people served.
- Responsibility to provide: who you are, what you do, how you do it, and funding sources
- Responsibility to provide accurate and unbiased information
- Maintain a positive attitude and focus on educational aspects to help dispel fears and promote better quality of life for patients affected by hepatitis C.
- All persons affected by hepatitis C should be treated with respect and dignity.

The Council will be working on a variety of issues in the future. A primary objective of the Council is to ensure that hepatitis public health policy is shaped to include funding for research and community-based organizations.

For more information on the Council, visit their Internet site at: http://www.hepcnetwork.org. The *Resource Directory* lists the members of the council, as well as many other great educational resources.

SUMMARY

Much has been learned about hepatitis C, but there is still so much we do not know. Luckily, for most people, HCV is not a death sentence. In fact, the majority of people affected by HCV will not die **from** the virus, but **with** the virus. Given enough time and financial support from the government and private sector, researchers will undoubtedly answer many of the questions nagging scientists today. How does the virus infect? Has western medicine really been successful in clearing the virus, or is it hidden in a reservoir somewhere in the body? Why do some people clear the virus on their own, while others develop a chronic infection that can have devastating consequences? Why does one form of treatment work for some and not for others?

Even if all of the scientific questions were answered tomorrow and effective treatments were available for everyone infected, there would still be hundreds of thousands of people worldwide who already have the disease, and hundreds of thousands more to whom it would be spread. Prevention is crucial if we want to achieve control of the spread of this disease. A critical need for information and education exists and will continue to exist for a very long time. We as individuals and as organizations have the opportunity to play a pivotal role in putting the spotlight on this slowly progressive, insidious, and potentially devastating disease. It will take a concerted effort on the part of everyone involved — researchers, government agencies, the private sector, patient advocates, and the public at large — if we are to win this battle.

> **"Never doubt that a small group of thoughtful committed citizens can change the world. Indeed, it is the only thing that ever has."**
> **— Margaret Mead**

APPENDIX I
Patients' Rights

Informed Consent: A Patient's Right to Know

It is your health care provider's responsibility to provide you with enough information about your treatment options for you to make an informed decision. This is referred to as informed consent. Your health care provider must have a consent form signed by you that reflects that this process has occurred before performing any non-emergency procedure or treatment. Your right to the informed consent process continues throughout your illness.

While the formal informed consent process is usually routine for procedures carried out in hospitals, clinics, and private offices, it may not be as routine in other environments. Although informed consent is your right as a patient, you and your health care providers share the responsibility for making sure you are adequately informed. It is important that you ask questions and learn what you can before you move forward with any health care option.

The requirement for informed consent has several purposes. Your health care provider is required to provide the following information to you about any treatment or procedure.

- what treatment will be given
- what the effects, both positive and negative, are likely to be
- why the treatment is being given or the procedure is being done
- what the expected outcome is, both with and without the treatment or procedure
- what your alternatives are to receiving the treatment or having the procedure

When you sign a consent form, you are saying you understand the reasons for the proposed treatment or procedure, and you are giving your consent to proceed with the treatment or procedure. Take time to carefully read the consent form. If there is **anything** you do not understand, ask questions until you understand everything on the form completely.

If you do not agree with something on the form, discuss the changes you wish to make with your health care provider. Along with other rights, you always have the right to refuse treatment.

American Hospital Association Patient Bill of Rights

The patient empowerment movement was started in the early 1970's when the American Hospital Association developed the following Patient Bill of Rights. This Bill of Rights has become the standard for the entire health care industry. You may find it helpful to keep these rights in mind throughout your experience with hepatitis C.

1. The patient has a right to considerate and respectful care.

2. The patient has a right to obtain from his or her physician complete current information about his or her diagnosis.

3. The patient has a right to obtain from his or her physician information necessary to give informed consent prior to the start of any procedure and/or treatment.

4. The patient has the right to refuse treatment to the extent permitted by law.

5. The patient has a right to every consideration of his or her privacy concerning his or

her own medical care program.

6. The patient has a right to expect that all communications and records pertaining to his or her care should be treated as confidential.

7. The patient has a right to expect that, within its capacity, a hospital must make a reasonable response to the request for patient services.

8. The patient has the right to obtain information as to any relationship of his or her hospital to any other health care and educational institutions insofar as his or her care is concerned.

9. The patient has a right to be advised if the hospital proposes to engage in human experimentation affecting his or her care and the right to refuse to participate in such research projects.

10. The patient has the right to expect reasonable continuity of care.

11. The patient has the right to examine and receive an explanation of his or her bill regardless of the source of payment.

12. The patient has the right to know what hospital rules and regulations apply to her or her conduct as a patient.

APPENDIX II

How To Cut Down On Your Drinking

National Institutes Of Health
National Institute On Alcohol Abuse And Alcoholism

How to Cut Down on Your Drinking

If you are drinking too much, you can improve your life and health by cutting down. How do you know if you drink too much? Read these questions and answer yes or no.

- Do you drink alone when you feel angry or sad?
- Does your drinking ever make you late for work?
- Does your drinking worry your family?
- Do you ever drink after telling yourself you won't?
- Do you ever forget what you did while you were drinking?
- Do you get headaches or have a hang-over after you have been drinking?

If you answered yes to any of these questions, you may have a drinking problem. Check with your doctor to be sure. Your doctor will be able to tell you whether you should cut down or abstain. **If you are alcoholic or have other medical problems, you should not just cut down on your drinking—you should stop drinking completely. Your doctor will advise you about what is right for you.**

If your doctor tells you to cut down on your drinking, these steps can help you.

1. Write your reasons for cutting down or stopping.

Why do you want to drink less? There are many reasons why you may want to cut down or stop drinking. You may want to improve your health, sleep better, or get along better with your family or friends. Make a list of the reasons you want to drink less.

2. Set a drinking goal.

Choose a limit for how much you will drink. You may choose to cut down or not to drink at all. If you are cutting down, keep below these limits:

Women: No more than one drink a day

Men: No more than two drinks a day

A drink is:

- a 12-ounce bottle of beer
- a 5-ounce glass of wine, or
- a 1 1/2-ounce shot of liquor.

These limits may be too high for some people who have certain medical problems or who are older. Talk with your doctor about the limit that is right for you.

Now—write your drinking goal on a piece of paper. Put it where you can see it, such as on your refrigerator or bathroom mirror. Your paper might look like this:

My drinking goal

- I will start on this day _____ .
- I will not drink more than _____ drinks in 1 day.
- I will not drink more than _____ drinks in 1 week.

or

    I will stop drinking alcohol.

---

3. Keep a diary of your drinking.

To help you reach your goal, keep a diary of your drinking. For example, write down every time you have a drink for 1 week. Try to keep your diary for 3 or 4 weeks. This will show you how much you drink and when. You may be surprised. How different is your goal from the amount you drink now? Use the drinking diary below to write down when you drink.

Week:			
	# of drinks	**type of drinks**	**place consumed**
Mon.			
Tues.			
Wed.			
Thurs.			
Fri.			
Sat.			
Sun.			
Week:			
	# of drinks	**type of drinks**	**place consumed**
Mon.			
Tues.			
Wed.			
Thurs.			
Fri.			
Sat.			
Sun.			

Now you know why you want to drink less and you have a goal. There are many ways you can help yourself to cut down. Try these tips:

Watch it at home.

Keep a small amount or no alcohol at home. Don't keep temptations around.

Drink slowly.

When you drink, sip your drink slowly. Take a break of 1 hour between drinks. Drink soda, water, or juice after a drink with alcohol. Do not drink on an empty stomach! Eat food when you are drinking.

Take a break from alcohol.

Pick a day or two each week when you will not drink at all. Then, try to stop drinking for 1 week. Think about how you feel physically and emotionally on these days. When you succeed and feel better, you may find it easier to cut down for good.

Learn how to say NO.

You do not have to drink when other people drink. You do not have to take a drink that is given to you. Practice ways to say no politely. For example, you can tell people you feel better when you drink less. Stay away from people who give you a hard time about not drinking.

Stay active.

What would you like to do instead of drinking? Use the time and money spent on drinking to do something fun with your family or friends. Go out to eat, see a movie, or play sports or a game.

Get support.

Cutting down on your drinking may be difficult at times. Ask your family and friends for support to help you reach your goal. Talk to your doctor if you are having trouble cutting down. Get the help you need to reach your goal.

Watch out for temptations.

Watch out for people, places, or times that make you drink, even if you do not want to. Stay away from people who drink a lot or bars where you used to go. Plan ahead of time what you will do to avoid drinking when you are tempted.

Do not drink when you are angry or upset or have a bad day. These are habits you need to break if you want to drink less.

DO NOT GIVE UP!

Most people do not cut down or give up drinking all at once. Just like a diet, it is not easy to change. That is okay. If you do not reach your goal the first time, try again. Remember, get support from people who care about you and want to help. Do not give up!

This information was provided by the National Institute on Alcohol Abuse and Alcoholism (NIAAA). If you would like more copies visit their website at:

http://www.niaaa.nih.gov/publications/handout.htm

APPENDIX III
Western (Allopathic) Medicine

The Hepatitis C Antiviral Long-Term Treatment Against Cirrhosis Trial, The HALT-C Trial

A clinical trial sponsored by the National Institutes of Health

Study Summary

This study will test whether long-term *antiviral* therapy with interferon can prevent liver disease from progressing in patients with *chronic hepatitis* C infection.

Patient Population for the Trial:
- Adult (18 years or older)
- *Nonresponder* to prior antiviral therapy (either monotherapy or combination treatment)
- Advanced *fibrosis* or *cirrhosis* on *liver biopsy*

Study Protocol:
- All patients receive 6 months of *pegylated* interferon alfa-2a plus *ribavirin.*
- Responders who clear virus on treatment receive an additional 6 months of therapy.
- Nonresponders are randomized to either no treatment or maintenance low-dose
    pegylated interferon alfa-2a for up to 4 years.

Clinical Effectiveness is Defined as Prevention of:
- Liver failure
- Transplant
- Death
- *Liver cancer*

Other Investigations:
- Effect of iron
- Effect of diet
- Quantitative assessment of liver function
- Studies of the virus
- Studies of the *immune system*
- Quality of life
- Serum fibrosis markers
- Tissue and blood repository

From: Living with Hepatitis C: A Survivor's Guide. Everson GT, Weinberg H. Hatherleigh Press, Inc. Copyright 2001.

For additional information on the HALT-C Trial, see the National Institutes of Health Internet site at: http://clinicalstudies.info.nih.gov/detail/A_2000-DK-0186.html.

APPPENDIX IV

AYURVEDIC MEDICINE

Ayurvedic herbs used to treat liver disorders

The most important herbs used in the formulas described in *Chapter 9: Ayurvedic Medicine* for the treatment of liver disorders are described below. Their botanical names, distribution, parts used, and medicinal uses are described. In addition, information on the dosage forms and side effects are provided.[1, 2, 3, 4]

Bhringaraj

Botanical Name:	*Eclipta alba, Eclipta erecta*
	The name means "ruler of the hair."
Family:	Compositae
Distribution:	This herb is found throughout India as well as the southwestern part of the United States.
Parts Used:	Herb, roots, and leaves
Actions:	Roots and leaves stimulate the flow of *bile* into the intestine. The root is used as an emetic and purgative (laxative). The leaf juice is used as a liver tonic. This is the main herb for the hair, and *cirrhosis*. It is believed to prevent aging, maintain and rejuvenate hair, teeth, bones, memory, sight, and hearing. It is a rejuvenative for pitta, kidneys, and liver. The root powder is used in Ayurvedic medicine for hepatitis, enlarged spleen, and skin disorders.
Dosage:	Infusions, *decoction*, powder, medicated oil, and ghee (clarified butter)
Safety Caution:	This herb can cause severe chills. **Do not use this herb without the supervision of a qualified health care provider**.

Bhuamalaki

Botanical Name:	*Phyllanthus niruri, Phyllanthus urinaria, Phyllanthus amarus*
Family:	Euphorbiaceae
Distribution:	This perennial herb is found from central and southern India to Sri Lanka. *Phyllanthus* species are also found in other countries including China (e.g., *Phyllanthus urinaria*), the Philippines, Cuba, Nigeria, and Guam.
Parts Used:	Leaves, roots, and whole plant
Active Compounds:	*Phyllanthus* primarily contains lignans (phyllanthine and hypophyllanthine), alkaloids, and bioflavonoids (quercetin). While it remains unknown which of these ingredients has an *antiviral* effect, research shows that this herb acts primarily on the liver. This action in the liver confirms its historical use as a remedy for *jaundice*.

Actions:	*Phyllanthus* has been used in Ayurvedic medicine for over 2,000 years and has a wide number of traditional uses. It is the main herb for treating liver disorders. Other uses include using the whole plant for jaundice, gonorrhea, frequent menstruation, and diabetes. It is also used topically as a poultice for skin ulcers, sores, swelling, and itchiness. The young shoots of the plant are administered in the form of an infusion for the treatment of chronic dysentery.
Dosage:	Infusion, juice, poultice, powder, or pill
Safety:	No side effects have been reported using *Phyllanthus* as recommended. Researchers have used the powdered form of *Phyllanthus* in amounts ranging from 900-2,700 mg per day for three months.

Guduchi

Botanical Name:	*Tinosporia cordifolia, Menisper mum cordifolium, Cocculuc cordifolia*
Family:	Menispermaceae
Distribution:	This herb is found in the Himalayas and in many parts of southern India.
Parts Used:	Whole plant, roots, and stems
Actions:	This herb is used to treat HIV/AIDS, other immune diseases, and pitta diseases. It is used as a blood purifier, to treat fever, and to aid recovery from fevers. It is also used for jaundice, digestion, constipation, hemorrhoids, dysentery, and cancer (strengthens persons before and after chemotherapy).
Dosage:	Extract, powder, concoctions for serious illnesses like cancer. Use one or more ounces daily.
Safety:	No information available.

Haritaki (Myrobalan)

Botanical Name:	*Terminalia chebula, Terminalia reticulata*
Family:	Combretaceae
Description:	This tree grows in many parts of India.
Parts Used:	Fruit
Actions:	This fruit is a blood purifier and is used to treat jaundice, colic, *anemia*, cough, asthma, hoarse voice, hiccups, vomiting, hemorrhoids, diarrhea, *malabsorption*, abdominal *distention*, gas, fevers, parasitic infections, tumors, and spleen and liver disorders. Small doses are good for constipation and diarrhea. It also improves digestion.
Dosage:	Decoction, powder, paste, and gargle

Safety Caution: **Do not take this fruit if you are pregnant or are suffering from dehydration, severe exhaustion, and/or emaciation**. No other infor mation about the safety of this plant is available.

Kalmegha (King of Bitters)

Botanical Name: *Andrographis paniculata*

Family: Acanthaceae

Distribution: This herb is found throughout India and southeast Asia.

Part used: Leaves

Active ingredient: Andrographolide

Actions: This herb is reported to possess astringent, anodyne, and tonic properties. The plant is bitter, acrid, and cooling. It is used as a laxative, anti-inflammatory, expectorant, and digestive. It is useful in treating dysentery, cholera, diabetes, influenza, bronchitis, hemorrhoids, gonorrhea, *hepatomegaly*, skin disorders, fever, worm infestations, burning sensations, wounds, ulcers, leprosy, itching, flatulence, colitis, and diarrhea.

Dosage: Powder, decoction, and extract

Safety: No information about the safety of this plant is available.

Katuka or Kutki

Botanical Name: *Picrorrhiza kurroa*

Description: This plant is found in the western Himalayas from Kashmir to Sikkim.

Parts Used: Dried rhizome

Actions: This herb is used with equal parts of licorice and raisins to treat constipation. It is also used with neem bark for bilious fever, and with aromatics to treat fevers, malaria, and worms in children.

Dosage: Tincture, extract, powder, or pills

Safety: No information about the safety of this plant is available

Musta (Nutgrass)

Botanical Name: *Cyperus rotundus*

Family Cyperaceae

Description: This plant is found in southern India.

Parts Used: Rhizome

Actions: This plant is used to treat poor appetite, diarrhea, dysentery, fevers, gastritis, indigestion, and sluggish liver. It is also used to harmonize the liver, spleen, and pancreas, and to treat malabsorption.

Dosage: Decoction or powder

Safety Caution: Prolonged use of this herb may cause constipation and excess *flatulence* or gas. No further information about the safety of this plant is available.

Pippali (Long Pepper)

Botanical Name: *Piper longum*

Distribution: This plant is indigenous to northeastern and southern India and Sri Lanka. It is cultivated in eastern Bengal.

Family: Piperaceae

Parts Used: Fruit

Actions: *Piper longum* is used to treat abdominal tumors and distention, and to improve the digestive fire. It is used to treat flatulence, gout, laryngitis, paralysis, rheumatic pain, sciatica, and worms. It is also used to enhance the *immune system*.

Dosage: Infusion, powder, and oil

Safety Caution: This herb causes high pitta. No information about the safety of this plant is available.

Punarnava (Red Hogweed)

Botanical Name: *Boerrhavia diffusa*

Family: Nyctaginae

Description: This herb is found throughout India. It can be white or red.

Parts Used: Herb or root

Actions: White and red species are used to treat *edema*, *anemia*, heart disease, cough, intestinal colic, jaundice, *ascites*, peritoneal concerns such as urethritis, and kidney disorders.

                         Other uses of red plant include hemorrhoids, skin diseases, rat and snake bites, alcoholism, wasting diseases, insomnia, rheumatism, eye diseases, and asthma (moderate doses). It induces vomiting in large doses. Leaf juice is used to treat jaundice. Root decoction or infusion is used to treat constipation, gonorrhea, and internal *inflammations*. It is used externally to treat *edema*, and rat and snake bites.

Dosage: Juice, decoction, infusion, powder, paste, oil, sugar water or honey paste

Safety Caution: No information about the safety of this herb is available. However, **large doses are known to cause vomiting**.

CURRENT AYURVEDIC RESEARCH ON PLANTS FOR THE TREATMENT OF LIVER DISORDERS

Research regarding plants traditionally used in Ayurveda for the treatment of liver disease has advanced significantly in the past 15 years. Much of what has been discovered supports traditional knowledge.

The following descriptions of some of these research studies are technical and may be somewhat difficult to understand. They are provided here for reference only. If you choose to incorporate Ayurvedic medicine into your treatment *protocol*, you should give this information to your non-Ayurvedic health care providers. It will help them understand what you are taking and how it may or may not affect any other treatments you are using.

The *hepatoprotective* effect of the ethanol to water (1:1) extract of *Eclipta alba* (Ea) has been studied at subcellular levels in rats against carbon tetrachloride-induced *hepatotoxicity*. Its hepatoprotective action is created by regulating the levels of hepatic microsomal drug metabolizing *enzymes*.[5]

Studies on *Phyllanthus niruri* have revealed that it blocks *DNA polymerase*, the enzyme needed for the *hepatitis B* virus to *replicate*. Fifty-nine percent of those infected with chronic viral hepatitis B lost one of the major blood markers of HBV infection (hepatitis B surface antigen) after using *Phyllanthus* for 30 days. While *clinical studies* on the outcome of *Phyllanthus* and HBV have been mixed, the species *P. urinaria* and *P. niruri* seem to work far better than *P. amarus*. Many previous studies on the hepatoprotective effects of *P. niruri* corroborated traditional knowledge of its role in liver disorders.[6, 7, 8, 9]

Turmeric has shown evidence of hepatoprotective effects in laboratory and animal studies. However, there are no human *clinical* studies. Like silymarin, turmeric has been found to protect animal livers from a variety of hepatotoxic substances including carbon tetrachloride, galactosamine, pentobarbitol, 1-chloro-2,4-dinitrobenzene, 7 4-hydroxy-nonenal, and *acetaminophen*. Giving curcumin along with piperine (long pepper) can enhance its absorption when taken orally. The hepatoprotective effects of turmeric may stem from its potent *antioxidant* effects. Turmeric contains several water and fat soluble antioxidant compounds. Curcumin was found to be the most active of these compounds. The antioxidant effects of other components of turmeric are also significant. A heat-stable *protein* isolated from the aqueous extract of turmeric was found to be more effective against superoxide than was curcumin, and more effective in inhibiting oxidative damage to DNA. In addition to its antioxidant effects, curcumin has also been shown to enhance liver detoxification by increasing the activity of glutathione S-transferase10,20. Glutathione S-transferase10,20 is an enzyme that joins *glutathione* with a wide variety of *toxins* to facilitate their removal from the body.[9, 10, 11, 12, 13]

Glycyrhhiza (licorice) has been shown to have a direct hepatoprotective effect. Glycyrhhiza flavonoids provide protection to *hepatocytes* exposed to carbon tetrachloride and galactosamine. Research points to the antilipid peroxidation effect of glycyrrhiza as the central mechanism contributing to its protective action against carbon tetrachloride-induced hepatotoxicity. Glycyrrhiza has also been shown to significantly quench *free radicals*. Recent studies have shown glycyrrhiza to enhance the detoxification of medications and toxins. Several mechanisms seem to be involved, one of which is increased liver glucuronidation. Glycyrrhiza exerts antiviral activity *in vitro* toward a number of viruses, including *hepatitis A*, varicella zoster, *HIV*, herpes simplex type 1, Newcastle disease, and vesicular stomatitis viruses. Intravenous glycyrrhizin has been shown to be effective in a double blind study against viral hepatitis, chronic viral hepatitis in particular. Administered in a physiologic saline solution in combination with cysteine and glycine (a product called Stronger Neo Minophagen-C, or SNMC), glycyrrhiza has been shown to stimulate *endogenous interferon* production in addition to its antioxidant and detoxifying effects.[14, 15, 16]

Picroliv, the active constituent isolated from the plant *Picrorhiza kurroa*, was evaluated as a hepatoprotective agent against ethanol-induced *hepatic* injury in rats. Alcohol feeding (3.75 g/kg x45 days) produced 20-114% alteration in selected *serum (AST, ALT* and ALP) and liver markers (lipid, *glycogen,* and protein). Further, it reduced the viability (44-48%) of isolated hepatocytes *ex vivo* as assessed by Trypan blue exclusion and rate of oxygen uptake. Its effect was also seen on specific alcohol-metabolizing enzymes (aldehyde dehydrogenase, 41%; *acetaldehyde* dehydrogenase, 52%) in rat hepatocytes. The levels of these enzymes were reduced in the cells following alcohol intoxication. Ethyl alcohol also produced *cholestasis* (41-53%), as indicated by reduction in bile volume, bile salts, and bile acids. Picroliv treatment (3-12 mg/kg p.o. x45 days) restored the altered parameters in a dose-dependent manner (36-100%).[17, 18]

Andrographolide, a chief constituent of *A. paniculata*, exhibits protective effects in *galactosamine* and paracetamol induced *toxicity* in rats.[19] Andrographolide was demonstrated to possess antihepatotoxic effects in carbon tetrachloride-induced *hepatotoxicity* in albino rats.[20] The LD50 of aqueous ethanolic extract of whole plant was determined to be >215 mg/kg, i.p. in mice.[21] *Andrographic paniculata* (Kalamegh) was used in an uncontrolled study at Kaya Chikitsa Dept. BHU, Varanasi, India. Average duration of treatment was 23 days. In 90% of patients, clinical as well as liver function parameters improved significantly.[22]

SAMPLE PANCHKARMA AND RASAYANA THERAPY FOR TREATMENT OF LIVER DISEASE

As noted in *Chapter 9: Ayurvedic Medicine*, panchakarma and rasayana are two treatments commonly used to treat chronic liver disorders. Following are sample protocols for each of these Ayurvedic treatments. However, keep in mind that Ayurvedic treatments are customized for each individual, and these are just sample protocols. Further, these treatments can only be done under the supervision of a qualified Ayurvedic practitioner.

If you are interested in adding Ayurvedic therapy to your hepatitis C treatment plan, you will need to see a qualified Ayurvedic practitioner. He or she can evaluate you, and then decide on the treatments that are appropriate for your unique situation.

Panchakarma Therapy (Body Cleansing)

Panchakarma is used in Ayurveda to eliminate excess doshas from the body. This therapy is widely used throughout India and the United States. It is used to balance humors and eliminate toxins from the body, thus treating various physical and psychiatric disorders.

Most liver disorders are typically aggravated conditions of pitta, which is also the predominant humor for the liver.

Panchakarma consists of three parts, *poorva karma*, *pradhana karma*, and *paschat karma*.

Poorva Karma (Pre-purification measures)

This procedure helps prepare the body for the main purification process. This treatment includes *abhyanga* (massage) and *pinda svedana* (warm massage with a small cotton bag containing warmed herbs).

Abhyanga: The term abhyanga is used as a synonym for oil bath. Oil is anointed all over the body, especially on the head and feet.

<u>Pinda Sveda</u> *(fomentation)*: This treatment is very efficacious wherever sweating is advised. The subject is massaged with warm oil all over the body. Then the subject is massaged with small bags containing cooked old rice that is warmed in a milk decoction mixture. The heat of the bags is maintained by re-warming them whenever necessary.

Medicaments for Panchakarma

<u>For abhyanga:</u>   *Balaguduchyadi taila*

Main Ingredients: *Sida cordifolia (bala), Tinospora cordifolia (guduchi), Santalum album (candana), Pluchea lanceolata (rasna), Valeriana wallichii (nata), Withania somnifera (ashwagandha)*

<u>For pinda sveda:</u> Old rice/rice powder cooked with milk and *Sida cordifolia* (bala) decoction

Pradhan Karma (Main Purification Measures)

Pradhan karma includes *virechana* (purgation), *pizhichil*, and *yapana vasti.*

Virechana (purgation)

This treatment is advised for the pitta disorders to eliminate aggravated pitta. Pitta disorders include liver disorders. The subject's physical constitution (prakruti) and strength will determine the dosage of the purgative herbs. Subjects are advised to consume purgative herbs in the early morning.

Pizhichil (medicated warm liquid oil massage)

This is a modified form of sarvangadhara. Warm liquid is poured from a certain height all over the body of the patient with unctuous liquids. After anointing the head with *ksheerabala* oil, warm *trivrit* oil is applied all over the body. The patient is then laid in a wooden compartment and again smeared with the warm unctuous fluid all over the body.

Yapana Vasti

This treatment is in the form of an enema. It helps improve strength and builds up muscle and tissue. It is intended to improve quality of life by alleviating ailments. This treatment is used only in subjects who can tolerate the procedure.

Medicaments for Pradhan Karma

For Virechana:

Based on the subject's physical constitution and strength either *Avipattikara choorna* (a mild powder laxative) or *triphala churna* powder (a combination of *Terminalia chebula, Terminalia bellirica,* and *Emblica officinals*) is administered.

For Yapana Vasti:

An herbal concoction is used along with milk and honey. The herbs used are *Glycyrrhiza glabra (yasti madhu), Tinospora cordifolia (guduchi), Picrorrhiza kurroa (katuki), Hemidesmus indicus (sariva),* and *Rubia cordifolia (manjista)*. The dose of each herb is 500 mg for a total treatment dose of 2.5 grams.

Paschat Karma

This treatment includes diet and lifestyle guidelines to bring about balance in the tridoshas after the subject has undergone the main purification procedure. Subjects are advised to follow the diet and lifestyle that will reestablish the balance of pitta. Paschat karma should be practiced during the entire treatment process.

Lifestyle: Patients should avoid sleeping in the afternoon, exposure to hot sun, exertion, anxiety, alcohol abuse, smoking, and irregular eating habits.

Diet: Vegetarianism is best for liver disorders. After mild purgation, subjects will be managed with a wholesome diet including non-spicy food, barley, wheat, basmati rice (old rice), and soup of lentils and green gram. The consistency of food should be gradually increased from a thin consistency on the first meal to a thicker one on seventh meal. A drink of warm water should follow each meal.

Rasayana Therapy (Rejuvenation Therapy)

Rasayana therapy is advised after the subject has undergone panchakarma therapy. Rasayana is a clinical specialty in Ayurveda wherein a specialized rejuvenating diet, herbs, and lifestyle are advised. Rasayana promotes tissue repair and the formation of healthy tissues. It alleviates exertion, lassitude, exhaustion, and debility. In other words, it builds up all the body tissues, improves immunity against diseases, and enhances the mental competence.

By its *immunomodulatory* and antioxidant effects, rasayana helps enhance the immune system, and prevents diseases and premature aging. The diet, herbs, and lifestyle also help alleviate already existing ailments and restore health. Therapy ensures proper transportation and absorption of nutrients, and builds normal tissues. Through rasayana, one attains longevity, memory, intelligence, youthful age, optimum strength of physique, and optimum sensory ability.

There are two types of rasayana treatments, *kutipravesika* (indoor) and *vataatapika* (outdoor). In this sample protocol, we discuss an outdoor rasayana.

People with liver disorders are prescribed rasayana therapy that is both hepatoprotective and immune enhancing. The therapy includes rejuvenation of the liver with herbs (mainly *Piper longum* in a powder formula, in a graded dose) and diet.

Pippali Rasayana

Mainly indicated for fever, fatigue, inflammation, liver and spleen enlargements, cough, and/or *dyspnea*.

Main Ingredient: *Pippali*

Dose: 1 tablespoon twice a day with warm water

Ashwagandha Rasayana

Mainly indicated in fatigue and immunodeficiency. It is an immune enhancer and a rejuvenator. Used when antioxidants are needed. Therapy is intended to decrease viral load.

Main Ingredients: *Withania somnifera (ashwagandha), Hemidesmus indicus (sariva), Cuminum cyminum (jiraka), Vitis vinifera (draksha)*

Dose: 1 tablespoon twice a day with warm water or milk

Triphala Rasayana

Mainly indicated in immunodeficiency and chronic illness.

Main Ingredients: *Terminalia chebula (haritaki), Terminalia bellirica (bibhitaki), Emblica officinals (amalaki), Madhuca indica (madhuka), Piper longum (pippali)*

Dose: 1 tablespoon at night with warm water

APPENDIX V

MODERN AND TRADITIONAL CHINESE MEDICINE

Chinese medicine herbs and formulas:
Pharmacology and clinical uses

COMPOSITION OF HERBAL THERAPIES

AI #3 Capsule

- *Mucunae caulis, Sargentodoxae caulis, Paederiae caulis*

Allicin Capsule

- *Allii sativum bulbus* (garlic)

BM Capsule

- *Momordica charantia, Fagophyrum tatarium*

Capillaris Combination

- *Artemisiae capillaris herba, Gardeniae fructus, Rhei rhizoma*

Capillaris Combination (plus blood cooling and toxin resolving herbs)

- *Artemisiae capillaris, Gardeniae fructus, Rhei rhizoma, Desmodii herba, Paeoniae rubra radix, Polygoni cuspidati, Plantaginis herba, Polyporus umbellatus, Scutellariae radix, Turmeric radix, Glycyrrhiza uralensis fisch*

Circulation No. 1 Tablet

- *Carthami flos, Persicae semen, Angelicae radix, Cnidii rhizoma, Rehmanniae radix, Paeoniae rubra radix, Achyranthis radix, Citri aurantii fructus, Bupleuri radix, Glycyrrhizae radix, Platycodi radix*

Coptin Tablet

- *Coptis chinensis franch*

Cordyceps Capsule

- *Cordyceps sinensis*

Gall No. 1 Tablets

- *Bupleuri radix, Artemisiae capillaris herba, Desmodii herba, Taraxaci herba, Gardeniae fructus, Saussureae radix, Citri pericarpium, Citri immaturi pericarpium, Salviae miltiorrhziae radix, Angelica radix, Scutellariae radix, Gentianae radix*

Ginseng and Atractylodes Formula

- *Ginseng radix, Dioscoreae rhizoma, Dolichoris album semen, Coicis semen, Nelumbinis semen, Atractylodis macrocephalae rhizoma, Poriae alba, Glycyrrhizae radix, Amomi fructus, Platycodi radix, and Zizipi jujubae fructus*

Glycyrrihzin Capsule

- *Glycyrrhiza uralensis fisch* (licorice root)

Hepa Formula No. 2 Capsule

- *Schizandrae fructus, Artemisiae capillaris herba, Alismatis rhizoma, Polyporus, Poria (Hoelen), Atractylodes rhizoma, Cinnamomi ramulus, Citri pericarpium, Magnoliae cortex, Zingiberis rhizoma* (ginger), *Glycyrrhizae radix* (licorice)

HerbSom Capsule

- *Corydalis yanhusao rhizoma, Zizyphus spinosi semen, Schizandrae fructus*

Modified Aconite, Ginseng, and Ginger Combination, and Gardenia and Hoelen Formula (Four Major Herb Combination and Rehmannia Eight Formula)

- *Aconiti praeparata raix, Cinnamomi ramulus, Zingiberis rhizoma, Atractylodes rhizoma, Dioscoreae batatis rhizoma, Polyporus, Poria (Hoelen), Polyporus umbellatus, Alismatis rhizoma, Arecae pericarpium, Glycyrrhiza uralensis fisch*

Modified Formulas of Bupleurum and Tang-kuei Formula, and Bupleurum and Peony and Six Major Herb Combination

- *Bupleuri radix polyporus, Poria (Hoelen), Atractylodes rhizoma, Paeoniae alba radix, Urantii fructus, Fructus oryzae germinatus, Fructus hordei germinatus, Endothelium corneum gigeriae galli, Fructus citri sarcodactylis, Glycyrrhiza uralensis fisch*

Modified Glehnia and Rehmannia Formula

- *Paeoniae alba radix, Aurantii fructus, Angelicae radix, Rehmanniae radix, Ophiopogonis radix, Fructus lycii, Glehniae radix, Cortex moutan radicis, Fructus meliae toosendan, Ligustri fructus, Polygoni multiflori radix, Zizyphi spinosi semen*

Modified Persica and Achyranthes Combination, and Persica and Cinidium Combination (Persica and Eupolyphaga Combination)

- *Carthami flos, Persicae semen, Cortex moutan radicis, Aurantii fructus, Leonuri herba, Cyperi rhizoma, Turmeric radix, Rhei rhizoma, Angelicae radix, Cnidii rhizoma, Rehmanniae radix, Paeoniae rubra radix, Achyranthis radix, Citri aurantii fructus, Bupleuri radix, Glycyrrhizae radix, Platycodi radix*

Ligustrin Capsule

- *Ligustrum lucidum ait*

Red Poeny Combination

- *Paeoniae rubra radix, Puerariae radix, Salviae miltiorrhziae radix, Persicae semen, Artemisiae capillaris herba, Aristolochiae fangchi radix*

Rhubarbin Tablet

- *Rhei rhizoma*

Tiao Ying Yin

- *Angelicae radix, Cnidii rhizoma, Paeoniae rubra radix, Rhei rhzoma, Polyporus, Poria (Hoelen), Corydalis yanhusao rhizoma, Dianthi herba, Zedoariae rhizoma, Mori radicis cortex, Leonuri fructus, Arecae pericarpipum*

PHARMACOLOGY OF HERBS AND FORMULAS

The following list of the *pharmacology* of the major herbal remedies is for reference only. If you choose to take any of these herbal remedies, it may be helpful to provide your western health care provider with this information. It will help him or her better understand what you are taking and how it may or may not affect any treatment he or she is prescribing.

HERBS

Allicin

- Allicin has a very wide spectrum of anti-infectious capabilities.
- It is effective against bacteria, mycobacteria, fungi, protozoa, and certain viruses.
- It is potent enough to treat many common infections such as bacillary dysentery, amebic dysentery, deep fungal infections, whooping cough, endobronchial tuberculosis, oxyuriasis (pinworms), trichomonas vaginitis, and others.
- It has been used in China for more than 20 years. For most of the above conditions, the cure rate is above 80%.
- It is virtually nontoxic. Its LD_{50} is 134.9 times higher than its therapeutic dose.

Artemisiae capillaris

- This is the main herb in TCM used to treat *jaundice*. It has the following pharmacological actions.
- It fosters *bile* secretion in both healthy or *carbon tetrachloride* liver damaged animals. The dry
  weight of the bile is increased with the increased secretion of the bile. Its *decoction* can decrease the tone of the sphincter of Oddi in anesthetized dogs.
- It has liver protective effects.
- It reduces carbon tetrachloride-induced liver damage and *ALT* elevation. It also helps recover liver *glycogen* and *RNA*.
- It lowers blood *lipids* and has fibrolytic effects.

Bupleuri Radix

- *Bupleuri radix* has the following liver-protective and biliary effects.
- It can protect the liver from *toxic* damage caused by galactosalmine, *Penicillium notatum* and carbon tetrachloride.
- It can increase bile secretion and the amount of bile salt in the bile.
- Its anti-inflammatory effect can be used to treat *inflammation* of the liver and gall bladder.

Coptis chinensis Franch

- *Coptis chinensis Franch* has antimicrobial properties.
- It can strongly suppress *Staphylococcus aureus, Streptococcus*, pneumococcus, *Vibrio comma*, anthrax bacillus, *Bacillus dysenteriae*, hay bacillus, pneumobacillus, *Bacillus diphtheriae, Bordetella pertussis, Brucellaceae*, and *Mycobacterium tuberculosis*.
- It can suppress influenza viruses and Newcastle disease virus *in vitro*.
- It can act against ameba, *Chlamydia trachomatis*, trichomonas, and *Leptospira*.
- It is virtually nontoxic. The LD_{50} is 205mg/kg.

Cordyceps Capsule (Cordyceps sinesis)

- In TCM, the various actions ascribed to Cordyceps Capsule are lung and kidney nourishing, vital essence and vital energy tonifying, hemostatic, and phlegm resolving or mucolytic.
- It is used in general debility after sickness, and for elderly persons.
- Its superior therapeutic effects have been confirmed in many controlled, well-designed studies carried out by medical schools in China including Beijing, Shanghai, and Nanjing.
- It is virtually nontoxic.
- The effects of this herb in *chronic* viral *hepatitis* have been studied. The efficacy rate was reportedly above 80% in a 256 patient clinical study. *Cordyceps sinesis* can lower ALT, improve liver function, relieve liver related *symptoms*, and increase *albumin*. It has also been used for *cirrhosis* caused by chronic viral hepatitis. In the previously mentioned study, 17 out of 22 patients had increased albumin levels after three months of treatment. Twelve of 17 patients with *ascites* experienced complete resolution of ascites while the other five had a reduction in ascites.[1]
- This herb is helpful for immunodeficiency caused by viral infection, *chemotherapy*, radiotherapy, major illness or surgery.
- *Cordyceps sinesis* is used to treat impotence, premature ejaculation, low libido, low sperm counts and/or activity, irregular menstruation, and leukorrhea.

Desmodii styracifolium Her

- This herb can facilitate bile secretion and help expel sandy gall stones.
- It can relax the sphincter of Oddi.
- It can abate biliary obstruction and pain.
- It prevents the precipitation of gallstone forming elements.

Glycyrrhizin (GL)

- GL has various pharmacological actions that can be useful in treating *hepatitis C*.
- GL has *antiviral* effects. It can induce the generation of interferon-gamma in test animals and humans. It can prolong the survival of mice after being injected with mouse hepatitis virus (MHV). In rabbits, it can inhibit vaccinia virus proliferation.
- GL protects liver cells from chemical injuries. It can alleviate *histological* changes due to carbon tetrachloride toxication, and lower ALT. It can reduce liver cell degeneration and *necrosis*, and help recover glycogen and RNA. Experimental hepatitis and cirrhosis studies in rats found GL can promote regeneration of liver cells and inhibit *fibrosis*. It can also reduce gamma-globulin and *interstitial* inflammation in the liver
- It has antiallergic, anti-inflammatory, and detoxifying activities that resemble those of glucocorticoid. GL also inhibits the release of histamine from mast cells.
- Although licorice is a nontoxic herb, long-term use of GL can cause adverse reactions in about 20% of patients. Adverse reactions include *edema*, rise in blood pressure, low blood potassium, dizziness, *fatigued* limbs, and others. **People with hypertension should not take GL**.
- The glycyrrhizin tablet used at Zhang's Clinic in New York City is a potassium salt of glycyrrhizic acid.

Ligustrum lucidum Ait

- Ligustrum is a highly purified extract of *Ligustrum lucidum fructus*. Its active chemical component is oleanolic acid. It can protect the liver from chemical and biological injuries.
- Ligustrum can lower ALT levels. In experimental cirrhosis studies, it has been found to inhibit degeneration and reduce necrosis of liver cells.[2] It can increase the glycogen in the liver, and accelerate the regeneration of liver cells. It can also inhibit inflammation and *collagen* formation.
- It can raise the white blood cell count, and is used to treat leukopenia caused by chemotherapy and radiotherapy.
- In *clinical trials* for hepatitis, ligustrum reduced ALT, *AST*, and jaundice.
- It promotes lymphoblast cell transformation and macrophage phagocytosis.
- Ligustrum can increase coronary blood flow.
- Acute and chronic *toxicity* tests have shown ligustrum has very low toxicity. After injecting dogs with 50mg/kg IV and mice with 5mg/20g IV, 24 hours of observation found no adverse reactions. After injecting rabbits with 50mg/kg IP daily for 6-12 weeks, there were no heart, liver, or kidney disorders found.

Marmodica charnatia (Bitter Melon)

- A 1981 clinical trial in England found that bitter melon (BM) can significantly improve *glucose* tolerance in type II diabetes.[3] A water soluble extract of BM can significantly reduce blood glucose concentrations during oral glucose tolerance tests.
- Animal studies with normal and diabetic rats and rabbits have shown BM has a hypoglycemic effect.[4] There are insulin-like molecules in the extract of BM that have physiological effects similar to those of *insulin*. The extract of BM can also stimulate the pancreas to secret insulin, so it can help type II diabetics produce more insulin. Some of the ingredients of BM can also prolong the effects of insulin. The blood sugar regulating effects of BM have different time phases, which make its blood sugar regulating effects gradual and steady. Comparative studies conducted in China found that its blood sugar reducing effects were similar to those of tolbutamide.[5]
- In China and southeast Asia, BM is a commonly consumed vegetable, which indicates that it is very safe.

Paederiae caulis

- In TCM, this herb is considered to be sweet with a slightly bitter aftertaste and a mild property.
- It is antirheumatic, digestant, antitussive, mucolytic, and analgesic. It also has sedative actions.
- It can elevate the pain threshold.
- *Paederiae caulis* inhibited spontaneous activity in mice experiments, and prolonged pentobarbital-induced sleep.[5]
- The total alkaloids of this herb inhibit the contraction of the isolated intestine, and antagonize spasm due to acetylcholine and histamine.
- *Paederiae caulis* has expectorant, antibacterial, hypotensive, and local anesthetic actions. It also has corticosteroid-like effects.
- *Paederiae caulis* has been used for many skin diseases such as eczema, neurodermatitis, and leprosy.

- This herb is also used to treat respiratory diseases such as bronchitis and whooping cough.
- It has a high LD50 and has virtually no toxicity.

Polygoni cuspidati rhizoma

- The 10% decoction of this herb inhibited Asian influenza virus type A, Jingke 68-1 strain, ECHO 11, and herpes simplex virus.[6]
- A stronger inhibitory action was exhibited by a 2% decoction against adenovirus type III,
  poliomyelitis virus type II, Coxsackie virus group A and B, ECHO 11 group, encephalitis B virus, and herpes simplex I strain. The MIC (minimal inhibitory concentration) against these viruses were 1:1600, 1:400, 1:400, 1:2560, 1:10240, 1:3200, and 1:51200, respectively. A 20% solution showed significant inhibitory action against the *hepatitis B* surface *antigen (HBsAg)*. The active principles I and II of the herb were able to decrease the HBsAg titer eight-fold.
- This herb has been used for chronic viral hepatitis, acute inflammatory diseases, neonatal
  jaundice, and leukopenia.

Rhei rhizoma (Rhubarb root)

- Extracts made by alcohol extraction of this herb contain aloe emodin, rhein, and chrysophanol.
- Pharmacological studies have found it has a wide antimicrobial spectrum. It can effectively suppress *Staphylococcus,* anthrax bacillu*s, Bacillus dysenteriae, Streptococcus*, and *E. coli*.[7] It is especially effective for *Staphylococcus* and *Streptococcus*.
- This herb also has antiviral effects. A strong inhibitory action against the influenza virus was exhibited by the herb decoction.[8] The minimum effective dose in chicken embryos was 5 mg per embryo.
- Clinically, rhubarb root has been used for indigestion, constipation, acute inflammatory diseases, infectious and parasitic diseases, hemorrhage, and thrombocytopenia (low platelets).
- Its strong purgative and laxative effects can be used to treat constipation.
- Chrysophanol has hemostatic effects (stops bleeding), and is often used for bleeding in the gastrointestinal system.
- The LD50 of rhubarb root is 250-500mg/kg. The LD50 of chrysophanol is 10grams/kg and is very safe.

Salviae miltiorrhziae radix (Salvia)

- Salvia improves the *microcirculation* in the liver. It markedly increases liver blood flow in acute and chronic carbon tetrachloride (CCl4) toxic models.[9] The fibrosis preventive effects of Salvia are mainly the result of its microcirculation improving effects.
- Salvia also improves microcirculation in people with coronary disease. In one study, 70% of the patients' conjunctiva and nail fold microcirculation improved with treatment.[10] In animal studies, the extract of this herb reversed the peripheral microcirculation blockage caused by intravenous infusion of 10% dextran.[10] It can increase blood supply to the heart and ischemic tissue.
- In the CCl4 toxic rat model, salvia can quickly lower ALT, and reduce inflammation, necrosis, and *steatosis* (fatty liver degeneration). In the control group, CCl4 caused liver collagen and globulin to increase from 19.8 mg/g to 51.4 mg/g, and 14.21 mg/

g to 23.04 mg/g, respectively. Every rat in the control group developed cirrhosis. In the salvia treated group, not a single rat developed cirrhosis, nor did the collagen and globulin increase.[11]

Schizandrae fructus

- Animal studies have shown the alcohol extract of the kernel of the fruit of schizandra (AEKFS) has many pharmacological activities such as:
  - lowering ALT caused by CCl4 induced liver damage
  - reducing fat deposits in liver cells caused by CCl4 intake
  - reducing the histological damage of the liver cells caused by CCl4
  - promoting glycogen and *serum* protein synthesis in the liver
  - promoting liver regeneration after partial removal of the liver, and
  - increasing metabolic *enzymes* in the liver.

- Clinical trials using tablets made from the whole AEKFS conducted in three hospitals in China found that of 107 chronic viral hepatitis cases, ALT was normalized for 73 with an associated improvement in clinical symptoms. There were no serious side effects reported.[12]

Sophorae subprostratae radix

- The active ingredient of this herb is oxymatrine. In three commonly used liver damage models (CCl4 induced rabbit, rat, and mouse liver damage models), oxymatrine prevented liver cell damage. Compared with the control group, the oxymatine treated group had much lower ALT, less liver cell necrosis, and much less inflammation.[13]
- Oxymatrine can increase cytochrome P-450 content and activity, and increase the amount of smooth surfaced endoplasmic reticulum of the liver cell.
- This herb is an inducer of the cytochrome P-450 system. Thus, it can strengthen the detoxification capability of the liver. It also has viral suppressive, anti-inflammatory, immunoregulatory, anticancer, and leukogenic (raising the white blood cell count) effects.

HERBAL FORMULAS

Capillaris Combination

- This is a very old and famous formula that was formulated by the Chinese medical sage Zhang Zhongjing about 2,000 years ago.
- Clinical Pharmacology
  - Clears dampness-heat type jaundice that manifests as bright yellowish coloration of the eyes and skin, oliguria with dark yellow urine, yellow and greasy fur on the tongue, a smooth and rapid pulse, and other signs and symptoms.
  - The whole formula has cholegogic and choleretic (facilitating bile secretion) effects. Intraduodenal administration of the alcohol extracts of this formula in rats markedly increased the bile collected by up to 51.28%, and increased the solid composition of the bile by 85%.[14] Its choleretic effects are mainly due to increasing the secretion of the bile in the micro bile ducts.
  - It has liver protective effects and can reduce the liver damage caused by a-naphthylisothiocyanate (ANIT). While using this formula, the ALP, total *bilirubin*, ALT, and AST elevations caused by ANIT all improved dramatically.[15]

- Histological examination revealed that hypertrophy of the micro bile duct cells, necrosis of liver cells, and inflammatory cell infiltration were much milder in treated animals compared with the untreated control group. The liver glycogen and RNA content were normalized, and the ALT activity was markedly reduced.[16]

Circulation No.1 Tablet

- This is a modified formula based on Persica & Achyranthes Combination and Persica & Cinidium Combination. Traditionally, these formulas were used for blood stagnancy or stasis that manifests with symptoms such as dark or purplish tongue, cold hands and feet, dark rings around the eyes, liver palm, spider moles, dry and itchy skin, rashes, lumps, and upper abdominal discomfort.
- Clinical Pharmacology
  - This formula can noticeably ameliorate the acute microcirculation disorder induced by macromolecular dextran in rats.[17] It dilates the microcapillaries, accelerates blood flow, and opens more micro-capillary networks. The result is to increase blood infusion to the tissues and stop the pathology caused by the microcirculation disorder. It can promote the phagocytosis by macrophages (Kupffer cells) in the liver. It can also clear the clotting factors in DIC (disseminated intravascular coagulation) and stop the progress of DIC.[18]
  - It will not prolong the PTT or *prothrombin time*. It can suppress the clustering of *platelets*.
  - It can improve phagocytosis by macrophages. It can also regulate cellular and humoral immunity.
  - It can noticeably suppress granuloma formation (a fibrotic activity).[19]

Ginseng and Atractylodes Formula

- This formula was first created by the National Medical Bureau of the Song Dynasty about 1,000 years ago.
- Clinical Pharmacology
  - This formula is used for strengthening digestion and vital energy. It is helpful for treating diarrhea, poor appetite, *emaciation*, and white and greasy fur on the tongue.
  - This formula can improve absorption in the intestinal tract. Giving the decoction of the formula increased water and chloride absorption in the intestine of rabbits under anesthesia.[20] It is an antagonist to the spastic effects of acetylcholine on the intestine.

HerSom Capsule

- Clinical Pharmacology
  - This formula has been studied in teaching hospitals in China. Randomized, controlled clinical trials have shown that this formula has sleep-inducing effects and improves the quality of sleep. In a study of 374 patients, improvement in sleep was found to be statistically equivalent to that of methaqualone.[21] HerbSom formula is not habit forming and has no hangover effect.
  - The pharmacological data of these herbs show that they may also have many beneficial effects on the cardiovascular and neurological systems of the body.

- These herbs have no harmful effects on the liver.
- **CAUTION: Keep this formula out of reach of children. This product should not be taken while driving a car or operating heavy machinery.**

Yunnan Paiyao Capsule

- This is a very famous traditional herbal medicine.
- Clinical Pharmacology
    - This formula can quickly stop bleeding in rat and rabbit liver injury models, and rabbit large artery injury models.[22] It has been shown to dramatically reduce clotting time in human and rabbit experiments.[23] The hemostatic effects begin 30 minutes after administration, and peaks 2-3 hours after administration. These effects can last for more than four hours. The hemostatic effect is due to a permeability change in the cell membranes of platelets. This causes the release of clotting factors from platelets that promote clotting.
    - This formula can suppress inflammation in various animal models.[24] The strength of its antiinflammatory effect is similar to that of corticosteroids.
    - It also has analgesic and antineoplastic (antitumor) effects.

APPENDIX VI

YOU AND YOUR HEALTH CARE

QUESTIONS TO ASK POTENTIAL HEALTH CARE PROVIDERS

There are a number of questions you might consider asking any potential health care provider. You may ask about his or her training, your level of participation in the decision-making process, his or her approach to treatment, and general issues such as insurance and how accessible he or she will be.

About Medical Training and Interests

- Are you board certified and/or licensed?

  Note: This question is relevant for all western doctors, but may not be for *complementary and alternative medicine (CAM)* providers. Some states require licensure for certain types of CAM practitioners while others do not.

- How much experience have you had with *hepatitis C* and how frequently do you treat people with this illness?
- Is hepatitis C one of your primary interests?
- [If you are having an invasive procedure such as a *liver biopsy*] How frequently do you perform the procedure? (Studies have shown the more experienced a health care provider is at a procedure, the better the outcome for the patient.)

About Approach to Treatment and Treatment Decisions

- How do you stay up-to-date on treatments?
- Do you have patients who participate in *clinical trials*?
- Which specialists, hospitals, and/or treatment centers do you work with?
- Are you comfortable with me seeking other medical opinions?
- Are you comfortable with me seeking information about hepatitis C and treatment options from other sources?
- If I decide to investigate and/or include CAM therapies in my treatment plan, will you work cooperatively with other practitioners such as acupuncturists, Chinese medicine specialists, herbalists, and naturopaths?

Other Concerns

- Do you accept my health insurance?
- Will you return my calls in a timely manner? How soon will someone answer my calls?
- Will I have access to you via e-mail? How soon will you answer my e-mail messages?

QUESTIONS TO HELP YOU COMMUNICATE EFFECTIVELY WITH YOUR HEALTH CARE PROVIDERS

Providing your health care practitioners with the answers to the following questions <u>about yourself</u> may help them work more effectively with you.

- Are you a cautious person or a risk taker?
- How do you approach decisions about your health?
- How much or how little do you want to participate in decisions about your treatment?

- Do you have any concerns about specific types of treatments?
- How much physical work does your job or other duties require?
- Is there anything significant going on in your life such as changes or problems in your family life or job that is causing you stress or that may interfere with your ability to follow a treatment plan?
- How much do you know about hepatitis C? How much do you want to learn?
- How do you feel about pain medication or mood altering drugs?
- How and when do you want to get information and in what form?

QUESTIONS TO HELP YOU GET THE INFORMATION YOU NEED FROM YOUR HEALTH CARE PROVIDERS

The following is a list of questions that people with hepatitis C often ask their health care providers. You may have many questions of your own to add to this list. Remember, there is no such thing as a stupid question. If you want to know, ask.

Your Diagnosis

- In understandable terms, what is wrong with me?
- How do you know that I have hepatitis C?
- What *genotype* of hepatitis C do I have?
- What is the *stage* of my hepatitis C?

Treatment Options

- What are the best treatment options for my stage of hepatitis C?
- Is watchful waiting or treatment more appropriate in my case?
- What is the goal of the treatment you have recommended? (Goals of treatment can include attempting a cure, slowing disease progression, and/or improving quality of life.)
- What will happen if I do not receive treatment?
- Are there treatments for my condition that are popular, but not approved? If they are not approved, why aren't they approved?
- What do you think of the unapproved treatments? (You may also want to ask about this if you hear about treatments your health care provider has not mentioned.)

Treatments Being Recommended

- What are the benefits of the treatment you are recommending?
- What are the names and dosages of the drugs/products/supplements you are recommending?
- How long and how often will I need to have treatment?
- What are the possible risks and side effects of the treatment being recommended?
- What will treatment cost?
- How can I expect my life to change during treatment, and how should I plan for this?
- Will I need to plan to rearrange work, childcare, travel, or other commitments if I go on this treatment and experience side effects?
- Once treatment ends, how often will I need follow-up visits?

How Treatment is Working

- How will we know if the treatment is working?
- If treatment is not successful, will the virus *mutate* or become resistant to potential future treatments?

Treatment Plan

- What should I do if I miss a treatment or dose?
- Are there foods or liquids I should eat or avoid?
- Are there prescription or over-the-counter medications or supplements I should take or avoid?
- What should I expect during treatment?
- How long will my treatment last?

After Treatment

- Is there any way to predict whether the hepatitis C virus is likely to return?
- If it does return, how will I know?
- If I respond to therapy, how often should I be tested for a *relapse*?

These questions are a guide. Other questions will most certainly come up for you. We encourage you to ask your health care providers whatever questions you need to have answered to feel comfortable with your treatment choices. Feeling comfortable and confident will ease your mind and help you adjust to whatever treatment protocol you choose.

APPENDIX VII

HCV/HIV COINFECTION

Liver-toxic medications and herbs

The following information is based on an appendix found in <u>The Hepatitis C Help Book</u> and is reprinted with the permission of the publisher, St. Martin's Press.

There is a great deal of research still to be done to identify those prescription medications, over-the-counter drugs, herbs and chemicals that are liver *toxic*. Some substances affect everyone negatively, some are dangerous for people who have liver disease. Others are hazardous when taken in too large a quantity, in combination with other substances or by people who have unusual immune responses.

The following list of suspected or confirmed liver-toxic medications and herbs should help guide anyone with hepatitis. It is not comprehensive, however, and any time a person with liver disease contemplates taking a drug or herb, even when prescribed by a health care practitioner, he or she should be on the lookout for negative reactions. Combining herbs with *interferon* and/or *ribavirin* demands particular care. Anyone with HCV should discuss potential reactions and drug interactions with both western and Chinese medicine practitioners before taking any medication or herbal remedy. Although liver-toxic substances are identifiable in the laboratory, liver hypersensitivity problems are not predictable. In some cases, hypersensitivity may result in organ failure. Although hypersensitivity is hard to anticipate, some indicators offer clues as to who may be vulnerable. Indicators of possible negative reactions to medical substances include:

- having multiple allergies and having had previous adverse reactions to drugs or herbs
- a history of chronic skin rashes
- current liver disease

Important! You should discontinue taking any drug or herb if you experience a skin rash, substantial nausea, bloating, fatigue and/or aching in the area of the liver, yellowing of the skin, or pale feces.

Dr. Gish has contributed information on liver-toxic drugs.

David L. Diehl, MD, FACP, an associate clinical professor of medicine at UCLA School of Medicine, focuses on herbal *toxicity*. He, Ken Flora, MD, formerly of the University of Oregon Health Sciences Center, and Misha Cohen are currently undertaking an extensive survey of the literature concerning the liver toxicity of herbal medicines.

PRESCRIPTION AND OVER-THE-COUNTER DRUGS

Patients who take the following medications regularly should undergo monthly laboratory testing for the first three months and then every three to six months to check on changes in liver function. Sample brand names are listed after the pharmaceutical name. Other products in addition to those mentioned may contain these drugs. Talk with your doctor and read all package inserts carefully.

- *acetaminophen* or APAP (Tylenol), particularly hazardous when taken with alcohol or anti-seizure medications
- alpha-methyldopa (Aldomet)
- amiodarone (Cordarone)
- azathioprine (Imuran, 6-mecaptopurine [6MP])
- carbamazapine (Tegretol, Epitol, Mazepine, Atretol, Carbatrol)
- chlorzoxazone (Parfon Forte DSC, Paraflex, Chlorzone Forte, Algisin)
- dantrolene (Dantrium)
- diclofenac (Voltaren, Cataflam)
- fluconazole or ketoconazole (Diflucan, Nizoral)
- flutamide (Drogenil, Euflex, Eulexin)
- hydralazine (Apresoline, Novo-Hylazin)
- ibuprofen (Advil, Motrin, Nuprin)
- isoniazid or INH (Laniazid, Nydrazid)
- long-acting nicotinic acid
- leukotriene synthase inhibitors (Zafirlukast, Accolate and Zileuton, Zyflo)
- methotrexate (Maxtrex)
- nitrofurantoin (Macrodantin)
- perihexilene maleate
- phenylbutazone (Mapap, Marnal, Lanatuss)
- phenytoin (Ethotoin, Mephenytoin, Dilantin)
- pravastatin, fluvastatin, simavastatin, lovastatin
- quinidine (Cardoquin, Cin-Quin, Duraquin)
- rifampin (Rifampicin, Rifadin, Rimactane)
- sulfa medications (especially Septra or Bactrim)
- tacrine (Cognex)
- ticlopidine (Ticlid)
- tolcapone (Tasmar)
- troglitzone (Rezulin)
- vitamin A (in doses greater than 5,000 units a day; beta-carotene is safe at all doses)

According to an article published in the April 1996 *New England Journal of Medicine*, the most common cause of acute liver failure in the United States is the negative interaction between *acetaminophen* (Tylenol) and alcohol. In addition, there are interactions that are less common but equally as serious. Research suggests individual genetic variations in *liver enzymes* may be the cause.

CHINESE HERBAL PREPARATION

Herbal patent medicines, tonics, elixirs and prepackaged solutions are particularly risky for anyone, whether they have liver disease or not. Ingredient labels may be incomplete or mistranslated. Herbs may be mistakenly used in the concoctions that are dangerous or inappropriate in combination with other herbs. Toxic herbs may be substituted for beneficial ones. The best bet is to avoid self-prescribed premixed preparations. Rely on the best-trained and most experienced herbalist available to individualize your herbal therapy and monitor your reactions. Some reportedly hazardous herbs and herb formulas:

Shosaikoto – a Japanese preparation used for improving *hepatic* dysfunction in *chronic hepatitis*. Its Chinese name is Xiao Chai Hu Tang. It may trigger *interstitial* pneumonia in people with chronic HCV who also are taking interferon, according to *Precautions* from the Pharmaceutical Affairs Bureau.

Jin Bu Huan – for insomnia and pain. This formula caused some liver problems but the exact trigger was never identified.

Aristolochia – used to treat fluid retention and rheumatic symptoms; has been banned in England after it was confused with an herb from the clematis plant that has the same name in Chinese as aristolochia: Mu Tong. The Mu Tong used was in fact the toxic species aristolochia rather than the other harmless herb. Aristolochia was part of a formula implicated in seventy cases of kidney failure in Belgium in 1993.

In addition, some Chinese patent medicines may contain heavy metals, poisons, and other potentially liver-toxic substances. In other cases, patent medicines contain western pharmaceutical agents that are not listed on the label.

Common Toxic Ingredients Found in Asian Patent Medicines: Be on guard for these ingredients.

- aconite or aconitum: causes paralysis and death if not highly processed before use
- acorus: causes convulsions and death
- borax: triggers severe kidney damage
- borneol: triggers internal bleeding and death
- cinnabar or calomel: a mercury compound
- litharge and minium: contain lead oxide
- myiabris: can trigger convulsions, vomiting and death
- orpiment or realgar: contains arsenic
- scorpion or buthus: causes paralysis of the heart and death
- strychnos nux vomica or semen strychni: strychnine-containing seeds cause respiratory failure
  and death
- toad secretion or bufonis: can paralyze heart muscle and lungs

TOXIC INDIVIDUAL HERBS

Dr. Diehl writes: "Herbal medicine is generally safe – safer than western pharmaceuticals. There are certain plants that are highly toxic. The most common examples are those that contain pyrolizidine alkaloids." Those that contain alkaloids or that reportedly have triggered toxic reactions include the following.

- Chaparral (creosote bush, greasewood)
- Comfrey (if taken internally)
- Crotalaria (Ye Bai He)
- Eupatorium
- Germander (This toxic herb is often substituted for skullcap, and skullcap is not toxic in well-formulated herbal remedies. However, always insist that any ingredient identified as skullcap be the genuine article and not germander.)
- Groundsel (senecio longilobus)
- Heliotropium
- Mentha pulegium
- Mistletoe

- Pennyroyal (squawmint) oil or Hedeoma pulegoides
- Sassafras
- Senicio species

SPECIAL CASES

Licorice: a mainstay of Chinese formulas, licorice is used in very small quantities to balance herbal action and often appears as glycyrrhizin (licorice root). However, licorice produces well-documented side effects such as hyperaldosteronism (an increase in levels of the adrenal hormone aldosterone, triggering imbalance of *electrolytes*) when taken in doses of more than 50 grams a day or for six weeks or longer. However, no side effects have been seen in smaller doses over thirty days or in higher doses for a very short period of time.

Skullcap: also called scutelleria or scute, this herb is used in many formulas to good effect. However, it appears that the toxic substance germander often is substituted for skullcap in formulas without being properly identified. As a result skullcap looks like the offending substance. Dr. Diehl found several mentions of skullcap toxicity in the literature, but those mentions may in fact refer to unidentified substitutions of germander. Further research is needed to clarify this. Until then, whenever skullcap appears in a formula, make sure that it, not germander, is in fact being used. If you cannot be sure, do not take the formula or herb.

Dr. Diehl has found one mention of toxicity in the literature for the following herbs. Further documentation of toxicity is needed.

- Calliepsis laureola
- Atractylis gunnifera
- margosa oil
- valerian (Valerian officinalis)

For more detailed information on substances toxic to the liver, please see:
The HIV Wellness Sourcebook, Henry Holt, Misha Cohen, 1998 and The Hepatitis C Help Book, Misha Cohen and Robert Gish, St. Martin's Press, 2000.

RESOURCE DIRECTORY

Disclaimer: The information contained in this Resource Directory is intended as reference material only. The Hepatitis C Caring Ambassadors Program makes no representation nor implies endorsement of any product or service, nor does it accept any responsibility for any claims made by any resources listed.

ORGANIZATIONS AND SUPPORT GROUPS

National Hepatitis C Advocacy Council
P.O. Box 1748
Oregon City, OR 97045
Phone: 503-632-9032
Fax: 503-632-9031
Internet address: http://www.hepcnetwork.org

The organizations listed below with an asterisk (*) are members of the National Hepatitis C Advocacy Council. The National Hepatitis C Advocacy Council is an association of organizations that creates a unified voice, promotes ethical guidelines, and improves the quality of services for people affected by hepatitis C. From this Internet address you can reach all member sites.

AIDS Community Research Consortium (ACRC)
1048 El Camino Real, Suite B
Redwood City, CA 94063-1633
Phone: 650-364-6563
Fax: 650-364-9001
Internet address: http://www.acrc.org

ACRC's mission it to improve health and quality of life through compassionate programs that address prominent and emerging public health concerns.

AIDS Treatment Data Network (The Network)
611 Broadway, Suite 613
New York, NY 10012
Phone: 212-260-8868 or (800)734-7104, ext. 16 (toll free in New York)
Fax: 212-260-8869
Internet address: http://www.atdn.org

The Network is an independent, nonprofit, community-based organization founded in 1988. The Network provides local and national services to people with HIV and coinfected with HCV/HIV. The Access Project (TheAccessProject@aol.com) is the agency's national treatment advocacy and access program. They advocate for patients and assist providers in obtaining treatments for hepatitis, HIV, and AIDS related conditions. The Network provides free, intensive case management services to people who are HIV positive. Specialized case management and treatment adherence programs are available for people in New York who are coinfected with HIV and HCV. National treatment information and counseling can be obtained via e-mail network@atdn.org or by phone.

American Liver Foundation *
75 Maiden Lane, Suite 603
New York, NY 10038-4810
Phone: 212-668-1000 or 800-676-9340
Fax: 212-483-8179
Internet address: http://www.liverfoundation.org

The American Liver Foundation is a national, voluntary, nonprofit health agency dedicated to preventing, treating, and curing hepatitis and all liver diseases.

The Ark Hepatitis C Support Group
719 Bakeway Court
Indianapolis, IN 46231
Phone: 317-838-0002
Internet address: http://www.hepatitis-central.com

The Ark is a hepatitis support group facilitated by people infected with the hepatitis C virus. The group seeks to help HCV patients gain a positive outlook through education and emotional support.

Back to Life
6252 Covington Way
Goleta, CA 93117
Phone: 805-692-2860
Fax: 805-964-0212

Back to Life
14252 Culver Drive A526
Irvine, CA 92604
Phone: 949-654-4250 or 888-85LIVER CA (toll-free)
Fax: 949-654-4251
Internet address: http://www.hepcCalifornia.org

Back to Life's missions are to increase public awareness, provide resources and education to the general public (including patients and groups at risk), and provide emotional and social support to patients with hepatitis C.

Connections
P.O. Box 4142
Bozeman, MT 59772-4142
Phone: 406-388-1262
E-mail: caseyconnections@msn.com

Connections' mission is to support and encourage positive life changes in all participants of our programs. Their goal is to lower the recidivism rate in Montana, and create healthier and safer communities in which to live. Connections believe in the power of knowledge and education, as well as supporting each other through life's journey. Support groups are open to people living with hepatitis C, their families, and interested members of the general public.

The First Year – Hepatitis C
2261 Market St. PMB 489
San Francisco, CA 94114
E-mail: cara@firstyearhepc.com and lisa@firstyearhepc.com
Internet address: http://www.firstyearhepc.com

This site is owned by Cara Bruce and Lisa Montanarelli, authors of the book The First Year - Hepatitis C published in March 2002 by Marlowe & Co. Both authors have hepatitis C. The site offers free excerpts from the book, a glossary of terms, links to hepatitis C resources, and other information.

Frontline Hepatitis Awareness *
701 West Elizabeth #54
Monroe, WA 98272
Phone: 360-805-1700
E-mail: Lama.Palmo@Verizon.net
Internet address: http://www.frontline-hepatitis-awareness.com

Frontline Hepatitis Awareness was founded in May 2000 on the Internet. Its goals are to provide people with information about hepatitis, bring together hepatitis support groups, patients, and organizations to work toward this common goal, offer services that otherwise might not be available, and give referrals.

Hep C Advocate Network (HepCAN) *
P.O. Box 3003
Longview, TX 75606
Phone: 903-291-9700
E-mail: hepcan1@aol.com
Internet address: http://www.hepcan.org

HepCAN is devoted to legislative changes for more testing and treatment of HCV infected individuals on the state and national level. They also work to increase professional education about hepatitis C.

Hep-C Alert *
660 Northeast 125th Street
North Miami, FL 33161
Phone: 877-HELP-4-HEP
Fax: 305-893-7998
Internet address: http://www.hep-c-alert.org

Hep C Alert is an educational, nonprofit organization working to raise public awareness and assist people affected by hepatitis C.

Hep C Connection *

1177 Grant Street, Suite 200
Denver, CO 80203
Phone: 303-860-0800 or 800-522-4372
Fax: 303-860-7481
Internet address: http://www.hepc-connection.org

Hep C Connection provides a hepatitis C network and support system to assist hepatitis C-challenged individuals and their families.

Hep C Education and Support Network *

PO Box 1231
Locust Grove, VA. 22508
Phone: 540-972-2856
Internet address: http://www.hepcesn.net

The Hep C Education and Support Network's mission is to educate the public and promote awareness through special events, programs, and the distribution of awareness pins. They provide support to patients living with hepatitis C through on-line support, educational brochures and posters, and a toll-free support line. They also work with methadone service providers to educate patients and staff about hepatitis C risks and management.

Hepatitis C Action & Advocacy Coalition (HAAC) *

James Learned
300 8th Avenue, # 5A
Brooklyn, NY 11215
E-mail: James_Learned@Prodigy.net

Brian Klein
530 Divisadero Street
Box 162
San Francisco, CA 94117
E-mail: HAAC_SF@hotmail.com

HAAC is a grassroots, all-volunteer group of individuals committed to nonviolent, direct action to end the hepatitis C crisis. They work to provide access to life-extending treatments to people with hepatitis C, foster effective prevention efforts, encourage sound public health policies, and ensure adequate funding and resources for the care, treatment, and prevention of hepatitis C. They do not accept money from pharmaceutical companies.

Hepatitis C Association*

1351 Cooper Road
Scotch Plains, NJ 07076
Phone: 866-437-4377
Fax: 908-561-4575
E-mail: info@hepcassoc.org
Internet address: http://www.hepcassoc.org

The Hepatitis C Association focuses on educating the public, creating awareness, promoting organ donation, and offering support to hepatitis patients. They do this through publications, an Internet site, a 24-hour toll-free support line, awareness pins, and educational programs.

Hepatitis C Awareness Project *

PO Box 41803
Eugene, OR 97404-0520
Phone: 541-607-5725
E-mail: hepcaware@aol.com

The Hepatitis C Awareness Project is an Oregon grassroots organization dedicated to increasing awareness about viral hepatitis, and educating the community about HCV prevention, diagnosis, and treatment. They are active in prison outreach and needle exchange. They produce a monthly newsletter for the state legislature and support group members.

Hepatitis C Caring Ambassadors Program *

PO Box 1748
Oregon City, OR 97045
Phone: 877-737-4372
Fax: 503-632-9031
Internet address: http://www.hepcchallenge.org

The Hepatitis C Caring Ambassadors Program is a privately funded nonprofit organization that was founded by a person with hepatitis C in search of treatment options. The Hepatitis C Caring Ambassadors Program has no drugs or products to sell, and no therapies or clinics to promote. The only philosophy promoted is that it is vitally important for people with hepatitis C to equip themselves with facts and information about the illness and the various treatment options available to them.

Hepatitis C Global Foundation *

1404 Madison Avenue
Redwood City, CA 94061-1550
Phone: 650-369-0330
Fax: 650-369-0331
Internet address: http://www.hcvglobal.org

The Hepatitis C Global Foundation is a grassroots, nonprofit organization dedicated to providing education and prevention programs for the millions of people worldwide who suffer with hepatitis C.

Hepatitis C Support Project *

P.O. Box 427037
San Francisco, CA 94142-7037
Phone: 415-587-8908
Internet address: http://www.hcvadvocate.org
The mission of the Hepatitis Support Project is to offer support to those who are affected by the hepatitis C virus (HCV). Support is provided through information and education, and access to support groups. The Project seeks to serve the HCV community and the general public.

Hepatitis Education Project *
4603 Aurora Ave
Seattle, WA 98103-6513
Phone: 206-732-0311
Internet address: http://www.scn.org/health/hepatitis

The Hepatitis Education Project is a nonprofit corporation that provides educational materials and support groups for hepatitis patients and their families.

Hepatitis Foundation International
504 Blick Drive
Silver Spring, MD 20904-2901
Phone: 301-622-4200
Internet address: http://www.hepfi.org/

Hepatitis Foundation International works to increase awareness of the worldwide problem of viral hepatitis, and to educate the public and health care providers about its prevention, diagnosis, and treatment.

Hepatitis Magazine *
523 N. Sam Houston Parkway East, Suite 300
Houston, TX 77060
Phone: 281-272-2744 Ext. 132
Fax: 281-847-5440
Internet address: http://www.hepatitismag.com/

Hepatitis magazine is the only national magazine dedicated to people with hepatitis B and C. The magazine is a bimonthly resource guide to assist hepatitis patients and their families in taking control of their health care by providing current, comprehensive information in one source.

Hepatitis Research Foundation *
RR 2 Box 12
Verbank, NY 12585
Internet address: http://www.heprf.org

The Hepatitis Research Foundation's mission is to raise money for research into new treatments for hepatitis.

Hepatitis United
765 North River Road
Oregon, IL 61061
Phone: 815-332-9600
Internet address: http://www.hepu.org

Hepatitis United is a nonprofit organization promoting wellness from within, including natural hepatitis treatments.

HepSource
P.O. Box 43653
Tucson, AZ 85733
Phone: 520-881-0141
Fax: 520-881-0141
E-mail: hepsource@earthlink.net

As southern Arizona's only hepatitis C centered agency, HepSource offers educational presentations and training opportunities on the local and national level. Carefully researched information is made available via individual counseling, support groups, referrals, and a 24-hour telephone helpline. Services are based on the notion that clear, fact-based information empowers the individual to make the best possible choices when facing the challenges of hepatitis C.

Hope4Heppers *
3353 Easton Road
Edgewater, MD 21037
Phone: 410-956-8191
Email: hope4heppers@aol.com

Hope4Heppers is a nonprofit organization providing emotional and financial support to people with hepatitis. Their goal is to help establish support groups, assist support group leaders to defray the cost of running support groups, and eventually be able to alleviate some of the financial burden of people with hepatitis.

Latino Organization for Liver Awareness (LOLA)
1560 Mayflower Avenue
Bronx, NY 10461
Phone: 718-892-8967
Internet address: http://www.lola-national.org

LiverHope, Inc.*
16807 Canterbury Drive
Minnetonka, MN 55345
Phone: 952-933-0932
Internet address: http://www.liverhope.com
LiverHope provides support, promotes education, generates awareness and advocates for quality medical care for all people with Hepatitis in the Metropolitan Minneapolis and St. Paul area of Minnesota.

Missouri Hepatitis C Alliance (MOCHA)*
10800 E. Walnut Dr.
Centralia, MO 65240
Phone: 573-682-1714
E-mail: bburkett@socket.net

MOHCA holds three area support group meetings on a regular basis. They also provide information for patients, families, and health care providers.

National Hepatitis C Coalition, Inc.

P.O. Box 921
Smyrna, TN 37167
Phone: 615-355-8604
Internet address: http://nationalhepatitis-c.org

The National Hepatitis C Coalition was the first nationwide coalition of hepatitis C patients and their families. It is a nonprofit tax exempt organization that provides education and support through on-line communication, a 24-hour HepLine, and grassroots support groups across America.

Nor-Cal Hepatitis C Task Force

1689 Torry Pine Drive
Yuba City, CA 95993
Phone: 530-671-7441
Fax: 530-671-7442
E-mail: ziegler@clear-cxn.net

The Nor-Cal Hepatitis C Task Force is a nonprofit organization that was founded in 1996. They offer educational classes to professionals, social workers, drug and alcohol counselors, CPS workers, drug and alcohol recovery programs, and correctional facilities. They are involved in many community service events such as health fairs, and back-to-school nights.

SAGE Project

1275 Mission Street
San Francisco, CA 94103
Phone: 415-905-5050
Internet address: http://www.sageinc.org

The SAGE Project is women working together to heal from the pain and trauma of abuse and to find alternatives to a life of drug addiction, violence, and prostitution.

United Foundation for Patient Humanities

1444 Hidden Creek South
Saline, MI 48176
Phone: 734-429-7374
Internet address: http://www.ufph.org

United Foundation for Patient Humanities is a nonprofit, volunteer organization operated by a blend of patients and health care professionals with the mission of restoring quality of life to those affected by HCV and related chronic diseases by providing resources and programs unique to the needs of patients and loved ones.

Veterans Aimed Toward Awareness *
111 West Main St.
Middletown, DE 19709
Phone: 302-378-1415
Fax: 302-633-5415
Internet address: http://www.veteranshepaware.com

Veterans Aimed Toward Awareness is committed to providing every veteran with what he or she needs to know about hepatitis C.

GENERAL MEDICAL INFORMATION INTERNET SITES THAT INCLUDE INFORMATION ABOUT HEPATITIS C

Aetna Intelihealth
Internet address: http://www.intelihealth.com

This site is sponsored by the Aetna, Inc., an insurance company that is part of a larger international conglomerate. This site features Harvard Medical School's Consumer Health Information.

The Alternative Health News On-line
Internet address: http://www.altmedicine.com

The Alternative Health News On-line site provides information on alternative and conventional medicine as it relates to various health issues including hepatitis.

The American Association of Naturopathic Physicians
Internet address: http://www.naturopathic.org

This official site of the American Association of Naturopathic Physicians offers a variety of resources on naturopathic medicine including a message board, library, and a naturopathic physician finder.

The American College for Advancement in Medicine (ACAM)
Internet address: http://www.acam.org

The American College for Advancement in Medicine (ACAM) is a nonprofit medical society dedicated to educating physicians and other health care professionals on the latest findings and emerging procedures in preventive/nutritional medicine. ACAM's goals are to improve skills, knowledge, and diagnostic procedures as they relate to complementary and alternative medicine, to support research, and to develop awareness of alternative methods of medical treatment.

The American Board of Medical Specialties (ABMS)
Internet address: http://www.certifieddoctor.org

The American Board of Medical Specialties (ABMS) site has a public education program, a physician locator, and information services. The board certification status, location by city and state, and specialty of any physician certified by one or more of 24 member boards of the ABMS can be checked through this site. This service is free to consumers. Listed physicians have subscribed to be included in this service.

The American Medical Association (AMA)
Internet address: http://www.ama-assn.org

The American Medical Association (AMA) site has a consumer health section that includes links to general health issues, specific conditions, your body, your family's health, Kids Health Club, Doctor Finder, Hospital Finder, and a Medical Group Practice Finder. The nutrition section has information on such things as vitamins and fitness. It also has a medical glossary. There is a link to recipes, and new ones are posted every two weeks. This link also has information on health oriented cookbooks and nutritional resources.

The British Medical Journal
Internet address: http://www.bmj.com

The British Medical Journal is a free publication with up-to-date information about hepatitis C, among many other topics.

CellMate Wellness Systems
Internet address: http://www.carbonbased.com/cbcblood.htm
A great site for understanding blood test results and blood chemistry definitions.

CenterWatch
Internet address: http://www.centerwatch.com

CenterWatch is a clinical trials listing service of industry and government sponsored trials including recently FDA approved drug therapies.

ClinicalTrials.gov
Internet address: http://www.clinicaltrials.gov

This site is sponsored by the National Cancer Institute, and provides current information on many clinical trials.

Doc Misha's Chicken Soup Chinese Medicine
Internet address: http://www.docmisha.com

This site has general information about Chinese medicine. There is specific information about HIV/AIDS and hepatitis C.

Dr. Koop.com
Internet address: http://www.drkoop.com

Dr. Koop is a former United States Surgeon General. This site provides up-to-date information on hepatitis C and available treatments.

Dr. Weil.com
Internet address: http://www.drweil.com

Dr. Andrew Weil is a leader in the integration of western medicine and the exploding field of alternative medicine. This site has extensive information about integrated medicine.

Dr. Zhang.com

Internet address: http://www.dr-zhang.com

This site provides information on modern Chinese medicine specifically related to hepatitis C. There is also information about some other diseases such as Lyme's disease and inflammatory bowel syndrome.

eBioCare.com

Internet address: http://www.eBioCare.com

This site provides information on risk factors, lifestyle, diet, and treatment options for people living with hepatitis C.

Healthfinder

Internet address: http://www.healthfinder.gov

The Healthfinder site is easy to navigate and has a tremendous amount of information. There is a lot of good information on hepatitis C and non-western medicine under the "Hot Topics" section. The non-western medicine information includes links for general information, therapies, nutrition and lifestyle information, quackery and fraud, training and associations, and other topics.

Health World On-line

Internet address: http://www.healthy.net

This comprehensive site provides access to information on a variety of therapies including acupuncture, Ayurveda, Chinese medicine, chiropractic medicine, homeopathy, and others. There are links to finding a health care provider for several different disciplines. This site has links to information on several diseases and conditions including hepatitis.

Hepatitis Awareness Center

Internet address: http://www.hepaware.com

This site is sponsored by Priority Healthcare Corporation. There is information on hepatitis C, and a free information packet is available.

The Hepatitis B Foundation

Internet address: http://www.hepb.org

The Hepatitis B Foundation is a national, nonprofit organization dedicated to finding a cure for hepatitis B and improving the quality of life of people affected by the illness. There are Chinese, Korean, and Vietnamese language versions of this site.

Hepatitis C Support Project
Internet address: http://www.hcvadvocate.org

The mission of the Hepatitis Support Project is to offer support to those who are affected by the hepatitis C virus (HCV). Support is provided through information and education, and access to support groups. The Project seeks to serve the HCV community and the general public. The Project also operates an informative Internet site that addresses HCV and HIV/HCV coinfection. The HCV Advocate Newsletter is available for download. Educational materials are available in English and Spanish. There is information on support groups, clinical trials, and regularly updated news items on HCV. The Medical Writers' Circle features articles written by respected and knowledgeable physicians in the field of liver disease.

Hepatitis C United Resource Exchange
Internet address: http://www.sci.ouc.bc.ca/gray/hepcure

The mission of the Hepatitis C United Resource Exchange is to cultivate an international network promoting hepatitis C education. There are sections on research, articles, links, and events.

Hepatology
Internet address: http://www.hepatology.org

This site provides access to *Hepatology,* the official journal of the American Association for the Study of Liver Diseases.

Herb Research Foundation
Internet address: http://www.herbs.org

The Herb Research Foundation is a source of accurate, science-based information on the health benefits and safety of herbs, and expertise in sustainable botanical resource development. The site has herb safety reviews and information packets.

Herbal Hall
Internet address: http://www.herb.com

This is the home of the professional herbalists' discussion list. Visit the HerbFiles for information about specific herbs. The site also has Herb News and frequently asked questions.

HIVandHepatitis.com
Internet address: http://www.HIVandHepatitis.com

The staff of HIVandHepatitis.com is a group of individuals closely linked to the communities of people living with HIV, hepatitis B, and hepatitis C. Their common objective is to create a quality, on-line publication that provides practical, reliable information about treatment and experimental vaccine options for these chronic conditions.

ITM On-line (Institute for Traditional Medicine)
Internet address: http://www.itmon-line.org

This is the site of the Institute for Traditional Medicine. The Articles section has a Disorders Index that will take you to articles on hepatitis C. The General Index has good basic information on a wide variety of topics including acupuncture, the best time of day to take herbs, qi gong, the immune system, pregnancy, and Chinese herbs. The Action Index has a Chinese herbal medicine primer designed for western health care providers. You may want to print it out and give it to your western health care provider if he or she has concerns about treatment options you are considering. In addition, the Action Index has information on Native American traditional medicine, Tibetan medicine resources, and other useful information.

The Lancet
Internet address: http://www.thelancet.com

Lancet is a peer-reviewed medical journal. You are able to search for articles on hepatitis C and are able to view the abstracts free, but there are fees if you want to view the full text of the articles.

Lab Tests Online
Internet address: http://www.labtestsonline.org/understanding/index.html
A public resource on clinical lab testing from the laboratory professionals who do the testing.

National AIDS Treatment Advocacy Project
Internet address: http://www.natap.org
NATAP posts new articles daily. From up to the minute conference reports, to the latest breaking news regarding HIV, HCV or HIV/HCV Coinfection information.

National Center for Complementary and Alternative Medicine (NCCAM)
Internet address: http://www.nccam.nih.gov

The National Center for Complementary and Alternative Medicine (NCCAM) at the National Institutes of Health (NIH) conducts and supports basic and applied research and training and disseminates information on complementary and alternative medicine to practitioners and the public. There are sections on health information, current and completed research, news and events, and alerts and advisories.

The New England Journal of Medicine
Internet address: http://www.nejm.org

This is the site of the medical journal, *The New England Journal of Medicine*. It provides access to the PubMed database from which you can search for and order medical journal articles on hepatitis C.

Net Wellness
Internet address: http://www.netwellness.com

This site is sponsored by the University of Cincinnati but is a joint project of Case Western Reserve University, Ohio State University, and the University of Cincinnati. The site is a consumer health information site and has sections on current health news, health topics, clinical trials and more.

Oasis, Inc.
Internet address: http://www.oasisclinic.org

The Organization to Achieve Solutions in Substance Abuse (Osais) is a nonprofit organization. The primary mission of Oasis is to provide low-cost, subsidized medical care, clinical research studies, and provision of and/or access to social and vocational rehabilitation services for medically marginalized former or current drug and alcohol users. They focus on people in the Oakland, California area.

United Network for Organ Sharing
Internet address: http://www.unos.org

This is the site of the United Network for Organ Sharing whose mission is to advance organ availability and transplantation. The site has news articles related to organ transplantation.

U.S. Pharmocopeia (USP)
Internet address: http://www.usp.org

In pursuit of its mission to promote public health, U.S. Pharmocopeia establishes state-of-the-art standards to ensure the quality of medicines for human and veterinary use. USP also develops authoritative information about the appropriate use of medicines. The site has prescription drug information and information about supplements.

WebMD
Internet address: http://www.webmd.com

This site is owned by WebMD Corporation. This is a comprehensive on-line resource committed to providing general health information and support. The site is extensive.

WellMed
Internet address: http://www.wellmed.com/wellmed

WellMed is owned by The Health Communication Company. The site is an on-line, personal health management service. Their services allow individuals to receive the accurate, personalized health information they need to maintain and improve their health. Tailored to the individual needs of each user, the health information that WellMed delivers can also help people communicate their health care requirements more effectively to employers, health plan, and care providers.

INTERNET RESOURCES FOR INFORMATION ON HEALTHCARE PROVIDERS

A Note About Fee-Based Referral Services

Many referral services are fee-based, which means that while they may be free for you to access, the health care providers pay a fee to be listed. Therefore, these services do not guarantee the experience level of the health care provider, they just provide general information. It will be up to you to find out if a health care provider listed with these services has experience with hepatitis C.

Information and Referral Resources on the Internet for Western (Allopathic and Osteopathic) Health Care Providers

American Medical Association
Internet address: http://www.ama-assn.org

The Doctor Finder link or AMA Physician Select allows you to search for a physician by name or medical specialty.

American Board of Medical Specialties (ABMS)
Internet address: http://www.certifieddoctor.org
This site has a public education program, a physician locator, and information services. You can verify the board certification status, location by city and state, and specialty of any physician certified by one or more of the 24 member boards of the ABMS. This service is free to consumers but physicians have subscribed to be listed in this service.

Information and Referral Resources on the Internet for Non-Western Health Care Providers

American Institute of Homeopathy
801 North Fairfax Street, Suite 306
Alexandria, VA 22314
Phone: 703-246-9501
E-mail: aih@bigplanet.com
Internet address: http://www.homeopathyusa.org

American Naturopathic Medical Association
P.O. Box 96273
Las Vegas, Nevada 89193
Phone: 702-897-7053
Internet address: http://www.anma.com
The American Naturopathic Medical Association will make referrals to naturopathic physicians and homeopathic practitioners.

HealthWorld On-line
Internet address: http://www.healthy.net
This comprehensive site provides links to resources for help in finding a health care provider in several different disciplines.

Institute for Traditional Medicine (ITM)
Internet address: http://www.itmon-line.org

This site has extensive information about CAM disciplines. There are also direct links to other sites on topics such as Chinese medicine, Tibetan medicine, Ayurvedic medicine, Native American medicine, western medicine, and others.

Healthfinder

Internet address: http://www.healthfinder.gov

Once on this site, look under Smart Choices for a link to Choosing Quality Care. You can find direct links to organizations such as:

- American Association of Acupuncture and Oriental Medicine
- American Holistic Health Association
- American Massage Therapy Association, and
- National Center for Homeopathy.

CONSUMER AND GOVERNMENT RESOURCES

Americans with Disabilities Act Information Line

Phone: 800-514-0301 (voice) or 800-514-0383 (TDD)

Centers for Disease Control and Prevention

Internet address: http://www.cdc.gov

Consumer Health Information Research

Phone: 816-228-4595

Department of Justice

Internet address: http://www.usdoj.gov

Equal Employment Opportunity Commission

For questions:
    Phone: 800-669-4000 (voice) or 800-669-6820 (TDD)
To request documents:
    Phone: 800-669-3362 (voice) or 800-800-3302 (TDD)

Food and Drug Administration (FDA)

Office of Special Health Issues
Parklawn Building, HF-12
5600 Fishers Lane
Rockville, MD
Phone: 800-FDA-1088
Internet address: http://www.fda.gov

Contact the FDA to report side effects or other problems with drug treatment.

Food and Nutrition Information Center

National Agricultural Library/USDA
10301 Baltimore Avenue, Room 304
Beltsville, MD 20705-2351
Internet address: http://www.nal.usda.gov/fnic/pubs/bibs/gen/dietsupp.html

This site provides a dietary supplement resource list.

National Center for Complementary and Alternative Medicine Clearinghouse

Phone: 888-644-6226
Internet address: http://www.nccam.nih.gov

You can request free information either on-line or by phone.

National Council Against Health Fraud
Phone: 909-824-4690

National Digestive Diseases Info Clearinghouse

Phone: 301-654-3810
Internet address: nddic@info.niddk.nih.gov

You can request free information either on-line or by phone.

National Foundation for Infectious Diseases

Phone: 301-656-0003
Internet address: http://www.nfid.org

National Institutes of Health

Phone: 301-496-1776
Internet address: http://www.nih.org

National Library of Medicine

Internet address: http://www.nlm.nih.gov

Social Security Disability Line
Phone: 800-772-1213

U.S. Department of Health and Human Services

Internet address: http://www.healthfinder.com

PHARMACEUTICAL COMPANIES

Roche Medical Services
Phone: 800-526-6367

Roche Hepline: 800-443-6676
Internet address: http://www.rocheusa.com

Schering "Be in Charge" Program
Phone: 888-437-2608
"Commitment to Care": 800-521-7157
Internet address: http://www.beincharge.com

RECOMMENDED READING

Books on Hepatitis C

Healing Hepatitis C with Modern Chinese Medicine, Qingcai Zhang, M.D., Sino-Med Institute, New York, NY. 2000.

Hepatitis and Liver Disease; What You Need to Know, Melissa Palmer, MD, Avery. Vonore, TN. 2000.

Hepatitis C, T.Liang, J. Hoofnagle, et al. Academic Press. San Diego, CA. 2000.

Living with Hepatitis C: A Survivor's Guide, Gregory T. Everson, Hedy Weinberg, John M. Vierling. Hatherleigh. Long Island City, NY. 1999.

My Mom Has Hepatitis C, Hedy Weinberg, and Shira Shump, Hatherleigh, Long Island City, NY. 2000.

The Hepatitis C Handbook, Matthew Dolan, Iain M. Murray-Lyon, John Tindall. North Atlantic Books. Berkeley, CA. 1999.

The Hepatitis C Help Book: : A Groundbreaking Treatment Program Combining Western and Eastern Medicine for Maximum Wellness and Healing, Misha Ruth Cohen, Robert G., M.D Gish, Kalia Doner (Contributor). St. Martins Press. New York, NY. 2000.

Other Health Care Books

Alternative Medicine: The Definitive Guide, Burton Goldberg Group. Future Medicine Publishing. Tiburon, CA. 1994.

Between Heaven and Earth: A guide to Chinese Medicine, Harriet Beinfield, LAc, Efrem Korngold, OMD, LAc. Ballantine Books. New York, NY. 1991.

Chinese Herbal Medicine, Formulas and Strategies, Compiled and translated by Dan Bensky and Andrew Gamble, with Ted Kaptchuk. Eastland Press. Vista, CA. 1986.

The Chinese Way to Healing: Many Paths to Wholeness, Misha Cohen, OMD, LAc. Penquin Putnam. New York, NY. 1996.

Complete Drug Reference, United States Pharmacopeia 2002. Rockville, MD. 2002. (This is an annual publication.)

Depression-Free, Naturally: 7 Weeks to Eliminating Anxiety, Despair, Fatigue, and Anger from Your Life, Joan Mathews-Larson, Ballantine Books, 2001

Discovering Homeopathy: Medicine for the 21st Century, Dana Ullman and Ronald W. Davey. North Atlantic Books. Berkeley, CA. 1991.

Eat, Drink and be Wary, T. Graedon. Rodale Inc. Emmaus, PA. 2000.

Eating Well for Optimum Health: The Essential Guide to Food, Diet, and Nutrition, Andrew Weil, Alfred A Knopf. New York, NY. 2000.

The Encyclopedia of Natural Medicine, M. Murray and J. Pizzorno. Prima Publishing. Roseville, CA. 1997.

The Green Pharmacy, J. Duke. St. Martin's Press. New York, NY. 1998.

The HIV Wellness Sourcebook, Misha Cohen. Henry Holt and Company. New York, NY. 1998.

Homeopathic Methodology: : Repertory, Case Taking, and Case Analysis: : An Introductory Homeopathic Workbook, Todd Rowe, Roger Morrison. North Atlantic Books. Berkeley, CA. 1998.

The Illustrated Encyclopedia of Healing Remedies; Over 1000 natural remedies for the prevention, treatment, and cure of common ailments and conditions. CN Shealy, Shaftsbury, Dorset. Elephant Books. Gilroy, CA. 1998.

Natural Health, Natural Medicine: A Comprehensive Manual for Wellness and Self-Care, Andrew Weil. Houghton Mifflin Co. Boston, MA. 1998.

PDR for Herbal Medicines, J. Gruenwald et al. Medical Economics Co. Montvale, NJ. 1998.

The People's Pharmacy to Home and Herbal Remedies, J. Graedon and T. Graedon. St. Martin's Press. New York, NY. 1999.

Physicians' Desk Reference (PDR®), Medical Economics Co. Montvale, NJ. 2002. (This is an annual publication.)

Pocket Manual of Meterica Medica with Repertory, Boericke, William, M.D., Jain. 1982.

Quantum Healing, Deepak Chopra. Bantam Books. New York, NY. 1989.

Repertory of the Homoeopathic Materia Medica, J.T. Kent. South Asia Books. Columbia, MO. 1994.

Return of the Rishi, Deepak Chopra. Houghton Mifflin Co. Boston, MA. 1988.

Seven Weeks to Sobriety, Joan Mathews Larson, Fawcett Books, 1997

The Web That Has No Weaver, Ted Kaptchuk. Contemporary Books. Chicago, IL. 1983.

GLOSSARY

Abstinence – the act or practice of refraining from something such as a food or alcohol

Acetaldehyde – a compound that is produced in the body from the breakdown of alcohol

Acetaminophen – an over-the-counter pain reliever; known by the trade name Tylenol®; found in many over-the-counter cold and sinus products

Acute hepatitis – a course of hepatitis (liver inflammation) that resolves in six months or less

Adjuvant – a substance that enhances the effect of a drug or treatment; a substance added to a vaccine to increase the immune response to the vaccine

Advocate – a person who works for the benefit and rights of others

Alanine aminotransferase (ALT) – an enzyme found in liver cells; measuring blood levels is an indicator of liver cell damage and/or death

Albumin – a protein made by the liver; blood levels are used to check liver function

Alpha-fetoprotein – a protein produced by liver cells normally found in only trace amounts in the body; the blood test for this substance is used as a screen for liver cancer (hepatocellular carcinoma)

Alpha glucosidase inhibitors – drugs that delay the digestion of sugars (carbohydrates); drugs used to treat type II or adult onset diabetes mellitus

ALT – see alanine aminotransferase

Amantadine – a drug used to prevent cells from being infected by a virus by interfering with the virus' ability to enter the cell

Amino acid – one of a group of substances that are the building blocks of proteins

Analogue – a molecule or substance that closely resembles another substance and may act like the original substance in some ways; sometimes called an isomer

Anasarca – generalized swelling (edema) of the body due to an abnormal accumulation of fluid in the tissues; can be seen in liver failure

Anecdotal – referring to an anecdote (see below)

Anecdote – in medicine, an account of one person's experience usually with a particular treatment

Anemia – a condition in which the blood is deficient in red blood cells and/or hemoglobin; a condition that reduces the blood's ability to carry oxygen to the tissues

Antibody – a protein produced by the immune system usually in response to infecting organisms such as bacteria or viruses; antibodies are one way the immune system tries to rid the body of infection

Antigen – a protein against which the immune system produces an antibody; derived from the words antibody generator

Anti-HCV antibody – any of a number of antibodies produced by the immune system in response to the hepatitis C virus; the presence of these antibodies in the blood mean that the person has been exposed to the hepatitis C virus; the screening test for hepatitis C (the anti-HCV test) detects these antibodies in the blood

Antioxidant – a substance that inhibits the chemical process called oxidation; in hepatitis C, antioxidants are used to limit damage done by high levels of free radicals present because of the ongoing inflammation caused by the virus

Antiproliferative – having the effect of decreasing the ability of something to rapidly grow and increase in number

Antisense – in drug development, a small molecule that binds to part of the genetic material of a target substance (such as the hepatitis C virus) to stop specific metabolic (life sustaining) functions; in hepatitis C, researchers are trying to develop antisense drugs that will prevent HCV replication (reproduction)

Antiviral – an agent that kills viruses or suppresses their replication (reproduction)

Apoptosis – a process of programmed cell death, which causes the cell to die within a specific timeframe

Arthralgia – pain in one or more joints

Ascites – abnormal accumulation of fluid in the abdomen; a common complication of portal hypertension

Aspartate aminotransferase (AST) – an enzyme found in liver cells; measuring blood levels is an indicator of liver cell damage and/or death

AST – see aspartate aminotransferase

Asymptomatic – without symptoms

B cell — (also called B lymphocyte) an immune cell that when activated produces antibodies; the cells responsible for the body's humoral (antibody) immune response

B cell lymphoma – a form of B cell cancer

Bile – a yellowish green fluid made by the liver from bile salts, bilirubin (broken down red blood cells), cholesterol, and other substances; the fluid stored in the gallbladder; the fluid released from the gallbladder into the intestine to help fat digestion

Bilirubin – a yellow-orange substance generated in the liver from the breakdown of hemoglobin from old red blood cells; the substance that causes jaundice when blood levels are abnormally high; blood levels are one indicator of liver function

Biofeedback – a way of monitoring small changes in the body with the aid of sensitive machines; a technique used to teach people to control bodily functions such as blood pressure, temperature, blood flow, gastrointestinal functioning, and brainwave activity

Bleeding esophageal varices – see varix

Blood serum – the liquid part of blood; the liquid that separates from blood when it clots completely

Body mass index (BMI) – a measure of weight in proportion to height; an indicator of being over or underweight; a number calculated by dividing your weight (in kilograms) by height (in meters squared); a healthy BMI for adults is between 18.5 and 24.9

Bone marrow suppression – inhibition of the body's ability to produce blood cells that are normally made in the bone marrow

Branched DNA test for HCV (b-DNA) – test used to check for the presence of the hepatitis C virus in the blood

Carbohydrate – a sugar (simple carbohydrate) or starch (complex carbohydrate); a food component found in sugars, certain vegetables, grains, and beans

Carbon tetrachloride-induced hepatotoxicity – liver damage resulting from exposure to carbon tetrachloride (CCl_4); liver damage caused by exposure to any of a number of substances containing CCl_4 such as dry cleaning fluid, solvents, rubber waxes, and resins

Carcinogenic – capable of causing cancer

Cardinal signs – signs that indicate the presence of a specific disease or condition

CD4 cell – (T4 cell, T-helper cell) an immune cell that participates in the body's cellular immune response; the cell that is the main target of the human immunodeficiency virus; immune cells that help turn on the body's immune response

CD4 count, absolute – the number of T-helper cells in a cubic millimeter of blood; also called a T4 count

CD8 – (T8 cell, T-suppressor cell, cytotoxic T-cell) an immune cell that participates in the body's cellular immune response; cells that destroy virus-infected cells and cause transplant rejection

CD81 – a protein on the surface of cells including liver cells; another term for TAPA-1 molecule (target of an antiproliferative antibody); may be a binding site for the hepatitis C virus that allows it to enter cells

Chemotherapy – the use of chemical agents to treatment or control disease; commonly refers to drugs used to kill cancer cells

Cholestasis – slowed or blocked bile flow; may be associated with elevated bilirubin levels

Chronic hepatitis – a course of hepatitis (liver inflammation) that lasts more than six months

Cirrhosis = scarring of the liver that has progressed to the point that the structure of the liver is abnormal; the stage of liver disease that follows if there is progressive fibrosis

cis – a chemical prefix that refers to a specific arrangement of chemical bonds; the opposite of this chemical arrangement is known as trans

Clinical – in medicine, anything related to disease that can be observed or diagnosed in a patient

Clinical trials – process used to evaluate the effectiveness and safety of new medications, procedures, or medical devices by monitoring their effects on large groups of people; the testing usually required by the Food and Drug Administration before approving a new drug, procedure or medical device

> **Phase I trial** – This is the first clinical trial for studying an experimental drug or treatment in humans. Phase I trials are usually small (10-100 people) and are used to determine safety and the best dose for a drug. These trials provide information about drug side effects, and how the body absorbs and handles the drug. The patients in these trials usually have advanced disease and have already received the best available treatment.

> **Phase II trial** – Phase II trials examine whether a drug or therapy is active against the disease it is intended to treat. Side effects are studied. A phase II trial is a noncomparative study, meaning the therapeutic effects and side effects of the experimental treatment are not compared to another drug or a placebo.

> **Phase III trial** – Phase III trials are conducted to find out how well a drug or therapy works compared to standard treatment or no treatment. Phase III trials are large studies and usually involve several hundred to thousands of patients.

> **Controlled clinical trial** – A controlled clinical trial divides participants into study groups to determine the effectiveness and safety of a new treatment. One group receives the experimental treatment; the other group receives placebo (an inactive substance) or the standard therapy. This group is called the control group. Comparison of the experimental group with the control group is the basis of determining the safety and effectiveness of the new treatment.

> **Randomized clinical trial** – A randomized clinical trial involves patients who are randomly (by chance) assigned to receive either the experimental treatment or the control treatment (placebo or standard therapy).

Collagen – fibrous protein that is one of the main components of scar tissue (fibrotic tissue); a component of bones, cartilage, tendons, and other connective tissues

Combination therapy – therapy that involves two or more components that can be drugs, procedures, or other specific treatments

Complementary and alternative medicine (CAM) – medical practices that are not routinely taught at western medical schools; medical disciplines other than allopathic medicine including traditional Chinese medicine, acupuncture, Ayurvedic medicine, naturopathy, homeopathy, chiropractic medicine, massage therapy, aromatherapy, and others

Complete blood count (CBC) – a blood test that includes measurements of white blood cells, red blood cells, hemoglobin, hematocrit, platelets, and possibly others

Conjunctiva – the lining of the inner surfaces of the eyelid and the exposed surface of the eyeball

Conjunctival capillaries – the tiny blood vessels of the conjunctiva (see above)

Contraindicate – (contraindication) in medicine, a condition or other reason not to use a particular drug or treatment

Cryoglobulin – abnormal blood protein formed when several antibody molecules (gamma globulins) clump together; protein in the condition cryoglobulinemia that can cause abnormal blood clots in the brain (stroke), eyes, and/or heart; can cause kidney damage and/or kidney failure

Cryoglobulinemia – the presence of abnormal proteins called cryoglobulins in blood; a condition that can cause kidney damage and possibly kidney failure; a condition that can accompany chronic hepatitis C

Cured – in hepatitis C, sustained viral clearance is considered a cure; undetectable hepatitis C virus in the blood for six or more months after the completion of treatment

Cytokine – small proteins released by cells that have specific effects on other cells; proteins that carry the signals for many of the immune system responses

Cytomegalovirus (CMV) – any of a group of viruses in the herpes virus family that cause infections in humans and animals; a virus that usually does not cause disease in healthy adults, but can cause disease in people with immune suppression such as those with HIV/AIDS or transplant recipients

Cytopathic – relating to disease or deterioration of cells; direct damage to cells

Decoction – in traditional Chinese medicine, a strong tea made by combining herbs with cold water, bringing the mixture to a boil, and simmering it for 10-20 minutes

Decompensation – in the liver, the inability of the liver to regenerate itself and compensate for damage it has sustained; liver damage that has progressed to the point that liver functions begin to deteriorate

Dehydration – in medicine, the condition when the body is deficient in water

Deoxyribonucleic acid (DNA) – the molecule human genes are made of; the molecule that carries all genetic information in humans

Depression – a mental condition characterized by apathy, lack of emotional expression, social withdrawal, changes in eating and sleep patterns, and fatigue; a mental condition that can accompany any life-changing event including being diagnosed with a chronic illness; a possible side effect of interferon/ribavirin therapy

Distend – (distention) to swell out or expand from internal pressure; in hepatitis C, ascites causes distention of the abdomen

Durable response – see sustained response

Dyspnea – difficult or labored breathing

Edema – swelling due to an excess fluid (water) in the body; most often seen in the lower legs and feet, but also seen in the hands

Electrolyte – in medicine, a dissolved chemical that carries either a positive or negative charge; commonly refers to sodium, potassium, chloride, bicarbonate, calcium and phosphate

Emaciation – extreme thinness; generally the result of starvation or severe illness

Encephalopathy – see hepatic encephalopathy

Endorphin – a substance produced in the brain, spinal cord, and other parts of the body that causes elevated mood, reduced pain, and reduced stress; the body's natural pain killer; a substance released by the body during exercise

Enzyme – a protein that starts and/or propels a specific chemical reaction

Enzyme immunoassay (EIA) – one of the tests used to detect antibodies to HCV (anti-HCV antibody)

Erythema nodosum – a type of skin inflammation that results in reddish, tender lumps most commonly located in the front of the legs below the knees

Exogenous – derived or produced outside the body

Extrahepatic – situated or originating outside the liver

Fatigue – the state of extreme tiredness that is usually not relieved by rest or sleep

Fatty Liver – a condition in which the liver cells contain an abnormal amount of fat

Ferritin – a protein that binds iron; tested to check the amount of iron in the body

Fibrinogen – a protein that when activated by the clotting (coagulation) system turns into fibrin, an essential component of a blood clot; measured in liver disease to check the liver's protein-making ability; a test of liver function

Fibroblastic – refers to cells or cell activities that lead to the formation of fibrous tissue or scarring

Fibrosis – in liver disease, the laying down of scar tissue in the liver; usually the result of ongoing inflammation

Fibrous – composed of or containing fibers; scar-like

Flatulence – excess gas in the lower intestinal tract

Flavinoid – a vitamin A-like substance found in many fruits and vegetables; many flavinoids are powerful antioxidants

Free radical – a highly reactive chemical that oxidizes other chemicals in the body; the chemicals that cause oxidative stress in the body; the chemicals that cause oxidative damage in the body; chemicals normally produced in the body and neutralized by antioxidants; chemicals produced in excessive amounts by chronic infection and/or inflammation

Fulminant liver failure – severe and rapidly progressive liver cell death

Galactosamine – a compound made in the body consisting of sugar and protein molecules that is used in the production of certain types of tissue; can be toxic to the liver; used in animal experiments to cause liver damage

Gamma-glutamyl transferase (GGT) — a liver enzyme (protein); blood GGT levels are measured to check for liver damage associated with slow or blocked bile flow; GGT is elevated in all forms of liver disease

Gastroenterologist – a doctor who specializes in diagnosing and treating diseases of the digestive system including the liver

Gastroesophageal varices – see varix

Gene – the material that encodes for all inherited traits and characteristics of a living thing; a piece of DNA (deoxyribonucleic acid) or RNA (ribonucleic acid) that carries the message for a particular trait or characteristic

Genome – all the genetic information of a particular organism

Genotype – in hepatitis C, one of several different species of the hepatitis C virus; different genotypes have different responses to interferon-based therapy; different genotypes have some differences in the genes they contain

Genotype test – a test to identify the specific genotype of the HCV virus

Glomerulonephritis – a kidney disease in which the filtering units of the kidney (the glomeruli) are damaged; the disorder is characterized by edema (swelling), elevated blood pressure, and excess protein in the urine

Glucose – (dextrose or blood sugar) the form of sugar found in the blood; the breakdown product of simple and complex carbohydrates that can be used by the body

Glutathione – a protein formed in the liver that plays an important role in the immune system; the body's most abundant natural antioxidant (protects against free radical damage)

Glycogen – a large molecule made up of smaller glucose molecules; the storage form of glucose primarily formed in the liver

Glycoprotein – (glucoprotein) a compound made of protein and carbohydrate (sugar)

Grade – in liver biopsy, a term used to describe the amount of inflammation in the liver; the higher the grade, the greater the inflammation

HBcAg – hepatitis B core antigen; a blood marker of active hepatitis B infection

HBeAg – hepatitis B envelope antigen; a blood marker of active hepatitis B infection

HBsAg – hepatitis B surface antigen; a blood marker of active hepatitis B infection

HCC – see hepatocellular carcinoma

HCV polymerase chain reaction (PCR) – test to check for the presence of the hepatitis C virus in the blood; a qualitative HCV PCR test determines the presence or absence of virus in the blood; a quantitative HCV PCR test measures the amount of detectable HCV in the blood

HCV RNA – hepatitis C virus ribonucleic acid; the genetic material of HCV

Helicase – an enzyme used in viral replication; it enables the genetic material to uncoil so it can be replicated; a potential target of antiviral drugs

Hematemesis – vomiting of blood

Heme – the iron-containing portion of hemoglobin, the substance in red blood cells that enables them to carry oxygen

Hemochromatosis – a hereditary disease caused by increased absorption and excessive storage of iron in the tissues, especially the liver; the untreated disorder can lead to cirrhosis of the liver, heart disease, diabetes mellitus, testicular atrophy, and arthritis

Hemoglobin – the protein in red blood cells that carries oxygen

Hemoglobinopathy – a group of hereditary disorders characterized by abnormal hemoglobin structure; sickle cell anemia is an example

Hemolytic anemia – anemia due to increased destruction of red blood cells; can be a side effect of ribavirin therapy

Hepatic – relating to the liver

Hepatic encephalopathy – a complication of liver failure that results from large amounts of ammonia that accumulate in the brain; symptoms include euphoria, depression, confusion, slurred speech, abnormal sleeping patterns, incoherent speech, tremors, rigid muscles, and eventually coma

Hepatitis – inflammation of the liver

Hepatitis A – a disease caused by the hepatitis A virus (HAV); transmitted by food or drink that has been contaminated by an infected person; symptoms include nausea, fever, and jaundice (yellowing of the skin and/or eyes); hepatitis A does not progress to chronic hepatitis

Hepatitis B – a disease caused by the hepatitis B virus (HBV); transmitted sexually or by contact with infected blood; hepatitis B may progress to chronic hepatitis and can be fatal

Hepatitis C – a disease caused by the hepatitis C virus (HCV) C; transmitted by contact with infected blood via contaminated needles and transfusion of infected blood products; rarely transmitted sexually; hepatitis C becomes chronic in 85% of people infected and can be fatal in a small percentage of cases

Hepatitis D – (delta hepatitis) a disease caused by the hepatitis D virus; transmitted via infected blood, contaminated needles, or sexual contact with an infected person; the virus only causes disease in patients who already have HBV

Hepatitis E – a disease caused by the hepatitis E virus; transmitted via food or drink handled by an infected person, or through infected water supplies in areas where fecal matter may get into the water; more common in tropical and subtropical regions of the world than in the United States and Canada

Hepatocellular carcinoma (HCC) – (liver cancer, hepatoma) the most common malignant tumor of the liver; chronic hepatitis B and C are risk factors for this cancer especially in those with cirrhosis

Hepatocyte – (hepatic cell) liver cells

Hepatologist – a doctor whose practice is limited to diseases and disorders of the liver

Hepatoma – see hepatocellular carcinoma

Hepatomegaly – liver enlargement

Hepatoprotective – protective of the liver

Hepatotoxic – toxic to the liver

Herbicide – a substance used to kill plants

Histologic – (histological) pertaining to study of the microscopic structure, composition, and function of tissues

Histology – the study of the form of cells and tissues that can only be seen with the microscope; also called microscopic anatomy

Hormone – a substance produced in the body that controls and regulates the activity of other cells or organs; most hormones are secreted by specialized glands such as the thyroid gland; they control digestion, metabolism, growth, reproduction, mood, and other essential body functions

Human immunodeficiency virus (HIV) – the virus that causes AIDS (acquired immunodeficiency syndrome); HIV infection weakens the body's immune defenses by destroying CD4 lymphocytes (T cells)

Hyperthyroidism – a condition caused by excess production of thyroid hormone resulting from an overactive thyroid gland

Hypoactivity – abnormally reduced activity

Hypochondrium – area of the upper abdomen below the ribs

Hypothyroidism – deficiency of the thyroid hormone from the thyroid gland

IL-10 – (interleukin 10) an anti-inflammatory and immunosuppressive cytokine; normally produced in the body at sites of injury and inflammation; controls the degree of inflammation

Immune globulin – (gamma globulin) a concentrated preparation of gamma globulins (antibodies) taken from a large group of human donors that is given by injection for the treatment of specific diseases; used to treat hepatitis A in people already infected with HBV and/or HCV

Immune system – a complex group of cells and organs that collectively protect the body from bacterial, parasitic, fungal, and viral infections and from the growth of tumor cells; includes T-helper cells (CD4 cells), T-suppressor cells, natural killer cells, B cells, granulocytes (polymorphonuclear leukocytes), macrophages, dendritic cells, the bone marrow, the thymus gland, the spleen, and the lymph nodes

Immunity — the condition of being protected from an infectious disease either by the action of the immune system or immunization (vaccines)

Immunoglobulin (Ig) – proteins that act as antibodies in the body; produced by plasma cells and B lymphocytes; part of the humoral immune response; antibodies that attach to foreign substances such as bacteria and viruses and assist in destroying them

Immunomodulator – a chemical agent that modifies the immune response or the functioning of the immune system

Immunopathic – (immunopathologic) substances or processes that are harmful to the immune system; damage caused by an abnormal or overactive immune response

Immunosuppressive – substances or processes that decrease the immune response

Immunotherapy – treatment to stimulate or restore the ability of the immune system to fight infection and disease; a treatment that acts by stimulating or working with the immune system

Inference – the act of drawing logical conclusions from known facts or facts assumed to be true

Inflammation – a localized tissue reaction to irritation, injury, or infection; usually characterized by swelling, redness, pain, with or without loss of function; abnormally intense inflammation can cause tissue damage as in chronic hepatitis C

Insulin — the hormone that controls the level of glucose in the blood; allows glucose to move from the blood into cells; produced in the pancreas by specialized cells called beta cells or islet cells

Integrated medicine – an approach to medicine that combines aspects of many medical disciplines; usually includes western medicine and any number of complementary and/or alternative medicine (CAM) approaches

Interferon – any of a group of glycoprotein cytokines that occur naturally in the body; they can have antiviral, and antibacterial actions; synthetic interferons are used to treat a number of diseases; interferons are the basis for current western therapy for chronic hepatitis C

Interferon-based therapy – any therapy that uses interferon as the main component; interferon-based therapy is currently the standard treatment for chronic hepatitis C in western (allopathic) medicine

Interstitial – in biology, pertaining to the small, narrow spaces between tissues or parts of an organ

In vitro – literally means in glass; something that is observed in a laboratory setting (as opposed to observations made in animals or people)

In vivo – something that is observed in a living organism, either animals or people

Jaundice – yellowish discoloration of the skin and whites of the eyes caused by abnormally high amounts of bilirubin in the body

Lassitude – weariness, listlessness, or reduced energy

Lethargy – a state of sluggishness, inactivity, and apathy

Lichen planus – a recurrent skin rash characterized by small, flat-topped, many-sided (polygonal) bumps that can grow together into rough, scaly patches on the skin; may occur in the lining (mucous membrane) of the mouth or vagina

Lipid – fat; there are many different types of fats in the diet and in the body such as cholesterol and triglyceride; some fats are healthy and necessary for good health; some fats are harmful and play a role in various diseases including hepatitis C; includes fatty acids, neutral fats, and waxes

Lipodystrophy – any of a group of conditions due to defective metabolism of fat that results in loss or redistribution of fat; believed to be a side effect of some HIV medications although the virus itself may also contribute to this condition; fat is usually redistributed from the face, arms, and legs into the abdomen and back

Lipoprotein – a lipid-protein complex; the form in which fats are transported in the blood; responsible for transporting cholesterol and triglycerides and other fats from the liver to other parts of the body

Liver biopsy – the removal and subsequent microscopic examination of small samples of liver tissue; the only reliable method to determine the amount of damage done to the liver by the hepatitis C virus; performed by inserting a long needle through the skin into the liver

Liver cancer – see hepatocellular carcinoma

Liver enzyme – any of the many enzymes present in liver cells including ALT, AST, GGT, LDH, alkaline phosphatase, and others; liver enzymes are monitored in chronic hepatitis C to determine the amount of ongoing damage occurring in the liver

Liver failure – a state in which the liver is unable to adequately perform its many functions; usually the result of end-stage cirrhosis; characterized by clotting abnormalities, protein abnormalities, abnormal electrolytes, and many other signs and symptoms

Liver function test(s) – any of a number of tests used to check for liver function; includes bilirubin, albumin, prothrombin time, total protein, and many others

Living donor liver transplantation – a new procedure involving the transplantation of a portion of a liver from a living donor to replace a failed liver; both livers can grow to normal size

Loins – the region of the hips, groin, and lower abdomen

Lymphatic fluid – the colorless, slightly opaque fluid that travels through vessels called lymphatics that connect the lymph nodes in the body; carries immune cells that help fight infection and disease

Lymphatic system – (lymph system) the network of lymph nodes and lymph vessels (lymphatics) in the body; lymph nodes are small, tightly packed collections of lymphocytes that filter, attack, and destroy organisms that cause infection; organs and tissues involved in the lymphatic system include bone marrow, thymus gland, liver, spleen, and collections of lymphatic tissue in the throat and small intestine

Lymphocyte – a specific type of white blood cell; a type of immune cell that specializes to perform different immune system activities; types of lymphocytes include T-cells, B-cells, and NK-cells (natural killer cells)

Malabsorption – (maldigestion) impaired or inadequate absorption of nutrients from the digestive tract

Manipulation – the application of manual force for healing; describes the techniques used in osteopathy, chiropractic medicine, massage, and other body work therapies

Meditation – any of many practices in which the mind is inwardly focused and quieted; the practice is a spiritual practice for many but is also used for stress reduction; meditation is known to lower levels of cortisol (a hormone released in response to stress), and is believed to enhance the immune system

Melena – the passage of dark, tarry stools containing decomposing blood; an indication of bleeding in the digestive tract

Meridians – in traditional Chinese medicine, the specific pathways through which vital energy (qi) and blood flow; acupuncture points are located along these meridians

Meta-analysis – statistical analysis that allows the results of several different studies of the same subject to be combined and analyzed

Metabolism – the collective biochemical processes that occur in a living organism; involves the balanced process of anabolism (building up or creating substances) and catabolism (breaking down or using substances); commonly used to refer the breakdown of food and its transformation into energy

Microcirculation – the flow of blood in the smallest blood vessels of the body; the part of the circulation where oxygen and nutrients pass into the tissues, and waste products are passed out of the tissues

Microorganism – a microscopic organism; includes bacteria, viruses, algae, fungi, protozoa, and some parasites

Modality – a form of therapy; usually refers to physical forms of therapy such as acupuncture, massage, chiropractic adjustments, etc.

Monogamous – having only one sexual partner

Monotherapy – the use of a single drug to treat a particular disorder or disease

Moxibustion – a technique that involves the stimulation of acupuncture points by burning a small cone of dried moxa (mugwort) leaves on the end of the needle, directly on protected skin, or above the body

Mutation – a permanent change in a gene or chromosome of an organism creating a new characteristic or trait not previously found; mutations can lead to new resistance to treatment

Myalgia – pain or ache in muscle(s)

Mycophenolate mofetil – drug marketed with trade name Cellcept® ; given to organ transplant recipients to prevent rejection of the new tissue; an immune system inhibitor

NAFL – abbreviation for nonalcoholic fatty liver

NAFLD – abbreviation for nonalcoholic fatty liver disease

NASH – abbreviation for nonalcoholic steatohepatitis

Necrosis – death of cells or tissues

Neurological – of or pertaining to the nervous system and the diseases that affect it

Neutrophil – (granulocyte) a type of granular white blood cell that attacks microorganisms such as bacteria

Nonresponder – a person who does not respond to therapy

Nonspecific – not due to any single known cause, such as a specific pathogen; a finding that cannot be linked to a specific disease or condition

Nonsteroidal analgesic — of, or pertaining to a substance that is not a steroid but has similar effects, such as the anti-inflammatory drug ibuprofen

Nucleocapsid – the coat (capsid) of a virus plus the enclosed genetic material (nucleic acid genome)

Nucleoside – (nucleotide) a subunit of DNA or RNA; to form a DNA or RNA molecule, thousands of nucleotides are joined in a long chain

Nucleoside reverse transcriptase inhibitor (NRTI) –_a group of drugs used primarily in the treatment of HIV/AIDs; these drugs are incorporated into the viral genome and block viral replication; examples include AZT (Retrovir®), 3TC®, ddC (Hivid®), ddI (Didanosine®), and d4T (Zerit®)

Nutritional supplement – any product such as a vitamin, mineral, or other substance that is taken to augment the amount of nutrients in the diet; used to improve overall health and/or to help correct specific health problems

OSHA – Occupational Safety and Health Administration, U.S. Department of Labor

Osteoporosis – thinning of the bones with reduction in bone mass due to depletion of calcium and bone protein; a condition that predisposes to bone fractures that are often slow to heal and/or heal poorly; more common in older adults, particularly postmenopausal women and people taking steroidal drugs

Oxidative stress – a condition that occurs when an overabundance of free radicals are present in the body; chronic infection and inflammation cause increased oxidative stress; high levels of free radicals can lead to tissue damage

Oxygenation — the chemical process of adding oxygen to something

Palpation – the act of feeling with the hand; the application of light pressure to the surfaces of the body to determine the consistency of the body parts as part of a physical diagnosis

Pathogen – an agent that causes disease, particularly a living microorganism such as a virus or bacterium

Pathogenesis – the processes that lead to the development of a disease or illness

Pathological – relating to or caused by disease

PCR – see HCV polymerase chain reaction

Pedal edema – swelling of the feet caused by an excess accumulation of fluid in the body

Pegylated interferon – a form of interferon in which polyethylene glycol molecules have been bound to the interferon molecule; pegylated interferon has a slower rate of breakdown and clearance from the body than standard interferon

Peptide – a compound containing two or more amino acids; groups of peptides form proteins

Peripheral blood mononuclear cell (PBMC) – (monocyte) a large white blood cell found in the blood; one of the cell types of the immune system

Pesticide – a chemical preparation used to kill insects or other plant/animals pests

Petechia – tiny, flat, round, purplish-red spots on the skin caused by bleeding between the layers of the skin or in the mucosal membranes

Pharmacology – the study of drugs; includes study of drug sources and their properties; also the study of the body's metabolism of and reaction to drugs

Phosphatidylcholine – a compound consisting of glycerol, fatty acids, and phosphorus; as a nutritional supplement, this compound has been shown to have a hepatoprotective effect

Phospholipid – the major form of lipids in the body; a principal structural material of living cells; the main component of cell membranes (the outer layer of cells)

Physiological – normal; not pathologic; characteristic of the normal functioning or state of the body, or a tissue or organ

Phytopharmacology – the study of compounds that are found in plants that have medicinal uses; the related terms phytochemical and phytonutrient are used interchangeably to describe those plant compounds that are thought to have medicinal properties

Pituitary – the main endocrine gland that controls endocrine functions in the body; called the master gland because it produces hormones that control other glands and many body functions

Placebo – an inactive substance, dummy medication, or sugar pill; widely used in clinical trials to test if an observed effect is truly due to the experimental drug; for a drug to be considered effective, it must show significantly better results than that produced by the placebo

Platelet – an irregular, disc-shaped element of the blood that assists in blood clotting; during normal blood clotting, platelets group together (aggregate); platelets are fragments of larger cells called megakaryocytes

Polyarteritis nodosa – a disorder of small and medium sized arteries characterized by inflammation and possible death of the blood vessel cells; usually affects adult males; can be associated with hepatitis C infection; the kidneys are most commonly involved, but muscles, the intestine, and the heart can also be affected

Polymer – a compound created by joining smaller molecules called monomers

Polymerase – any enzyme that catalyzes polymerization, the successive joining together of smaller monomers to make a polymer

Polymyalgia – pain or aching in many muscles; sometimes short for polymyalgia rheumatica (PMR), a disorder of the muscles and joints of older persons characterized by pain and stiffness

Porphyria cutanea tarda (PCT) – an inherited disorder of porphyrin metabolism; the liver uses porphyrins to make hemoglobin, the iron-containing portion of red blood cells; PCT can be acquired with certain types of chemical poisoning

Porphyrin – pigmented (colored) compounds that are found in heme (the iron containing molecule in hemoglobin), bile, and cytochromes; blood levels of the various porphyrins can be affected by liver failure

Portal hypertension – increased blood pressure in the portal vein that brings blood into the liver; usually occurs because scarring in the liver resists the free flow of blood into the liver; the increased pressure in the portal vein also causes increased pressure in the veins of the abdomen, intestines, stomach, and esophagus; portal hypertension causes many of the complications associated with liver cirrhosis

Portal vein – the large vein that carries blood from the intestines to the liver for processing before returning it to circulation via the hepatic veins

Prodromal symptom – symptom that starts before the onset of an illness

Prognosis – the probable outcome or course of a disease; a person's chance of recovery from a disease or injury

Protease inhibitor – any of a class of anti-HIV drugs designed to inhibit the HIV protease enzyme; protease inhibitors prevent the replication of viruses

Protein – a large molecule composed of one or more chains of amino acids (peptides); proteins are required for the structure, function, and regulation of the body's cells, tissues, and organs; the liver is responsible for making many of the body's proteins

Proteinase – (protease) any enzyme that breaks down proteins by splitting them into chains of peptides

Prothrombin time (PT) – the time it takes for blood to form a clot; monitored in liver disease to assess liver function; many of the proteins needed for clotting are produced in the liver

Protocol – a detailed plan for medical treatment or an experiment

Pruritus – intense itching of the skin

Psoriasis – a reddish, scaly rash often located on the elbows, knees, scalp, and around or in the ears, navel, genitals or buttocks; caused by the body making too many skin cells; some cases are believed to be autoimmune conditions

Psychosocial – having aspects of social and psychological behavior

Qi – in traditional Chinese medicine, the energy that flows through everything and is the organizing force of the universe; the most important substance circulating through the body

Qi gong – qi means energy, and gong means skill; a self-healing art that combines movement and meditation; visualizations are employed to enhance the mind/body connection and assist healing

Quasispecies – species of viruses that are very similar but have genetic differences; quasispecies are the result of a virus mutation; mutation can cause several quasispecies to exist in the same person

RA (rheumatoid arthritis) factor – a specific antibody present in the blood of 60-80% of people with rheumatoid arthritis

Rebetron® – a combination of interferon alfa 2b and ribavirin used to treat hepatitis C infection; ribavirin is taken by mouth and interferon alfa 2b is administered subcutaneously (beneath the skin)

Recombinant immunoblot assay (RIBA) – blood test used to check for antibodies against the hepatitis C virus; a test to determine exposure to HCV

Relapse – the return of signs and symptoms of a disease following a period of remission (absence of the disease); in hepatitis C, a relapse is the reappearance of the virus after an period of it being undetectable; less frequently used to mean a spike in the liver enzymes after a period of being normal

Relapser – someone who has experienced a relapse (see above)

Remission – the resolution of the signs and symptoms of a disease; can be temporary or permanent

Renal – having to do with the kidneys

Replication – process of duplicating or reproducing; viral reproduction is called replication

Reservoir – in chronic viral illnesses (such as HIV) a place in the body where the virus exists but is not detectable by usual medical means; some researchers believe there is a possibility there is one or more reservoirs of HCV in the body, at least in some people with the infection

Retrovirus – an RNA virus; a virus with an RNA genome instead of a DNA genome

Rheumatoid arthritis – an autoimmune disease that causes chronic inflammation of the joints, the tissue around the joints, and other organs in the body

RIBA – see recombinant immunoblot assay

Ribavirin – a nucleoside analogue drug; it has no activity against HCV when used alone, but is effective in some people when used in combination with interferon; ribavirin is believed to act against HCV not as an antiviral but as an immune enhancer

Ribonucleic acid (RNA) - one of two types of molecules that encode genetic information (the other is DNA)

Ribozyme – an RNA molecule that also acts as an enzyme; ribozymes bind to RNA and cut (cleave) it

RNA – see ribonucleic acid

Secondary condition – condition that develops as a consequence of another condition that preceded it

Serum – see blood serum

Sign – in medicine, any objective (observable) evidence of a disease or condition

Sjögren's syndrome – (Sicca syndrome) an autoimmune disease characterized by dry eyes and mouth, purple spots on the face or inside the mouth, and swollen salivary glands; often seen in people with rheumatoid arthritis; a condition that is sometimes seen in people with chronic hepatitis C

Spontaneous clearing – in hepatitis C, the ability to rid the body of virus without treatment; this occurs in 15-20% of people infected with HCV

Stage – in hepatitis C, the degree of fibrosis present on liver biopsy; the higher the stage, the more fibrosis present

Steatohepatitis – the presence of fat in the liver cells with inflammation (hepatitis)

Steatosis – accumulation of fat in the liver that can cause inflammation and lead to fibrosis and/or cirrhosis

Sustained responder – in hepatitis C, a person who has no detectable virus in his or her blood and whose liver enzyme tests continue to be normal six months after completing therapy

Sustained response – see sustained responder (above)

Symptom – any subjective change (something experienced by the patient) that may indicate a disease process such as fatigue, pain, thirst, etc.

T-cell – (T lymphocyte) a type of white blood cell that is a crucial part of the immune system; they activate the rest of the immune system and directly attack invading organisms

Tai chi – a system of gentle, flowing exercises designed to keep the body's qi (energy) moving

Thymus gland – the organ in which T lymphocytes (such as CD4 and CD8 T cells) mature; part of the immune system

Thyroid gland — the organ that produces thyroid hormones that control the metabolic rate of every cell in the body

Thyroiditis – inflammation of the thyroid gland; can cause the release of excess of thyroid hormones into the blood stream

Tinnitus – ringing in the ears; can be caused by certain medications (such as aspirin and other anti-inflammatory drugs), aging, trauma, and other disorders

Toxic – poisonous; capable of causing injury or harm, especially by chemical means

Toxicity – the quality of being toxic

Toxin – a poisonous substance, particularly a protein produced by living cells or organisms; certain toxins are capable of inducing the immune system to produce neutralizing antibodies called anti-toxins

trans – a chemical prefix that refers to a specific arrangement of chemical bonds; the opposite of the trans chemical arrangement is known as cis

Transcription mediated amplification (TMA) – a testing technique used to measure the amount of HCV in the blood

Transient ischemic attack (TIA) – also called a mini-stroke; a neurological event that has the signs and symptoms of a stroke but that resolves in a short period of time; due to a temporary lack of adequate oxygen (ischemia) in the brain

Triglyceride – a form of fat that exists in many foods and in the body; triglycerides in blood come from fats in foods and can also be made in the body

Tui-na – Chinese massage therapy

Tumor – an abnormal mass of tissue that can be either benign (noncancerous) or malignant (cancerous)

Ultrasonography – (sonography) diagnostic imaging technique that uses sound waves to construct a picture (sonograph) of an internal organ or body structure

Ultrasound – high-frequency sound waves; an ultrasound test (sonography) bounces sound waves off internal organs of the body to construct images of the target organ; liver ultrasound is used to screen for liver cancer

Urticaria — (hives) raised, itchy areas of skin that are usually a sign of an allergic reaction

Vaccination – the introduction of vaccine into the body for the purpose of inducing immunity to a specific disease or group of diseases

Vaccine – a suspension of weakened or killed microorganisms, or other substances that are introduced into the body to induce an immune reaction; the immune reaction is intended to protect the recipient from getting the illness associated with a specific microorganism; newer vaccines are being developed to alter the course of infectious diseases

Varix – (*pl.* varices) an abnormally dilated or swollen vein; portal hypertension can cause esophageal varices that can rupture and cause vomiting of large amounts of blood; bleeding esophageal varices are a medical emergency

Vascular – relating to the blood vessels of the body

Vasculitis – a general term for a group of diseases that feature inflammation of the blood vessels

Vertigo – the sensation of dizziness or spinning

Viral clearance – elimination of a virus or reducing it to the point that it cannot be detected in the blood

Viral load – the amount of virus present in the blood

Virologist – a scientist who specializes in the study of viruses

Virology – the branch of microbiology that is concerned with viruses and viral diseases

HEPATITIS C: CHOICES
CITATIONS AND REFERENCES

Chapter 1
OVERVIEW OF HEPATITIS C
Robert G. Gish, MD

1. Alter MJ, Kruszon-Morgan D, Nainan OV, et al. The prevalence of hepatitis C virus infection in the United States, 1988 through 1994. *N Engl J Med.* 1999;341(8):556-562.
2. Alter MJ. Epidemiology of hepatitis C. *Hepatology.* 1997;26(3 Suppl 1):62-65S.
3. EASL: International Consensus Conference on Hepatitis C Consensus Statement. *J Hepatol.* 1999;30:956-961.
4. Amarapurkar D. Natural history of hepatitis C virus infection. *J Gastroenterol Hepatol.* 2000;15(Suppl E):105-110.
5. Lucidarme D, Dumas F, Arpurt JP, et al. Rapid progress of cirrhosis in hepatitis C: the role of age at the time of viral contamination. *Presse Med.* 1998;27(13):608-611.
6. Bortolotti F, Faggion S, Con P. Natural history of chronic viral hepatitis in childhood. *Acta Gastroenterol Belg.* 1998;61(2):198-201.
7. Datz C, Cramp M, Haas T, et al. The natural course of hepatitis C virus infection 18 years after an epidemic outbreak of non-A, non-B hepatitis in a plasmapheresis centre. *Gut.* 1999;44(4):563-567.
8. Poynard T, Bedossa P, Opolon P. Natural history of liver fibrosis progression in patients with chronic hepatitis C. The OBSVIRC, METAVIR, CLINIVIR, and DOSVIRC groups. *Lancet.* 1997;349(9055):825-832.
9. Kuboki M, Shinzawa H, Shao L, et al. A cohort study of hepatitis C virus (HCV) infection in an HCV epidemic area of Japan: age and sex-related seroprevalence of anti-HCV antibody, frequency of viremia, biochemical abnormality and histological changes. *Liver.* 1999;19(2):88-96.
10. Alric L, Fort M, Izopet J, et al. Study of host- and virus-related factors associated with spontaneous hepatitis C virus clearance. *Tissue Antigens.* 2000;56(2):154-158.
11. Inoue G, Horiike N, Michitaka K, Onji M. Hepatitis C virus clearance is prominent in women in an endemic area . *J Gastroenterol Hepatol.* 2000;15(9):1054-1058.
12. Yamakawa Y, Sata M, Suzuki H, Noguchi S, Tanikawa K. Higher elimination rate of hepatitis C virus among women. *J Viral Hepat.* 1996;3(6):317-321.
13. Alberti A, Chemello L, Benvegnù L. Natural history of hepatitis C. *J Hepatol.* 1999;31(Suppl 1):17-24.
14. Hourigan LF, Macdonald GA, Purdie D, et al. Fibrosis in chronic hepatitis C correlates significantly with body mass index and steatosis. *Hepatology.* 1999;29(4):1215-1219.
15. de Medina M, Schiff ER. Hepatitis C: diagnostic assays. *Semin Liver Dis.* 1995;15(1):33-40.
16. Atrah HI, Ahmed MM. Hepatitis C virus seroconversion by a third generation ELISA screening test in blood donors. *J Clin Path.* 1996;49:254-255.
17. Gretch DR. Diagnostic tests for hepatitis C. *Hepatology.* 1997;26(3 Suppl 1):43-47S.
18. Dienstag JL. Non-A, non-B hepatitis. I. Recognition, epidemiology and clinical features. *Gastroenterology.* 1983; 85(2):439-462.
19. Marcellin P. Hepatitis C: the clinical spectrum of the disease. *J Hepatol.* 1999;31(Suppl 1):9-16.

20. Seeff LB. Natural history of hepatitis C. *Hepatology.* 1997;26(3 Suppl 1):21-28S.

21. Hoofnagle JH. Hepatitis C: the clinical spectrum of disease. *Hepatology.* 1997;26(3 Suppl 1):15-20S.

22. Yuki N, Hayashi N, et al. Relation of disease activity during chronic hepatitis C infection to complexity of hypervariable region 1 quasispecies. *Hepatology.* 1997;25(2):439-444.

23. Detre KM, Belle SH, Lombardero M. Liver transplantation for chronic viral hepatitis. *Viral Hepatitis Reviews.* 1996;2:219-228.

24. Seeff LB, Buskell-Bales Z, Wright EC, et al. Long-term mortality after transfusion-associated non-A, non-B hepatitis. The National Heart, Lung, and Blood Institute Study Group. *N Engl J Med.* 1992;327(27):1906-1911.

25. Koretz RL, Stone O, Mousa M, Gitnick GL. Non-A, non-B posttransfusion hepatitis - a decade later. *Gastroenterology.* 1985;88(5 Pt 1):1251-1254.

26. Takahashi M, Yamada G, Miyamoto R, et al. Natural course of chronic hepatitis C. *Am J Gastroenterol.* 1993;88(2):240-243.

27. National Institutes of Health Consensus Development Conference Panel. Statement: management of hepatitis C. *Hepatology.* 1997;26(Suppl 1):2-10S.

28. Yano M, Kumada H, Kage M, et al. The long-term pathological evolution of chronic hepatitis C. *Hepatology.* 1996;23(6):1334-1340.

29. Di Bisceglie AM. Hepatitis C and hepatocellular carcinoma. *Hepatology.* 1997;26(Suppl 1):34-38S.

Chapter 2
ALCOHOL and HEPATITIS C
Douglas R. LaBrecque, MD and Lorren Sandt

1. Wiley TE, McCarthy M, Breidi L, McCarthy M, Layden TJ. Impact of alcohol on the histological and clinical progression of hepatitis C infection. *Hepatology.* 1998;28(3):805-809.

2. Poynard T, Bedossa P, Opolon P. Natural history of liver fibrosis progression in patients with chronic hepatitis C. The OBSVIRC, METAVIR, CLINIVIR, and DOSVIRC groups. *Lancet.* 1997;349(9055):825-832.

3. Regev A, Jeffers LJ. Hepatitis C and alcohol. *Alcohol Clin Exp Res.* 1999;23(9):1543-1551.

4. Schiff ER. The alcoholic patient with hepatitis C virus infection. *Am J Med.* 1999;107(6B):95-99S.

5. Ohta S, Watanabe Y, Nakajima T. Consumption of alcohol in the presence of hepatitis C virus is an additive risk for liver damage. *Prev Med.* 1998;27(3):461-469.

6. Caldwell SH, Jeffers LJ, Ditomaso A, et al. Antibody to hepatitis C is common among patients with alcoholic liver disease with and without risk factors. *Am J Gastroenterol.* 1991;86(9):1219-1223.

7. Pares A, Barrera JM, Caballeria J, et al. Hepatitis C virus antibodies in chronic alcoholic patients: association with severity of liver injury. *Hepatology.* 1990;12(6):1295-1299.

8. Coelho-Little ME, Jeffers LJ, Bernstein DE, et al. Hepatitis C virus in alcoholic patients with and without clinically apparent liver disease. *Alcohol Clin Exp Res.* 1995;19(5):1173-1176.

9. Mendenhall CL, Seeff L, Diehl AM, et al. Antibodies to hepatitis B virus and hepatitis C virus in alcoholic hepatitis and cirrhosis: their prevalence and clinical relevance. The VA Cooperative Study Group 119. *Hepatology.* 1991;14(4 Pt 1):581-589.

10. Mendenhall CL, Moritz T, Rouster S, et al. Epidemiology of hepatitis C among veterans with alcoholic liver disease. The VA Cooperative Study Group 275. *Am J Gastroenterol.* 1993;88(7):1022-1026.

11. Corrao G, Arico S. Independent and combined action of hepatitis C virus infection and alcohol consumption on the risk of symptomatic liver cirrhosis. *Hepatology.* 1998;27(4):914-919.

12. Pessione F, Degos F, Marcellin P, et al. Effect of alcohol consumption on serum hepatitis C virus RNA and histological lesions in chronic hepatitis C. *Hepatology.* 1998;27(6):1717-1722.

13. Ostapowicz G, Watson KJ, Locarnini SA, Desmond PV. Role of alcohol in the progression of liver disease caused by hepatitis C virus infection. *Hepatology.* 1998;27(6):1730-1735.

14. Khan MH, Thomas L, Byth K, et al. How much does alcohol contribute to the variability of hepatic fibrosis in chronic hepatitis C? *J Gastroenterol Hepatol.* 1998;13(4):419-426.

15. Kondili LA, Tosti ME, Szklo M, et al. The relationships of chronic hepatitis and cirrhosis to alcohol intake, hepatitis B and C, and delta virus infection: a case-control study in Albania. *Epidemiol Infect.* 1998;121(2):391-395.

16. Frieden TR, Ozick L, McCord C, et al. Chronic liver disease in central Harlem: the role of alcohol and viral hepatitis. *Hepatology.* 1999;29(3):883-888.

17. Nevins CL, Malaty H, Velez ME, Anand BS. Interaction of alcohol and hepatitis C virus infection on severity of liver disease. *Dig Dis Sci.* 1999;44(6):1236-1242.

18. Loguercio C, Di Pierro M, Di Marino MP, et al. Drinking habits of subjects with hepatitis C virus-related chronic liver disease: prevalence and effect on clinical, virological and pathological aspects. *Alcohol Alcohol.* 2000;35(3):296-301.

19. Roudot-Thoraval F, Bastie A, Pawlotsky JM, Dhumeaux D. Epidemiological factors affecting the severity of hepatitis C virus- related liver disease: a French survey of 6,664 patients. The Study Group for the Prevalence and the Epidemiology of Hepatitis C Virus. *Hepatology.* 1997;26(2):485-490.

20. Bellentani S, Tiribelli C, Saccoccio G, et al. Prevalence of chronic liver disease in the general population of northern Italy: the Dionysos Study. *Hepatology.* 1994;20(6):1442-1449.

21. Takase S, Tsutsumi M, Kawahara H, et al. The alcohol-altered liver membrane antibody and hepatitis C virus infection in the progression of alcoholic liver disease. *Hepatology.* 1993;17(1):9-13.

22. Donato F, Tagger A, Chiesa R, et al. Hepatitis B and C virus infection, alcohol drinking, and hepatocellular carcinoma: a case-control study in Italy. Brescia HCC Study. *Hepatology.* 1997;26(3):579-584.

23. Mori M, Hara M, Wada I, et al. Prospective study of hepatitis B and C viral infections, cigarette smoking, alcohol consumption, and other factors associated with hepatocellular carcinoma risk in Japan. *Am J Epidemiol.* 2000;151(2):131-139.

24. Khan KN, Yatsuhashi H. Effect of alcohol consumption on the progression of hepatitis C virus infection and risk of hepatocellular carcinoma in Japanese patients. *Alcohol Alcohol.* 2000;35(3):286-295.

25. Noda K, Yoshihara H, Suzuki K, et al. Progression of type C chronic hepatitis to liver cirrhosis and hepatocellular carcinoma - its relationship to alcohol drinking and the age of transfusion. *Alcohol Clin Exp Res.* 1996;20(1 Suppl):95-100A.

26. Oshita M, Hayashi N, Kasahara A, et al. Increased serum hepatitis C virus RNA levels among alcoholic patients with chronic hepatitis C. *Hepatology.* 1994;20(5):1115-1120.

27. Cromie SL, Jenkins PJ, Bowden DS, Dudley FJ. Chronic hepatitis C: effect of alcohol on hepatitic activity and viral titre. *J Hepatol.* 1996;25(6):821-826.

28. Sherman KE, Rouster SD, Mendenhall C, Thee D. Hepatitis C RNA quasispecies com-

plexity in patients with alcoholic liver disease. *Hepatology.* 1999;30(1):265-270.

29. Ohnishi K, Matsuo S, Matsutani K, et al. Interferon therapy for chronic hepatitis C in habitual drinkers: comparison with chronic hepatitis C in infrequent drinkers. *Am J Gastroenterol.* 1996;91(7):1374-1379.

30. Okazaki T, Yoshihara H, Suzuki K, et al. Efficacy of interferon therapy in patients with chronic hepatitis C. Comparison between non-drinkers and drinkers. *Scand J Gastroenterol.* 1994;29(11):1039-1043.

31. Ma X, Svegliati-Baroni G, Poniachik J, et al. Collagen synthesis by liver stellate cells is released from its normal feedback regulation by acetaldehyde-induced modification of the carboxyl-terminal propeptide of procollagen. *Alcohol Clin Exp Res.* 1997;21(7):1204-1211.

32. McClain C, Shedlofsky S, Barve S, Hill D. Cytokines and alcoholic liver disease. *Alcohol Health Res World.* 1997;21(4):317-320.

33. Lands WE. Cellular signals in alcohol-induced liver injury: a review. *Alcohol Clin Exp Res.* 1995;19(4):928-938.

34. Maher J, Friedman S. Pathogenesis of hepatic fibrosis. In: Hall P (Ed.). <u>Alcoholic Liver Disease: Pathology and Pathogenesis</u>. Oxford University Press. London, England. 1995.

35. Lieber CS. Hepatic and other medical disorders of alcoholism: from pathogenesis to treatment. *J Stud Alcohol.* 1998;59(1):9-25.

36. Lieber CS. Alcoholic liver disease: new insights in pathogenesis lead to new treatments. *J Hepatol.* 2000;32(1 Suppl):113-128.

37. Kurose I, Higuchi H, Kato S, Miura S, Ishii H. Ethanol-induced oxidative stress in the liver. *Alcohol Clin Exp Res.* 1996;20(1 Suppl):77-85A.

38. Gavaler J, Arria A. Increases susceptibility of women to alcoholic liver disease: Artifactual or real? In: Hall P (Ed.). <u>Alcoholic Liver Disease: Pathology and Pathogenesis</u>. Oxford University Press. London, England. 1995.

39. Tuyns AJ, Pequignot G. Greater risk of ascitic cirrhosis in females in relation to alcohol consumption. *Int J Epidemiol.* 1984;13(1):53-57.

40. Nicholls P, Edwards G, Kyle E. Alcoholics admitted to four hospitals in England. II. General and cause-specific mortality. *Q J Stud Alcohol.* 1974;35(3):841-855.

41. Patwardhan RV, Desmond PV, Johnson RF, Schenker S. Impaired elimination of caffeine by oral contraceptive steroids. *J Lab Clin Med.* 1980;95(4):603-608.

42. Johnson RD, Williams R. Genetic and environmental factors in the individual susceptibility to the development of alcoholic liver disease. *Alcohol Alcohol.* 1985;20(2):137-160.

43. Frezza M, di Padova C, Pozzato G, et al. High blood alcohol levels in women. The role of decreased gastric alcohol dehydrogenase activity and first-pass metabolism. *N Engl J Med.* 1990;322(2):95-99.

44. Taylor JL, Dolhert N, Friedman L, et al. Alcohol elimination and simulator performance of male and female aviators: a preliminary report. *Aviat Space Environ Med.* 1996;67(5):407-413.

45. Kwo PY, Ramchandani VA, O'Connor S, et al. Gender differences in alcohol metabolism: relationship to liver volume and effect of adjusting for body mass. *Gastroenterology.* 1998;115(6):1552-1557.

46. Li T, Beard J, Orr W, et al. Gender and ethnic differences in alcohol metabolism. *Alcohol Clin Exp Res.* 1998;22(3):771-772.

47. Levitt MD, Li R, DeMaster EG, et al. Use of measurements of ethanol absorption from stomach and intestine to assess human ethanol metabolism. *Am J Physiol.* 1997;273(4 Pt 1):G951-957.

48. Mochida S, Ohnishi K, et al. Effect of alcohol intake on the efficacy of interferon

therapy in patients with chronic hepatitis C as evaluated by multivariate logistic regression analysis. *Alcohol Clin Exp Res*. 1996;20(95):371-377A.

49. Fleming M, Manwell LB. Brief intervention in primary care settings. A primary treatment method for at-risk, problem, and dependent drinkers. *Alcohol Res Health*. 1999;23(2):128-137.

50. Alcohol Alert No. 43. Brief intervention for alcohol problems. National Institute on Alcohol Abuse and Alcoholism. Bethesda, Maryland. 1999.

51. DiClemente CC, Bellino LE, Neavins TM. Motivation for change and alcoholism treatment. *Alcohol Res Health*. 1999;23(2):86-92.

52. Steinglass P. Family Therapy: Alcohol. In: Galanter M, Kleber H, (Eds.). The American Psychiatric Press Textbook of Substance Abuse Treatment. American Psychiatric Press. Washington, DC. 1999.

53. O'Farrell TJ. Marital and family therapy in alcoholism treatment. *J Subst Abuse Treat*. 1989;6(1):23-29.

54. Matching Alcoholism Treatments to Client Heterogeneity: Project MATCH posttreatment drinking outcomes. *J Stud Alcohol*. 1997;58(1):7-29.

55. Miller WR, Zweben A, DiClemente CC, Rychatrik R. Motivational Enhancement Therapy Manual. NIH Pub. No. 94-3723. National Institutes of Health. Rockville, Maryland. 1995.

56. Humphreys K, Mankowski ES, Moos RH, Finney JW. Do enhanced friendship networks and active coping mediate the effect of self-help groups on substance abuse? *Ann Behav Med*. 1999;21(1):54-60.

57. Tonigan JS, Toscova R, Miller WR. Meta-analysis of the literature on Alcoholics Anonymous: sample and study characteristics moderate findings. *J Stud Alcohol*. 1996;57(1):65-72.

58. Longabaugh R, Wirtz PW, Zweben A, Stout RL. Network support for drinking, Alcoholics Anonymous and long-term matching effects. *Addiction*. 1998;93(9):1313-1333.

59. Morgenstern J, Labouvie E, McCrady BS, et al. Affiliation with Alcoholics Anonymous after treatment: a study of its therapeutic effects and mechanisms of action. *J Consult Clin Psychol*. 1997;65(5):768-777.

60. Schiffman S, Balabanis M. Associations between alcohol and tobacco. In: Fertig J, Allen J (Eds.). Alcohol and Tobacco: From Basic Science to Clinical Practice. NIH Pub No. 95-3531. National Institutes of Health. Bethesda, Maryland. 1995.

61. Hurt RD, Eberman KM, Croghan IT, et al. Nicotine dependence treatment during inpatient treatment for other addictions: a prospective intervention trial. *Alcohol Clin Exp Res*. 1994;18(4):867-872.

Chapter 3
PROGRESSION OF LIVER DISEASE
Lorren Sandt

1. Datz C, Cramp M, Haas T, Dietze O Nitschko H. The natural course of hepatitis C virus infection 18 years after an epidemic outbreak of non-A, non-B hepatitis in a plasmapheresis centre. *Gut*. 1999;44(4):563-567.

2. Persico M, Persico E, Suozzo R, et al. Natural history of hepatitis C virus carriers with persistently normal aminotransferase levels. *Gastroenterology*. 2000;118(4):760-764.

3. Knodell R, Ishak K, Black W, et al. Formulation and application of a numerical scoring system for assessing histological activity in asymptomatic chronic active hepatitis. *Hepatology*. 1981;1(5):431-435.

4. Ishak K, Baptista A, Bianchi L, et al. Histological grading and staging of chronic hepati-

tis. *J Hepatol.* 1995;22(6):696-699.

5. The French METIVIR Cooperative Study Group. Intraobserver and interobserver variations in liver biopsy interpretation in patients with chronic hepatitis C. *Hepatology.* 1994;20(1 Pt 1):15-20.

6. Desmet V, Gerber M, Hoofnagle J, et al. Classification of chronic hepatitis: diagnosis, grading and staging. *Hepatology.* 1994;19(6):1513-1520.

Chapter 4
SIGNS AND SYMPTOMS THAT MAY BE ASSOCIATED WITH HEPATITIS C
Tina M. St. John, MD

1. Dolan, M. The Hepatitis C Handbook, 2nd Edition. North Atlantic Books. Berkely, California. 1999.

2. Fauci A, Braunwald E, Isselbacher K, Wilson J, Martin J, Kasper D, Hauser S, Longo D (Eds.). Harrison's Principles of Internal Medicine, 14th Edition. McGraw Hill Companies. New York, New York. 1998.

3. Mandell G, Bennett J, Dolin R (Eds.). Principles and Practice of Infectious Diseases, 4th Edition. Churchill Livingstone. New York, New York. 1995.

Chapter 5
LABORATORY TESTS AND PROCEDURES
Tina M. St. John, MD

1. Burtis CA, Ashwood ER (Eds.). Tietz Textbook of Clinical Chemistry, 3rd Edition. W.B. Saunders Company. Philadelphia, Pennsylvania. 1999.

2. Cotran RS, Kumar V, Robbins SL, Schoen FJ (Eds.). Robbins Pathological Basis of Disease, 5th Ed. W.B. Saunders Company. Philadelphia, Pennsylvania. 1994.

3. Dolan M. The Hepatitis C Handbook, 2nd Edition. North Atlantic Books. Berkeley, California. 1999.

4. Fauci AS, Braunwald E, Isselbacher KJ, Wilson JD, Martin JB, Kasper DL, Hauser SL, Longo DL (Eds.). Harrison's Principles of Internal Medicine, 14th Edition. McGraw-Hill Companies. New York, New York. 1998.

5. Mandell GL, Bennett JE, Dolin R (Eds.). Principles and Practice of Infectious Diseases, 4th Edition. Churchill Livingstone Inc. New York, New York. 1995.

Chapter 6
PROMOTING LIVER HEALTH
Lorren Sandt

1. Waitley D. The Psychology of Winning. Simon & Schuester. New York, New York. 1995.

2. Pearsall P. Superimmunity: Master Your Emotions and Improve Your Health. McGraw-Hill. New York, New York. 1987.

3. Hobson, A. Chemistry of Conscious States. MIT Press. Cambridge, Mass. 1999.

4. Coren S. Sleep Thieves: An Eye-Opening Exploration into the Science and Mysteries of Sleep. Free Press. New York, New York. 1997.

5. Palmer M. Hepatitis and Liver Disease; What you Need to Know. Avery. Venore, TN. 2000.

6. Clouston A, et al. Weight reduction in patients with chronic hepatitis C improves liver

histology and biochemistry. Meeting of the American Association for the Study of Liver Diseases. Dallas, Texas. Abstract 593. *Hepatology.* 2000;32(4).

7. Charnetski CJ, Brennan FX. The effect of sexual behavior on immune system function. Eastern Psychological Association Convention. Providence, Rhode Island. 1999. [At the time of publication, a report on this study was available on the Internet at: http://www.altmedicine.com/Article.asp?ID=1867.]

8. Recommendations for prevention and control of hepatitis C virus (HCV) infection and HCV-related chronic disease. *MMWR.* 1998;47(No.RR19);1-39.

9. Dolan M. The Hepatitis C Handbook, 2nd Ed. North Atlantic Books. Berkeley, California. 1999.

Chapter 7
NUTRITION AND HEPATITIS C
Lark Lands

1. Yu MW, Horng IS, Hsu KH, et al. Plasma selenium levels and risk of hepatocellular carcinoma among men with chronic hepatitis virus infection. *Am J Epidemiol.* 1999;150(4):367-374.

2. Corraro G, Ferrari PA, Galatola G. Exploring the role of diet in modifying the effect of known disease determinants: application to risk factors of liver cirrhosis. *Am J Epidemiol.* 1995;142(11):1136-1146.

3. Willett WC, Ascherio A. Trans fatty acids: are the effects only marginal? *Am J Public Health.* 1994;84(5):722-724.

4. Alter H, Seef L. Recovery, persistence and sequelae in hepatitis C infection: a perspective on long-term outcome. *Sem Liver Disease.* 2000;20(1):17-35.

5. Pessione F, Degos F, Marcellin P. Effect of alcohol consumption and serum hepatitis C virus RNA and histological lesions in chronic hepatitis C. *Hepatology.* 1998;27(6):1717-1722.

6. Palmer BF. Pathogenesis of ascites and renal salt retention in cirrhosis. *J Investig Med.* 1999;47(5):183-202.

7. Tandon N, Thakur V, Guptan RK, Sarin SK. Beneficial influence of an indigenous low-iron diet on serum indicators of iron status in patients with chronic liver disease. *Br J Nutr.* 2000;83(3):235-239.

Chapter 8
WESTERN (ALLOPATHIC) MEDICINE
Section 1
OVERVIEW OF THE WESTERN (ALLOPATHIC) APPROACH TO
THE TREATMENT OF HEPATITIS C
Douglas LaBrecque, MD

1. Bonkovsky HL, Woolley JM. Reduction of health-related quality of life in chronic hepatitis C and improvement with interferon therapy. The Consensus Interferon Study Group. *Hepatology.* 1999;29(1):264-270.

2. McHutchison JG, Gordon SC, Schiff ER, et al. Interferon alfa-2b alone or in combination with ribavirin as initial treatment for chronic hepatitis C. Hepatitis Interventional Therapy Group. *N Engl J Med.* 1998;339(21):1485-1492.

3. EASL: International Consensus Conference on Hepatitis C Consensus Statement.. *J Hepatol.* 1999;30(5):956-961.

4. Schalm SW, Weiland O, Hansen B, et al. Interferon-ribavirin for chronic hepatitis C with

and without cirrhosis: analysis of individual patient data of six controlled trials. Eurohep Study Group for Viral Hepatitis. *Gastroenterology.* 1999;117(2):408-413.

5. Zeuzem S, Feinman SV, Rasenack J, et al. Peginterferon alfa-2a in patients with chronic hepatitis C. *N Engl J Med.* 2000;343(23):1666-1672.

6. Heathcote EJ, Shiffman ML, Cooksley WG, et al. Peginterferon alfa-2a in patients with chronic hepatitis C and cirrhosis. *N Engl J Med.* 2000;343(23):1673-1680.

7. Serfaty L, Aumaitre H, Chazouilleres O, et al. Determinants of outcome of compensated hepatitis C virus-related cirrhosis. *Hepatology.* 1998;27(5):1435-1440.

8. Giannini E, Fasoli A, Botta F, et al. Long-term follow up of chronic hepatitis C patients after alpha-interferon treatment: a functional study. *J Gastroenterol Hepatol.* 2001;16(4):399-405.

9. Foster GR, Goldin RD, Thomas HC. Chronic hepatitis C virus infection causes a significant reduction in quality of life in the absence of cirrhosis. *Hepatology.* 1998;27(1):209-212.

10. Rodger AJ, Jolley D, Thompson SC, et al. The impact of diagnosis of hepatitis C virus on quality of life. *Hepatology.* 1999;30(5):1299-1301.

11. Ware JE, Jr., Bayliss MS, Mannocchia M, Davis GL. Health-related quality of life in chronic hepatitis C: impact of disease and treatment response. The Interventional Therapy Group. *Hepatology.* 1999;30(2):550-555.

12. Nishiguchi S, Kuroki T, Nakatani S, et al. Randomized trial of effects of interferon-alpha on incidence of hepatocellular carcinoma in chronic active hepatitis C with cirrhosis. *Lancet.* 1995;346(8982):1051-1055.

13. Fattovich G, Giustina G, Degos F, et al. Effectiveness of interferon-alfa on incidence of hepatocellular carcinoma and decompensation in cirrhosis type C. European Concerted Action on Viral Hepatitis (EUROHEP). *J Hepatol.* 1997;27(1):201-205.

14. Fattovich G, Giustina G, Degos F, et al. Morbidity and mortality in compensated cirrhosis type C: a retrospective follow-up study of 384 patients. *Gastroenterology.* 1997;112(2):463-472.

15. Mazzella G, Accogli E, Sottili S, et al. Alpha-interferon treatment may prevent hepatocellular carcinoma in HCV- related liver cirrhosis. *J Hepatol.* 1996;24(2):141-147.

16. Camma C, Giunta M, Andreone P, Craxi A. Interferon and prevention of hepatocellular carcinoma in viral cirrhosis: an evidence-based approach. *J Hepatol.* 2001;34(4):593-602.

17. Baffis V, Shrier I, Sherker AH, Szilagyi A. Use of interferon for prevention of hepatocellular carcinoma in cirrhotic patients with hepatitis B or hepatitis C virus infection. *Ann Intern Med.* 1999;131(9):696-701.

18. Ikeda K, Saitoh S, Kobayashi M, et al. Long-term interferon therapy for 1 year or longer reduces the hepatocellular carcinogenesis rate in patients with liver cirrhosis caused by hepatitis C virus: a pilot study. *J Gastroenterol Hepatol.* 2001;16(4):406-415.

19. Marcellin P, Boyer N, Gervais A, et al. Long-term histologic improvement and loss of detectable intrahepatic HCV RNA in patients with chronic hepatitis C and sustained response to interferon-alpha therapy. *Ann Intern Med.* 1997;127(10):875-881.

20. Lau DT, Kleiner DE, Ghany MG, Park Y, Schmid P, Hoofnagle JH. 10 year follow-up after interferon-alpha therapy for chronic hepatitis C. *Hepatology.* 1998 Oct;28(4):1121-1127.

21. Bailar JC, III. The powerful placebo and the Wizard of Oz. *N Engl J Med.* 2001;344(21):1630-1632.

22. Hrobjartsson A, Gotzsche PC. Is the placebo powerless? An analysis of clinical trials comparing placebo with no treatment. *N Engl J Med.* 2001;344(21):1594-1602.

23. Shiffman ML, Hofmann CM, Contos MJ, et al. A randomized, controlled trial of mainte-

nance interferon therapy for patients with chronic hepatitis C virus and persistent viremia. *Gastroenterology*. 1999;117(5):1164-1172.

24. Balart L, Lee S, Schiffman M, et al. Histologic improvement following treatment with once weekly pegylated interferon alfa-2a (Pegasys) and thrice weekly interferon alfa-2a (Roferon) in patients with chronic hepatitis C and compensated cirrhosis. *Gastroenterology*. 2000;118:A961 (abstract). [Note: This abstract is not available on the National Library of Medicine database PubMed.]

25. Poynard T, McHutchison J, Davis GL, et al. Impact of interferon alfa-2b and ribavirin on progression of liver fibrosis in patients with chronic hepatitis C. *Hepatology*. 2000;32(5):1131-1137.

26. Poynard T, Ratziu V, Benmanov Y, et al.. Fibrosis in patients with chronic hepatitis C: detection and significance. *Semin Liver Dis*. 2000;20(1):47-55.

27. Muriel P. Alpha-interferon prevents liver collagen deposition and damage induced by prolonged bile duct obstruction in the rat. *J Hepatol*. 1996;24(5):614-621.

28. Fort J, Pilette C, Veal N, et al. Effects of long-term administration of interferon alpha in two models of liver fibrosis in rats. *J Hepatol*. 1998;29(2):263-270.

29. Reeves HL, Dack CL, Peak M, Burt AD, Day CP. Stress-activated protein kinases in the activation of rat hepatic stellate cells in culture. *J Hepatol*. 2000 Mar;32(3):465-72.

Section 2
TREATMENT OPTIONS FOR THOSE
WHO HAVE NOT HAD PRIOR TREATMENT
Douglas LaBrecque, MD

1. Hoofnagle JH, Mullen KD, Jones DB, et al. Treatment of chronic non-A,non-B hepatitis with recombinant human alpha interferon. A preliminary report. *N Engl J Med*. 1986;315(25):1575-1578.

2. Di Bisceglie AM, Martin P, Kassianides C, et al. Recombinant interferon alfa therapy for chronic hepatitis C. A randomized, double-blind, placebo-controlled trial. *N Engl J Med*. 1989;321(22):1506-1510.

3. Davis GL, Balart LA, Schiff ER, et al. Treatment of chronic hepatitis C with recombinant alfa-interferon. A multicenter randomized, controlled trial. The Hepatitis Interventional Therapy Group. *J Hepatol*. 1990;11(Suppl 1):S31-35.

4. Causse X, Godinot H, Chevallier M, et al. Comparison of 1 or 3 MU of interferon alfa-2b and placebo in patients with chronic non-A, non-B hepatitis. *Gastroenterology*. 1991;101(2):497-502.

5. Marcellin P, Boyer N, Giostra E, et al. Recombinant human alpha-interferon in patients with chronic non-A, non-B hepatitis: a multicenter randomized controlled trial from France. *Hepatology*. 1991;13(3):393-397.

6. Lee WM. Therapy of hepatitis C: interferon alfa-2a trials. *Hepatology*. 1997;26(3 Suppl 1):89-95S.

7. Chemello L, Bonetti P, Cavalletto L, et al. Randomized trial comparing three different regimens of alpha-2a- interferon in chronic hepatitis C. The TriVeneto Viral Hepatitis Group. *Hepatology*. 1995;22(3):700-706.

8. Rumi M, Del Ninno E, Parravicini ML, et al. A prospective, randomized trial comparing lymphoblastoid to recombinant interferon alfa 2a as therapy for chronic hepatitis C. *Hepatology*. 1996;24(6):1366-1370.

9. Diodati G, Bonetti P, Noventa F, et al. Treatment of chronic hepatitis C with recombinant human interferon- alpha 2a: results of a randomized controlled clinical trial. *Hepatology*. 1994;19(1):1-5.

10. Douglas DD, Rakela J, Lin HJ, et al. Randomized controlled trial of recombinant alpha-2a-

interferon for chronic hepatitis C. Comparison of alanine aminotransferase normalization versus loss of HCV RNA and anti-HCV IgM. *Dig Dis Sci.* 1993;38(4):601-607.

11. Keeffe EB, Hollinger FB. Therapy of hepatitis C: consensus interferon trials. Consensus Interferon Study Group. *Hepatology.* 1997;26(3 Suppl 1):101-107S.

12. Tong MJ, Reddy KR, Lee WM, et al. Treatment of chronic hepatitis C with consensus interferon: a multicenter, randomized, controlled trial. Consensus Interferon Study Group. *Hepatology.* 1997;26(3):747-754.

13. Poynard T, Leroy V, Cohard M, et al. Meta-analysis of interferon randomized trials in the treatment of viral hepatitis C: effects of dose and duration. *Hepatology.* 1996;24(4):778-789.

14. Lin R, Roach E, Zimmerman M, et al. Interferon alfa-2b for chronic hepatitis C: effects of dose increment and duration of treatment on response rates. Results of the first multicentre Australian trial. Australia Hepatitis C Study Group. *J Hepatol.* 1995;23(5):487-496.

15. Manesis EK, Papaioannou C, Gioustozi A, et al. Biochemical and virological outcome of patients with chronic hepatitis C treated with interferon alfa-2b for 6 or 12 months: a 4-year follow- up of 211 patients. *Hepatology.* 1997;26(3):734-739.

16. Poynard T, Bedossa P, Chevallier M, et al. A comparison of three interferon alfa-2b regimens for the long-term treatment of chronic non-A, non-B hepatitis. Multicenter Study Group. *N Engl J Med.* 1995;332(22):1457-1462.

17. Reichard O, Foberg U, Fryden A, et al. High sustained response rate and clearance of viremia in chronic hepatitis C after treatment with interferon-alpha 2b for 60 weeks. *Hepatology.* 1994;19(2):280-285.

18. Carithers RL, Jr, Emerson SS. Therapy of hepatitis C: meta-analysis of interferon alfa-2b trials. *Hepatology.* 1997;26(3 Suppl 1):83-88S.

19. EASL: International Consensus Conference on Hepatitis C Consensus Statement. *J Hepatol.* 1999;30(5):956-961.

20. Schalm SW, Weiland O, Hansen BE, et al. Interferon-ribavirin for chronic hepatitis C with and without cirrhosis: analysis of individual patient data of six controlled trials. Eurohep Study Group for Viral Hepatitis. *Gastroenterology.* 1999;117(2):408-413.

21. Recommendations for prevention and control of hepatitis C virus (HCV) infection and HCV-related chronic disease. *MMWR.* 1998;47(No. RR-19):1-39.

22. Poynard T, Marcellin P, Lee SS, et al. Randomised trial of interferon alpha2b plus ribavirin for 48 weeks or for 24 weeks versus interferon alpha2b plus placebo for 48 weeks for treatment of chronic infection with hepatitis C virus. International Hepatitis Interventional Therapy Group (IHIT). *Lancet.* 1998;352(9138):1426-1432.

23. McHutchison JG, Gordon SC, Schiff ER, et al. Interferon alfa-2b alone or in combination with ribavirin as initial treatment for chronic hepatitis C. Hepatitis Interventional Therapy Group. *N Engl J Med.* 1998;339(21):1485-1492.

24. Poynard T, McHutchison J, Goodman Z, et al. Is an "a la carte" combination interferon alfa-2b plus ribavirin regimen possible for the first line treatment in patients with chronic hepatitis C? The ALGOVIRC Project Group. *Hepatology.* 2000;31(1):211-218.

25. Schalm SW, Hansen BE, Chemello L, et al. Ribavirin enhances the efficacy but not the adverse effects of interferon in chronic hepatitis C. Meta-analysis of individual patient data from European centers. *J Hepatol.* 1997;26(5):961-966.

26. Reddy KR. Controlled-release, pegylation, liposomal formulations: new mechanisms in the delivery of injectable drugs. *Ann Pharmacother.* 2000;34(7-8):915-923.

27. Kozlowski A, Harris JM. Improvements in protein PEGylation: pegylated interferons for treatment of hepatitis C. *J Control Release.* 2001;72(1-3):217-224.

28. Zeuzem S, Feinman SV, Rasenack J, et al. Peginterferon alfa-2a in patients with chronic hepatitis C. *N Engl J Med.* 2000;343(23):1666-1672.

29. Heathcote EJ, Shiffman ML, Cooksley W, et al. Peginterferon alfa-2a in patients with chronic

hepatitis C and cirrhosis. *N Engl J Med.* 2000;343(23):1673-1680.

30. Glue P, Rouzier-Panis R, Raffanel C, et al. A dose-ranging study of pegylated interferon alfa-2b and ribavirin in chronic hepatitis C. The Hepatitis C Intervention Therapy Group. *Hepatology.* 2000;32(3):647-653.

31. Fried M, Shiffman M, Reddy R, et al. Pegylated (40 kDa) interferon alfa-2a (PEGASYS) in combination with ribavirin: efficacy and safety results from a phase III, randomized, actively-controlled, multicenter study. *Gastroenterology.* 120 (Suppl), A55. 2001. (Abstract).

32. Manns M, McHutchison J, Gordon S, et al. Peginterferon alfa-2b plus ribavirin compared with interferon alfa-2b plus ribavirin for initial treatmentof chronic hepatitis C: a randomized trial. *Lancet.* 2001;358(9286):958-965.

33. Trepo C, Lindsey K, Niederau C, et al. Pegylated interferon alfa-2b (PEG-INTRON) monotherapy is superior to interferon alfa-2b (INTRON A) for the treatment of chronic hepatitis C. *J Hepatol.* 2000;32(S2):29.

34. Sulkowski M, Reindollar R, Yu J. Pegylated interferon alfa-2a (PEGASYS) and ribavirin combination therapy for chronic hepatitis C: a phase II open-label study. *Gastroenterology.* 188(S2), A950. 2000. (Abstract).

35. Jacobson IM, Russo M, Brown R, et al. Pegylated interferon alfa-2b plus ribavirin in patients with chronic hepatitis C: a trial in prior nonresponders to interferon monotherapy or combination therapy, and in combination therapy relapsers. *Gastroenterology.* 120(S1). 2001. (Abstract).

36. Fried MW, Shiffman ML, Reddy KR, et al. Peginterferon alfa-2a plus ribavirin for chronic hepatitis C virus infection. *N Engl J Med.* 2002;347(13):975-982.

37. Reddy KR, Wright TL, Pockros PJ, et al. Efficacy and safety of pegylated (40-kd) interferon alpha-2a compared with interferon alpha-2a in noncirrhotic patients with chronic hepatitis C. *Hepatology.* 2001;33(2):433-438.

38. Hassanein T, et.al. Treatment with 40kda peginterferon alfa-2a (Pegasys) in combination with ribavirin significantly enhances quality of life compared with interferon alpha-2b plus ribavirin. *Hepatology.* 2001;34:243A (abstract). [Note: This abstract is not available on the National Library of Medicine database PubMed.]

39. Perrillo RP, Rothstein K, Alam I, et al. Efficacy, safety, and tolerability in patients switched to PEG (40 kDa) IFN alfa-2a (PEGASYS) after discontinuation from interferon alfa-2b plus ribavirin (REBETRON) combination therapy for chronic hepatitis C. *Gastroenterology.* 120(S1), A567. 2001. (Abstract).

40. Rothstein K, Perrillo RP, Imperial J, et al. Efficacy, quality of life, safety, and tolerability in patients with chronic hepatitis C treated with PEG (40 kDa) IFN alfa-2a (PEGASYS) or standard interferon alfa-2b/ribavirin (REBETRON) combination therapy. *Gastroenterology.* 120(S1), A77. 2001. (Abstract).

41. Bernstein D, Cooksley G, Fried MW, et al. Correlation of health-related quality of life with virological response and early treatment discontinuation in patients treated with pegylated (40 kDa) interferon alfa-2a (PEGASYS) compared with standard interferon alfa-2a. *Gastroenterology.* 120(S1), A382. 2001. (Abstract).
Jaeckel E, Cornberg M, Wedemeyer H, et al. Treatment of acute hepatitis C with interferon alfa-2b. *N Eng J Med.* 2001;345(20):1452-1457.

42. National Institutes of Health Consensus Development Conference: Management of Hepatitis C: 2002. *Hepatology.* 2002;36(5):Suppl 1. [Note: This is not available on the National Library of Medicine database PubMed. At the time of publication, the final consensus statement was available at: http://consensus.nih.gov/cons/116/Hepc091202.pdf.]

43. Sjogren M, Holtzmuller K, Smith M, Sjogren, Jr R. Sustained antiviral response with consensus interferon (CIFN) plus ribavirin or interferon alfa-2b (IFN alfa-2b) plus ribavirin in treatment-naïve subjects with chronic hepatitis C. A pilot study. *Hepatology.* 2002;36:311A (abstract).

[Note: This abstract is not available on the National Library of Medicine database PubMed.]

44. Kaiser S, Hass H, Gregor M. High dose induction therapy with consensus interferon and ribavirin for treatment-naïve patients with hepatitis C. *Hepatology*. 2002:36:362A (abstract). [Note: This abstract is not available on the National Library of Medicine database PubMed.]

45. Kaiser S, Hass H, Gregor M. High viral response rates in previous interferon/ribavirin nonresponder patients with chronic hepatitis C retreated with consensus interferon induction therapy and ribavirin. *Hepatology*. 2002;36:358A (abstract). [Note: This abstract is not available on the National Library of Medicine database PubMed.]

46. Marcellin P, Levy S, Erlinger S. Therapy of hepatitis C: patients with normal aminotransferase levels. *Hepatology*. 1997;26(3 Suppl 1):133-136S.

47. Zeuzem S. Treatment of chronic hepatitis C virus infection in patients with cirrhosis. *J Viral Hepat*. 2000;7(5):327-334.

48. Gumber SC, Chopra S. Hepatitis C: a multifaceted disease. Review of extrahepatic manifestations. *Ann Intern Med*. 1995;123(8):615-620.

49. Cacoub P, Poynard T, Ghillani P, et al. Extrahepatic manifestations of chronic hepatitis C. MULTIVIRC Group. Multidepartment Virus C. *Arthritis Rheum*. 1999;42(10):2204-2212.

50. Darby SC, Ewart DW, Giangrande PL, et al. Mortality from liver cancer and liver disease in haemophilic men and boys in UK given blood products contaminated with hepatitis C. UK Haemophilia Centre Directors' Organisation. *Lancet*. 1997;350(9089):1425-1431.

51. Benhamou Y, Bochet M, Di Martino V, et al. Liver fibrosis progression in human immunodeficiency virus and hepatitis C virus coinfected patients. The Multivirc Group. *Hepatology*. 1999;30(4):1054-1058.

52. Daar ES, Lynn H, Donfield S, et al. Relation between HIV-1 and hepatitis C viral load in patients with hemophilia. *J Acquir Immune Defic Syndr*. 2001;26(5):466-472.

53. Nishiguchi S, Kuroki T, Nakatani S, et al. Randomised trial of effects of interferon-alpha on incidence of hepatocellular carcinoma in chronic active hepatitis C with cirrhosis. *Lancet*. 1995;346(8982):1051-1055.

54. Fattovich G, Giustina G, Degos F, et al. Effectiveness of interferon alfa on incidence of hepatocellular carcinoma and decompensation in cirrhosis type C. European Concerted Action on Viral Hepatitis (EUROHEP). *J Hepatol*. 1997;27(1):201-205.

55. Fattovich G, Giustina G, Degos F, et al. Morbidity and mortality in compensated cirrhosis type C: a retrospective follow-up study of 384 patients. *Gastroenterology*. 1997;112(2):463-472.

56. Mazzella G, Accogli E, Sottili S, et al. Alpha interferon treatment may prevent hepatocellular carcinoma in HCV-related liver cirrhosis. *J Hepatol*. 1996;24(2):141-147.

57. Camma C, Giunta M, Andreone P, Craxi A. Interferon and prevention of hepatocellular carcinoma in viral cirrhosis: an evidence-based approach. *J Hepatol*. 2001;34(4):593-602.

58. Baffis V, Shrier I, Sherker AH, Szilagyi A. Use of interferon for prevention of hepatocellular carcinoma in cirrhotic patients with hepatitis B or hepatitis C virus infection. *Ann Intern Med*. 1999;131(9):696-701.

59. Ikeda K, Saitoh S, Kobayashi M, et al. Long-term interferon therapy for 1 year or longer reduces the hepatocellular carcinogenesis rate in patients with liver cirrhosis caused by hepatitis C virus: a pilot study. *J Gastroenterol Hepatol*. 2001;16(4):406-415.

60. Sulkowski M, et al. Changes in hemoglobin during therapy with interferon alfa-2b plus ribavirin in IFN-naïve and experienced patients. *Hepatology*. 2000;32:368A (abstract). [Note: This abstract is not available on the National Library of Medicine database PubMed.]

61. Sulkowski M, et al. Once weekly recombinant human erythropoietin facilitates optimal ribavirin dosing in hepatitis C virus-infected patients receiving interferon alfa-2b/ribavirin therapy. Poster 18. Annual Meeting of the American Association for the Study of Liver Diseases. Chicago, Illinois. 2001.

62. Wasserman R, et al. Once weekly Epoetin Alfa increases hemoglobin and decreases RBV

discontinuation among HCV patients who develop anemia on RBV/IFN therapy. *Hepatology.* 2000;32:368A (abstract). [Note: This abstract is not available on the National Library of Medicine database PubMed.]

63. Lau DT, Kleiner DE, Ghany MG, Park Y, Schmid P, Hoofnagle JH. 10 year follow-up after interferon-alpha therapy for chronic hepatitis C. *Hepatology.* 1998 Oct;28(4):1121-1127.

Section 3
OPTIONS FOR THOSE WHOSE INITIAL TREATMENT FAILED
TO CLEAR THE HEPATITIS C VIRUS
Gregory T. Everson, MD

1. Fried MW, Shiffman ML, Reddy RK, et al. Peginterferon alfa-2a plus ribavirin for chronic hepatitis C virus infection. *N Engl J Med.* 2002;347:975-982.

2. Carithers RL Jr, Emerson SS. Therapy of hepatitis C: Meta-analysis of interferon alfa-2b trials. *Hepatology.* 1997;26(3 Suppl 1):83-88S.

3. Manns MP, McHutchison JG, Gordon SC,et al and the International Hepatitis Interventional Therapy Group. Peginterferon alfa-2b plus ribavirin compared with interferon alfa-2b plus ribavirin for initial treatment of chronic hepatitis C: A randomized trial. *Lancet.* 2001;358(9286):958-965.

4. Lau DT, Kleiner DE, Ghany MG, et al. 10 years follow-up after interferon alfa therapy for chronic hepatitis C. *Hepatology.* 1998;28(4):1121-1127.

5. Imai Y, Kawata S, Tamura S, et al. Relation of interferon therapy and hepatocellular carcinoma in patients with chronic hepatitis C. Osaka Hepatocellular Carcinoma Prevention Study Group. *Ann Intern Med.* 1998;129(2):94-99.

6. Schalm SW, Fattovich G, Brouwer JT. Therapy of hepatitis C: Patients with cirrhosis. *Hepatology.* 1997;26 (Suppl 1):128-132S.

7. Trotter JF, Wachs M, Everson GT, Kam I. Adult-to-adult transplantation of the right hepatic lobe from a living donor. *N Engl J Med.* 2002;346(14):1074-1082.

8. Everson GT, Weinberg H. Living with Hepatitis C: A Survivor's Guide, 3rd Ed. Hatherleigh Press, Inc. New York, New York. 2001.

9. Cheng SJ, Bonis PA, Lau J, et al.. Interferon and ribavirin for patients with chronic hepatitis C who did not respond to previous interferon therapy: A meta-analysis of controlled and uncontrolled trials. *Hepatology.* 2001;33:231-240.

10. Di Bisceglie AM, Thompson J, Smith-Wilkaitis N, et al. Combination of interferon and ribavirin in chronic hepatitis C: re-treatment of nonresponders to interferon. *Hepatology.* 2001;33:704-707.

11. Everson GT, Folan R, Goff J, et al. The Colorado hepatitis treatment group: Early results of the use of combination interferon-alfa-2B (Intron A) plus ribavirin (Rebetrol) in the treatment of nonresponders. *Hepatology.* 1998; 476A (abstract).

12. Shiffman ML, Hofmann CM, Contos MJ, et al. A randomized, controlled trial of maintenance interferon therapy for patients with chronic hepatitis C virus and persistent viremia. *Gastroenterology.* 1999;117(5):1164-1172.

13. Pestka SS. Langer JA, Zoon KC, Samual KC. Interferons and their actions. *Annu Rev Biochem.* 1987;56:727-777.

14. Fattovich G, Giustina G, Degos F, et al. Effectiveness of inteferon alfa on incidence of hepatocellular carcinoma and decompensation in cirrhosis type C. *J Hepatol.* 1997;27(1):201-205.

15. Everson, GT. Maintenance interferon for chronic hepatitis C: More issues than answers? *Hepatology.* 2000;32(2):436-438.

Section 4:
THE FUTURE OF WESTERN TREATMENT FOR HEPATITIS C
Robert G. Gish, MD

1. Xu ZX, Hoffman J, Patel I, Joubert P. Single-dose safety/tolerability and pharmacokinetics/pharmacodynamics (PK/PD) following administration of ascending subcutaneous doses of pegylated-interferon (PEG-IFN) and interferon alpha-2a (IFN alpha-2a) to healthy subjects. *Hepatology.* 1998;28:A702.

2. Heathcote EJ, Fried MW, Bain MA, DePamphilis J, Modi M. The pharmacokinetics of pegylated-40K interferon alpha-2A (PEG-IFN) in chronic hepatitis C (CHC) patients with cirrhosis. *Gastroenterology* 1999;116:A735.

3. Reddy KR, Wright TL, Pockros PJ, et al. Efficacy and safety of pegylated (40-kd) interferon alpha-2a compater with interferon alpha-2a in noncirrhotic patients with chronic hepatitis C. *Hepatology.* 2001;33(2):433-438.

4. Lindsay KL, Trepo C, Heintges T, et al. A randomized, double-blind trial comparing pegylated interferon alfa-2b to interferon alfa-2b as initial treatment for chronic hepatitis C. *Hepatology.* 2001;34(2):395-403.

5. Healthcote EJ, Shiffman ML, Cooksley WG, et al. Peginterferon alfa-2a in patients with chronic hepatitis C and cirrhosis. *N Engl J Med.* 2000;343(23):1673-1680.

6. Zeuzem S, Herrmann E, Lee JH, et al. Viral kinetics in patients with chronic hepatitis C treated with standard or perinterferon alpha-2a. *Gastroenterology.* 2001;120(6):1438-1447.

7. Abrignani S, Houghton M, Hsu HH. Perspectives for a vaccine against hepatitis C virus. *J Hepatology* 1999;31(Suppl 1):259-263.

8. Tyrell DL, et al. Development of a mouse model to support hepatitis C viral replication. Frontiers for Drug Development. Abstract 024. HepDART 2001. Maui, Hawaii. 2001.

9. Caselmann WH, Eisenhardt S, Alt M. Synthetic antisense oligodeoxynucleotides as potential drugs against hepatitis C. *Intervirology* 1997;40(5-6):394-399.

10. Fattovich G, Giustina G, Alberti A, et al. A randomized controlled trial of thymopentin therapy in patients with chronic hepatitis B. *J Hepatol.* 1994;21:361-366.

11. Eichberg JW, Seeff LB, Lawlor DL, et al. Effect of thymosin immunostimulation with and without corticosteroid immunosuppression on chimpanzee hepatitis B carriers. *J Med Virol.* 1987;21(1):25-37.

12. Davis GL. Treatment of chronic hepatitis B. *Hepatology.* 1991;14(3):567-569.

13. Rasi G, DiVirgilio D, Mutchnick MG, et al. Combination thymosin alpha 1 and lymphoblastoid interferon treatment in chronic hepatitis C. *Gut.* 1996;39(5):679-683.

14. Mutchnick MG, Lindsay KL, Schiff ER, et al. Thymosin a-1 treatment of chronic hepatitis B: a multicenter randomized, placebo-controlled double blind study. *Gastroenterology.* 1995;108:A1127.

15. Holzmayer TA, Pestov DG, Roninson IB. Isolation of dominant negative mutants and inhibitory antisense RNA sequences by expression selection of random DNA fragments. *Nucleic Acids Res.* 1992;20(4):711-717.

16. Endres CL, Bergquam EP, Axthelm MK, Wong SW. Suppression of simian immunodeficiency virus replication by human immunodeficiency virus type 1 trans-dominant negative rev mutants. *J Virol.* 1995;69(8):5164-5166.

17. Purcell R. The hepatitis C virus: overview. *Hepatology.* 1997;26(3 Suppl 1):11-14S.

18. Major ME, Feinstone SM. The molecular virology of hepatitis C. *Hepatology.* 1997;25:1527-1538.

19. Behrens SE, Tomei L, De Francesco R. Identification and properties of the RNA-dependent RNA polymerase of hepatitis C virus. *EMBO J.* 1998;15(1):12-22.

20. Mehta A, Zitzmann N, Rudd PM, Block TM, Dwek RA. Alpha-glucosidase inhibitors as potential broad based anti-viral agents. *FEBS Lett.* 1998;430(1-2):17-22.
21. Flint M, Maidens C, Loomis-Price LD, et al. Characterization of hepatitis C virus E2 glycoprotein interaction with a putative cellular receptor, CD81. *J Virol.* 1999;73(8):6235-6244.
22. Higginbottom A, Quinn ER, Kuo CC, et al. Identification of amino acid residues in CD81 critical for interaction with hepatitis C virus envelope glycoprotein E2. *J Virol.* 2000;74(8):3642-3649.

Chapter 9
AYURVEDIC MEDICINE
Shri K. Mishra MD, MS, Bharathi Ravi, BAMS (Ayurveda) and Sivaramaprasad Vinjamury, MD (Ayurveda)

1. Chatterjee P. Physiology of Gastrointestinal Tract: Human Physiology, Part I. Popular Publishers. Calcutta, India. 1997.
2. Seef LB. The A, B, C, D, E's of viral hepatitis. Annual Postgraduate Gastroenterology Course, Section 2A: Liver. College of Gastroenterology 64th Annual Scientific Meeting. Phoenix, Arizona. 1999.
3. Thomas DL, Astemborski J, Rai RM, et al. The natural history of hepatitis C virus infection: host, viral, and environmental factors. *JAMA.* 2000;284:450-456.
4. Patrick, L. Hepatitis C: Epidemiology and review of complementary alternative medicine treatment. *Altern Med Rev.* 1999;4(4):220-238.
5. National Institutes of Health Consensus Development Conference Panel Statement: management of hepatitis C. *Hepatology.* 1997;26(3 Suppl 1):2-10S.
6. Laksmipathi A. History of Ayurveda. Ayurvedic Encyclopaedia, Vol 1, 16th Edition. Vavilla Ramaswamy Sastrulu and Sons. Madras, India. 1965.
7. Laksmipathi A. Treatises of Ayurveda. Ayurvedic Encyclopaedia, Vol 1. Vavilla Ramaswamy Sastrulu and Sons. Madras, India. 1965.
8. Sharma PV (Ed.). Charaka Samhita: Sutrasthanam, 23rd Edition. Chapter 30, stanza 23. Chaukambha Orientalia. Varanasi, India. 1981.
9. *Ibid,* stanzas 26, 47.
10. *Ibid,* stanza 41.
11. Varier, PS. Principles of Ayurveda, Chikitsa Samgraham. Arya Vaidya Sala, Kottakkal, India. 1989.
12. *Ibid,* ref 8, chapter 12.
13. Vagbhata, D. Ashtanga Hridayam. Chaukambha Orientalia. Varanasi, India. 1980.
14. *Ibid,* stanza 1-8.
15. *Ibid,* ref 8, chapter 20, stanzas 11-13.
16. Sharma PV (Ed.). Charaka Samhita: Vimanasthanam. Chapter 5. Chaukambha Orientalia. Varanasi, India. 1981.
17. Susruta Samhita: Sutrasthanam. Chapter 21, stanza 9. Motilal Banarasidas Publishers. New Delhi, India. 1983.
18. *Ibid,* ref 16, chapter 5, stanzas 6-10.
19. *Ibid,* ref 13, chapter 13, stanza 25.
20. *Ibid,* ref 8, chapter 30, stanzas 6-11.
21. *Ibid,* ref 16, chapter 8, stanzas 112 -115.
22. Susruta Samhita: Sutrasthanam. Motilal Banarasidas Publishers. New Delhi, India. 1983.
23. *Ibid,* chapter 24, stanza 10.

24. *Ibid*, chapter 21.
25. Ibid, ref 8, chapter 20.
26. Sharma PV (Ed.). <u>Charaka Samhita: Nidanasthanam</u>. Chapter 1, stanzas 6-11. Chaukambha Orientalia. Varanasi, India. 1981.
27. <u>Yogaratnakara: Vol ume I, Pradhamakanda</u>. Verse 35. Chaukambha Prakashan. Varanasi, India. 1989.
28. <u>Sarangadhara Samhita</u>. Chapter 1, verses 1-3. Chaukambha Orientalia. Varanasi, India. 1987.
29. *Ibid*, ref 22.
30. *Ibid*, ref 16, chapter 7, stanzas 33, 43.
31. *Ibid*, ref 13, chapter 13.
32. *Ibid*, ref 8, chapter 2.
33. Mishra,Shri K. Recent advances in liver diseases in Ayurvedic medicine in complementary and alternative medicine in chronic liver disease. National Institutes of Health Conference on Complementary and Alternative Medicine in Chronic Liver Diseases. Bethesda, Maryland. 1999 p.67.

AYURVEDIC APPENDIX
Shri K. Mishra MD, MS and Sivaramaprasad Vinjamury, MD

1. Mishra ,Shri,K. Recent advances in liver diseases in Ayurvedic medicine in complementary and alternative medicine in chronic liver disease. National Institutes of Health Conference on Complementary and Alternative Medicine in Chronic Liver Diseases. Bethesda, Maryland. 1999.
2. Nadkarni KM, Nadkarni KA. <u>Indian Materia Medica</u>. Popular Prakashan. Bombay, India. 1993.
3. Luper S. A review of plants used in the treatment of liver disease: part two. *Altern Med Rev.* 1999;4(3):178-188.
4. <u>Madhava Nidanam.</u> Kaamala roga. Vavilla Ramaswamy Sastrulu & Sons. Madras, India. 1975.
5. Sharma PV (Ed.). <u>Charaka Samhita</u>. Vimanasthanam. Chapter 7, stanzas 33, 43. Chaukambha Orientalia. Varanasi, India. 1981.
6. Vagbhata, D. <u>Ashtanga Hridayam</u>. Sutrasthanam. Chapter 13. Chaukambha Orientalia. Varanasi, India. 1980.
7. *Ibid*, ref 5, chapter 16, stanzas 12-48.
8. Frawley, D. <u>Ayurvedic Healing</u>. Motilal Banarasi Das Publishers. New Delhi, India. 1992.
9. <u>Susruta Samhita</u>. Sutrasthanam. Motilal Banarasidas Publishers. New Delhi, India. 1983.
10. Saxena AK, Singh B, Anand KK. Hepatoprotective effects of Eclipta alba on subcellular levels in rats. *J Ethnopharmacol.* 1993;40(3):155-61.
11. Wang M, Cheng H, Li Y, Meng L, Zhao G, Mai K. Herbs of the genus phyllantus in the treatment of chronic heptatitis B: observations with three preparations from different geographic sites. *J Lab Clin Med.* 1995;126(4):350-352.
12. Xiang ZX, He XQ, Zhou GF, et al. Protective effects of an ethanolic extract and essential oil of Curcuma kwangsinensis s. against experimental liver lesions in mice. *Chung Kuo Chung Yao Tsa Chih.* 1989;14(5):303-305, 320.
13. Piper JT, Singhal SS, Salameh MS, et al. Mechanisms of anticarcinogenic properties of curcumin: the effect of curcumin on glutathione linked detoxification enzymes in rat liver. *Int J Bioch Cell Biol.* 1998;30(4):445-456.

14. Wang BE. Treatment of chronic liver diseases with traditional Chinese medicine. *J Gastroenterol Hepatol.* 2000;15(May 15 Suppl):E67-70.

15. Visen PKS, Saraswat B, Patnaik GK, Agarwal DP, Dhawan BN. Protective activity of picroliv isolated from *Picrorhiza kurrooa* against ethanol toxicity in isolated rat hepatocytes. *Indian J Pharmacol.* 1996;28:98-101.

16. Saraswat B, Visen PK, Patnaik GK, Dhawan BN. Ex vivo and in vivo investigations of picroliv from *Picrorhiza kurroa* in an alcohol intoxication model in rats. *J Ethnopharmacol.* 1999;66(3):263-269.

17. Deshpande UR, Gadre SG, Raste AS, Pillai D, Bhide SV, Samuel AM. Protective effect of turmeric (Curcuma longa L.) extract on carbon tetrachloride-induced liver damage in rats. *Indian J Exp Biol.* 1998;36(6):573-77.

Chapter 10
HOMEOPATHIC MEDICINE
Sylvia Flesner, ND

1. Ferley JP, Zmirou D, D'Adhemar D, Balducci F. A controlled evaluation of a homoeopathic preparation in the treatment of influenza-like syndromes. *Br J Clin Pharmacol.* 1989;27(3):329-335.

2. Reilly DT, Taylor MA, McSharry C, Aitchison T. Is homoeopathy a placebo response? Controlled trial of homoeopathic potency, with pollen in hayfever as model. *Lancet.* 1986;2(8512):881-886.

3. Linde K, Clausius N, Ramirez, et al. Are the clinical effects of homeopathy placebo effects? A meta-analysis of placebo-controlled trials. *Lancet.* 1997;350(9081):834-843.

4. Fisher P, Greenwood A, Huskisson EC, Turner P, Belon P. Effect of homeopathic treatment on fibrositis (primary fibromyalgia). *BMJ.* 1989;299(6695):365-366.

Additional References
Wagner H, Wiesenauer M. <u>Phytotherapie and Pflazliche Homoopathika</u>. Fischer-Verlag. Jena, New York. 1995.

Boericke, W. <u>Homeopathic Materia Medica with Repertory, 9th Edition</u>. Boericke and Runyon. Philadelphia, Pennsylvania. 1927.

Clarke, JH. <u>The Prescriber</u>. The CW Daniel Company. Essex, United Kingdom. 1987.

Johnson, J. <u>Homeopathic Family Guide</u>. Boericke & Hahnemann Publishing House. Philadelphia, Pennsylvania. 1886.

Chapter 11
MIND/BODY MEDICINE AND SPIRITUAL HEALING
Peggy McCarthy, MBA

1. Cousins, N. <u>Anatomy of an Illness as Perceived by the Patient</u>. Bantam Books. New York, New York. 1991.

2. Cassileth B. <u>The Alternative Medicine Handbook</u>. W.W. Norton & Co. New York, New York. 1998.

3. Hammar M, Frisk J, Grimas O, et al. Acupuncture treatment of vasomotor symptoms in men with prostatic carcinoma: a pilot study. *J Urol.* 1999;161(3):853-856.

4. Komori T, Fujiwara R, Tanida M, et al. Effects of citrus fragrance on immune function and depressive states. *Neuroimmunomodulation.* 1995;2(3):174-180.

5. Cawthorn A. A review of the literature surrounding the research into aromatherapy. *Complement Ther Nurs Midwifery.* 1995;1(4):118-120.

6. Rose JE, Behm FM. Inhalation of vapor from black pepper extract reduces smoking withdrawal symptoms. *Drug Alcohol Depend.* 1994;34(3):225-229.

7. Alternative medicine: expanding medical horizons. A report to the National Institutes of Health on alternative medical systems and practices in the United States. NIH Pub. No. 94-066. US Government Printing Office. Washington, DC. 1994.

8. Ezzone S, Baker C, Rosselet R, Terepka E. Music as an adjunct to antiemetic therapy. *Oncol Nurs Forum.* 1998;25(9):1551-1556.

9. Watkins GR. Music therapy: proposed physiological mechanisms and clinical implications. *Clin Nurse Spec.* 1997;11(2):43-50.

10. Lane D. Music therapy: a gift beyond measure. *Oncol Nurs Forum.* 1992;19(6):863-867.

11. Fields of practice: mind-body control. National Institutes of Health Internet site available at the time of publication at: http://nccam.nih.gov/health/whatiscam/.

12. Mathewson-Chapman M. Pelvic muscle exercise/biofeedback for urinary incontinence after prostatectomy: an education program. *J Cancer Educ.* 1997;12(4):218-223.

13. NIH Technology Assessment Panel. Integration of behavioral and relaxation approaches into the treatment of chronic pain and insomnia. *JAMA.* 1996:276(4):313-318.

14. Shekelle PG, Adams AH, Chassin MR, et al. Spinal manipulation for low-back pain. *Ann Intern Med.* 1992;117(7):590-598.

15. Assendelft WJ, Koes BW, Knipschild PG, Bouter LM. The relationship between methodological quality and conclusions in reviews of spinal manipulation. *JAMA.* 1995;274(24):1942-1948.

16. *Ibid*, ref 2

17. Green C, Martin CW, Bassett K, Kazanjian. A systematic review of craniosacral therapy; biological plausibility, assessment reliability and clinical effectiveness. *Complement Ther Med.* 1999;7(4):201-207.

18. Complementary and Alternative Methods. Crystal healing. American Cancer Society Internet site available at the time of publication at: http://www.cancer.org/eprise/main/docroot/ETO/content/ETO_5_3X_Crystals?sitearea=ETO.

19. Monsour AA, Beuche M, Laing G, Leis A. A study to test the effectiveness of placebo Reiki standardization procedures developed for a planned Reiki efficacy study. *J Altern Complement Med.* 1999;5(2):153-164.

20. Rosa L, Rosa E, Sarner L, Barrett S. A close look at therapeutic touch. *JAMA.* 1998;279(13):1005-1010.

21. Launso L, Brendstrup, E, Arnberg S. An exploratory study of reflexological treatment for headache. *Altern Ther Health Med.* 1999;5(3):57-65.

22. *Ibid*, ref 2

23. Cousins N, Dubos R. Anatomy of an Illness as Perceived by the Patient.:Reflections on Healing and Regeneration. W. W. Norton & Co. New York, New York. 1995.

24. Berk LS, Tan SA, Fry WF, et al. Neuroendocrine and stress hormone changes during mirthful laughter. *Am J Med Sci.* 1989;298(6):390-396.

25. Weisenberg M, Tepper I, Schwarzwald, J. Humor as a cognitive technique for increasing pain tolerance. *Pain.* 1995;63(2):207-212.

26. Ziegler J. Immune system may benefit from the ability to laugh. *J Natl Cancer Inst.* 1995;87(5):342-343.

27. Seaward BL. Humor's healing potential. *Health Prog.* 1992;73(3):66-70.

28. *Ibid*, ref 13

29. Morrow GR, Hickok JT. Behavioral treatment of chemotherapy-induced nausea and vomiting. *Oncology*. 1993;7(12):83-89.

30. Levitan AA. The use of hypnosis with cancer patients. *Psychiatr Med*. 1992;10(1):119-131.

31. *Ibid*, ref 2

32. Field TM. Massage therapy effects. *Am Psychol*. 1998;53(12):1270-1281.

33. Cawley N. A critique of the methodology of research studies evaluating massage. *Eur J Cancer Care*. 1997;6(1):23-31.

34. *Ibid*, ref 2

35. Benson H. Timeless Healing: The Power of Biology and Belief. Scribner. New York, New York. 1996.

36. Spencer JW, Jacobs JJ. Complementary/Alternative Medicine: An Evidence-Based Approach. Mosby, Inc. St. Louis, Missouri.1999.

37. Mind-Body Practice: Meditation. National Institutes of Health Internet site available at the time of publication at: http://www.cancer.org/eprise/main/docroot/ETO/content/ ETO_5_3X_Meditation?sitearea=ETO.

38. Coker KH. Meditation and prostate cancer: integrating a mind/body intervention with traditional therapies. *Semin Urol Oncol*. 1999;17(2):111-118.

39. Massion AO, Teas J, Hebert JR, et al. Meditation, melatonin and breast/prostate cancer: hypothesis and preliminary data. *Med Hypotheses*. 1995;44(1):39-46.

40. Wu H, Chen H, Hua X, et al. Clinical therapeutic effect of drug-separated moxibustion on chronic diarrhea and its immunologic mechanisms. *J Tradit Chin Med* 1997;17(4):253-258.

41. Marwick C. Should physicians prescribe prayer for health? Spiritual aspects of well-being considered. *JAMA*. 1995;273(20):1561-1562.

42. Byrd RC. Positive therapeutic effects of intercessory prayer in a coronary care unit population. *South Med J*. 1998;81(7):826-829.

43. Mytko JJ, Knight SJ. Body, mind and spirit: towards the integration of religiosity and spirituality in cancer quality of life research. *Psychooncology*. 1999;8(5):439-450.

44. Harris WS, Gowda M, Kolb JW, et al. A randomized, controlled trial of the effects of remote, intercessory prayer on outcomes in patients admitted to the coronary care unit. *Arch Intern Med*. 1999;159(19):2273-2278.

45. *Ibid*, ref 36

46. Spiegel D, Bloom JR, Kraemer HC, Gottheil E. Effect of psychosocial treatment on survival of patients with metastatic breast cancer. *Lancet*. 1989;2(8668):888-891.

47. Fawzy FI, Fawzy NW, Arndt LA, Pasnau RO. Critical review of psychosocial interventions in cancer care. *Arch Gen Psychiatry*. 1995;52(2):100-113.

48. Cassileth BR. The aim of psychotherapeutic intervention in cancer patients. *Support Care Cancer*. 1995;3(4):267-269.

49. Wu WH, Bandilla E, Ciccone DS, et al. Effects of qi gong on late-stage complex regional pain syndrome. *Altern Ther Health Med*. 1999;5(1):45-54.

50. Sancier KM. Medical applications of qigong. *Altern Ther Health Med*. 1996;2(1):40-46.

51. Cohen K. Native American medicine. *Altern Ther Health Med*. 1998;4(6):45-57.

52. Mehl-Madrona LE. Native American medicine in the treatment of chronic illness: developing an integrated program and evaluating its effectiveness. *Altern Ther Health Med*. 1999;5(1):36-44.

53. Channer KS, Barrow D, Barrow R, Osborne M, Ives G. Changes in haemodynamic parameters following Tai Chi Chuan and aerobic exercise in patients recovering from acute myocardial infarction. *Postgrad Med J*. 1996;72(848):349-351.

54. Kutner NG, Barnhart H, Wolf SL, et al. Self-report benefits of tai chi practice by older

adults. *J Gerontol B Psychol Sci Soc Sci.* 1997;52(17):242-246.

55. Ross MC, Presswalla JL. The therapeutic effects of tai chi for the elderly. *J Gerontol Nurs.* 1998;24:45-47.

56. Province MA, Hadley EC, Hornbrook MC, et al. The effects of exercise on falls in elderly patients. A preplanned meta-analysis of the FICSIT trials. Frailty and injuries: cooperative studies of intervention techniques. *JAMA.* 1995;273(17):1341-1347.

57. Lan C, Lai JS, Wong MK, Yu ML. Cardiorespiratory function, flexibility, and body composition among geriatric tai chi chuan practitioners. *Arch Phy Med Rehabil.* 1996;77(6):612-616.

58. Schaller KJ. Tai chi chih: an exercise option for older adults. *J Gerontol Nurs.* 1996;22(10):12-17.

59. *Ibid,* ref 7

60. Garfinkel MS, Schumacher HR Jr, Husain A, Levy M, Reshetar RA. Evaluation of a yoga-based regimen for treatment of osteoarthritis of the hands. *J Rheumatol.* 1994;21(12):2341-2343.

61. Garfinkel MS, Singhai A, Katz WA, Allan DA, Reshetar R, Schumacher HRJ. Yoga-based intervention for carpal tunnel syndrome: a randomized trial. *JAMA.* 1998;280(18):1601-1603.

62. Taylor E. Yoga and meditation. *Altern Ther Health Med.* 1995;1:77-78.

Chapter 12
MODERN AND TRADITIONAL CHINESE MEDICINE
Qing Cai Zhang, MD (China), LicAc

Note: Many of these citations come from medical journals and reference texts that are published in Chinese. The titles have been translated by Dr. Zhang.

1. Peng WW, et al. The Studies of Viral Hepatitis. Guong Dong Science and Technology Press. Guongzhou, China. 1999.

2. Chen KJ. Some thoughts on advancement of Chinese medicine. *Chinese Journal of Integrated Traditional and Western Medicine.* 2000;20(4P):294.

3. Wang, BJ. TCM Hepatology. Chinese Medical Technology Press. Beijing,China. 1993.

4. Hong JH. Practical TCM Hepatology. TCM College Press. Shanghai, China. 1993.

5. Mathurin P, Moussalli J, Cadranel JF, et al. Slow progression rate of fibrosis in hepatitis C virus patients with persistently normal alanine transaminase activity. *Hepatology.* 1998;27(3):868-872.

6. Ye WF, et al. The Therapy of Liver Diseases. Tianjin Science and Technology Press. Tianjin, China. 1993.

7. Jie YB. Pharmaceutical Action and Application of Available Composition of Chinese Materia Medica. Helongjian Science and Technology Press. Harbin, China. 1992.

8. Wang JT, et al. A review on treating hepatitis B with Chinese medicinal herbs. *Chinese Journal of Infectious Disease.* 1991;9(4):208.

9. Zhang Z, et al. Anti-HBV effects of 60 Chinese medicinal herbs. *Academic Journal of Beijing Medical University.* 1988;20(3):211.

10. Li D, et al. Chinese medicinal herbal treatments for hepatitis B. *New Medicine.* 1985;(6):297.

11. Wang CB. Integrated TCM-WM research of viral hepatitis. *Chinese Journal of Integrated Traditional and Western Medicine.* 1988;8(2):152.

12. Jan CH, et al. The treatment and study of chronic hepatitis. *Chinese Journal of Integrated Traditional and Western Medicine.* 1984;4(2):73.

13. Smaglik P. Reservoirs dog AIDS Therapy. *Nature*. 2000;405(6784):270-272.

14. Zhang, QC. AIDS and Chinese Medicine. OHAI Press. Long Beach, California. 1990.

15. Schiff ER, Sorrell M, Maddrey W (Eds.). Schiff's Diseases of the Liver. Lippincott-Raven Publishers. Philadelphia, Pennsylvania. 1999.

MODERN AND TRADITIONAL CHINESE MEDICINE APPENDIX
Qing Cai Zhang, MD (China), LicAc

Note: Many of these citations come from medical journals and reference texts that are published in Chinese. The titles have been translated by Dr. Zhang.

1. Zheng FR. The current clinical applications of cultured Cordyceps. *Chinese Journal of Hospital Pharmacy*. 1992;12:84.

2. Jie YB. Pharmacological Action and Application of Available Composition of Chinese Materia Medica. Helongjian Science and Technology Press. Harbin, China. 1992.

3. Leatherdale BA, Panesar RK, Singh G, et al. Improvement in glucose tolerance due to Momordica charantia (karela). *British Medical Journal*. 1981;282(6279):1823-1824.

4. Day C, Cartwright T, Provost J, Bailey CJ. Hypoglycaemic effect of Momordica charantia extracts. *Planta Medica*. 1990;56(5):426-429.

5. The Great Dictionary of Chinese Materia Medica. Shanghai Science and Technology Press. Shanghai, China. 1985.

6. Ying J, et al. Modern Studies and Clinical Applications of Chinese Materia Medica, Vol. 1. Xue Huan Press. Beijing, China. 1994:1214-1215.

7. Chen ZB. The anti-microbial effects of Rhei rhizoma. *Academic Journal of Chinese University of Pharmacy*. 1990;21(6):373.

8. Chen JH, et al. Anti-viral effects of Rhei rhizoma. *Journal of New Medicine*. 1974;(5):34.

9. Wang BJ, et al. Blood activating and stasis expelling herbs for chronic hepatitis: Salvia miltiorrhiza. TCM Hepatology. Chinese Medical Technology Press. Beijing, China. 1993:96-97.

10. Pathophysiology Department of Shanghai First Medical College. The effects of Salvia miltiorrhiza on microcirculation. *Chinese Journal of Integrated Traditional and Western Medicine*. 1977;2(4):203.

11. Ma XH, et al. The liver-protective effects of Salvia miltiorrhiza. *Chinese Journal Integrated Traditional and Western Medicine*. 1983;3:180.

12. Bao TT, et al. Modern Studies of Chinese Materia Medicia, Vol. 1. Beijing Medical University and Union Medical University Press. Beijing, China. 1995:371.

13. Sa JM. Treating chronic viral hepatitis with Sophorae subprostratae radix. *Pharmaceutical Bulletin*. 1983;18(10):37.

14. Kimura M. The choleretic effects of Capillaris combination. *Proc Symp WAKAN-YAKU*. 1977;(10):121.

15. Bai G, et al. The Basic Studies and Clinical Applications of TCM Formulas. Chinese Science and Technology Press. Beijing, China. 1995:745.

16. Zheng SX. The study of treating acute jaundice in rat model with Capillaris combination. *Chinese Journal of Integrated Traditional and Western Medicine*. 1985;(6):356.

17. Fan QL. The effects of Persica and Achyranthes combination on microcirculation. *TCM Patent Medicine*. 1988;(7):29.

18. Tianjin First Central Hospital. Treating DIC with Persica and Achyranthes combination. *Chinese Journal of Internal Medicine*. 1977;2(2):79.

19. Liang YJ. Treating nodular vasculitis with Persica and Achyranthes combination. *Journal of TCM*. 1984;(4):44.

20. Liu WX. The effects of Ginseng and Atractylodes combination on intestinal functions on experimental rabbits model. *The Study of TCM Patent Medicine*. 1982;(8):25.

21. Ma YD, et al. Observation on efficacy and experimental study with compound Suanzaoren Ansen capsules for insomnia. *Chinese Journal of Integrated Traditional and Western Medicine*. 1989;9(2):85.

22. Zhou JM. Observation of Yunan paiyao's bleeding-stopping effects. *The Study of TCM Patent Medicine*. 1980;(2):43.

23. Ogle CW, Dai S, Ma JC. The haemostatic effects of the Chinese herbal drug Yunnan Bai Yao: a pilot study. *American Journal Chinese Medicine*. 1976;4(2):147-152.

24. He GM. Yunan pai yao's anti-inflammatory effects. Proceedings of First National Conference of the Association of TCM Materia Medica of China. Beijing, China. 987:949.

Chapter 13
NATUROPATHIC MEDICINE
Lyn Patrick ND

1. Pizzorno J. Total Wellness. Prima Communications. Rocklin, California. 1996: 95-102.

2. Droge W, Pottmeyer-Gerber C, et al. Glutathione augments the activation of cytotoxic T lymphocytes in vivo. *Immunobiology*. 1986;172(2):151-156.

3. White AC, et al. Glutathione deficiency in human disease. *J Nutr Biochem*. 1994;5:218-226.

4. Burgunder JM, Lauterburg BH. Decreased production of glutathione in patients with cirrhosis. *Eur J Clin Invest*. 1987;17:408-414.

5. Loguercio C, Blanco FD, De Girolamo V. Ethanol consumption, amino acid and glutathione blood levels in patients with and without chronic liver disease. *Alcohol Clin Exp Res*. 1999;23(11):1780-1784.

6. Barbaro G, Di Lorenzo G, Soldini M. Hepatic glutathione deficiency in chronic hepatitis C: quantitative evaluation in patients who are HIV positive and HIV negative and correlations with plasmatic and lymphocytic concentrations and with the activity of the liver disease. *Am J Gastroenterol*. 1996;91(12):2569-2573.

7. Staal FJ, Roederer M, Anderson MT, et al. Glutathione deficiency and human immunodeficiency virus infection. *Lancet*. 1992;339:909-912.

8. Alter H, Seef L. Recovery, persistence and sequelae in hepatitis C infection: a perspective on long-term outcome. *Sem Liver Disease*. 2000;20(1):17-35.

9. Pessione F, Degos F, Marcellin P. Effect of alcohol consumption on serum hepatitis C virus RNA and histological lesions in chronic hepatitis C. *Hepatology*. 1998;27(6):1717-1722.

10. Dienstag JL. Management of hepatitis C: a consensus. *Gastroenterology*. 1997;113(2):375.

11. McClain CJ, Price S, et al. Acetaminophen hepatotoxicity: an update. *Curr Gastroenterol Rep*. 1999;1(1):42-49.

12. Mori M, Hara M, Wada I. Prospective study of hepatitis B and C viral infections, cigarette smoking, alcohol consumption, and other factors associated with hepatocellular carcinoma risk in Japan. *Am J Epidemiol*. 2000;151(2):131-139.

13. Urgert R, Meyboom S, Kuilman M, et al. Comparison of the effect of cafetiere and flitered coffee on serum concentrations of liver aminotransferases and lipids: six-month randomized controlled trial. *BMJ*. 1996;313(7069):1362-1366.

14. Urgert R, Schultz AGM, Katan et al. Effects of cafestol and kahweol from coffee grounds on serum lipids and serum liver enzymes in humans. *Am J Clin Nutr*.

1995;61(1):149-154.

15. Etherton GM, Kochar MS. Coffee. Facts and Controversies. *Arch Fam Med*. 1993;2(3):317-322.

16. Michalek JE, Ketchum NS, Alchtar FZ. Postservice mortality of US Air Force veterans occupationally exposed to herbicides in Vietnam: 15-year follow-up. *Am J Epidemiol*. 1998;148(8):786-792.

17. Longnecker MP, Rogan WJ, Lucier G. The human health effect of DDT and PCBs and an overview of organochlorines in public health. *Annu Rev Public Health*. 1997;18:211-244.

18. Redlich CA, Beckett WS, Sparer J, et al. Liver disease associated with occupational exposure to the solvent dimethylformamide. *Ann Int Med*. 1988;108(5):680-686.

19. Pizzorno J, Murray M. Encyclopedia of Natural Medicine. Prima Communications. Rocklin, California. 1998.

20. Sanchez A, Reeser J, Lau HS, et al. Role of sugars in human neutrophilic phagocytosis. *Am J Clin Nutr*. 1973;26(11):1180-1184.

21. Ringsdorf W, Cheraskin E, et al. Sucrose, neutrophil phagocytosis and resistance to disease. *Dent Surv*. 1976;52(12):46-48.

22. Lirussi F, Sanchez B, et al. Natural killer cells in patients with chronic hepatitis C (CHC). *Gut*. 1998;42 (Supp 1):A32.

23. Corrao G, Ferrari PA, Galatola G. Exploring the role of diet in modifying the effect of known disease determinants: application to risk factors of liver cirrhosis. *Am J Epidemiol*. 1995;142(11):1136-1146.

24. Niederau C, Strohmeyer G, Heintges T, et al. Polyunsaturated phosphatidylcholine and interferon alpha for treatment of chronic hepatitis B and C: a multi-center, randomized, double-blind, placebo-controlled trial. Leich Study Group. *Hepatogastroenterology*. 1998;45(21):797-804.

25. Lieber CS. Alcoholic liver disease: new insights in pathogenesis lead to new treatments. *J Heptatol*. 2000;32(1 Suppl):113-128.

26. Flora K, Hahn M, Rosen H, et al. Milk thistle (*Silybum marianum*) for the therapy of liver disease. *Am J Gastroenter*. 1998;93(2):139-143.

27. Strader D, Bacon B, Hoofnagle J, et al. Use of CAM by patients in liver disease clinics. NIH Conference on Complementary and Alternative Medicine in Chronic Liver Disease. Bethesda ,Maryland. 1999.

28. Bosisio E, Benelli C, Pirola O. Effect of the flavanolignans of Silybum marianum L. on lipid peroxidation in rat liver microsomes and freshly isolated hepatocytes. *Pharmacol Res*. 1992;25:147-154.

29. Boigk G, Stroeder L, Herbst H, et al. Silymarin retards collagen accumulation in early and advanced biliary fibrosis secondary to complete bile duct obliteration in rats. *Hepatology*. 1997;26:643-649.

30. Campos R, Garrido A, Guerra A, et al. Silybin dihemisuccinate protects against glutathione depletion and lipid peroxidation induced by acetaminophen on rat liver. *Planta Med*. 1989;55:417-419.

31. Bernhard MC, Junker E, Hettinger A, et al. Time course of total cysteine, glutathione, and homocysteine in plasma of patients with chronic hepatitis C treated with interferon-alpha with and without supplementation with N-acetylcysteine. *J Hepatol*. 1998;28(5):751-755.

32. Magliulo E, Gagliardi B, Fiori GP. Results of a double blind study on the effect of silymarin in the treatment of acute viral hepatitis, carried out at two medical centres. *Med Klin*. 1978;73(28-29):1060-1065.

33. Feher J, Deak G, Muzes G, et al. Hepatoprotective activity of silymarin (Legalon) therapy in patients with chronic liver disease. *Orv Hetil*. 1989;130(51):2723-2727.

34. Ferenci P, Dragosics B, Dittrich H, et al. Randomized controlled trial of silymarin treatment in patients with cirrhosis of the liver. *J Hepatol (Netherlands).* 1989;9(1):105-113.

35. Pares A, Planas R, Torres M, et al. Effects of silymarin in alcoholic patients with cirrhosis of the liver: results of a controlled, double-blinded, randomized and multi-center trial. *J Hepatol.* 1998;28:615-621.

36. Moscarella S, Giusti A, Marra F. Therapeutic and antilipoperoxidant effects of silybin-phosphatidylcholine complex in chronic liver disease: preliminary results. *Curr Ther Res.* 1993;53:98-102.

37. Alschuler L. Milk thistle: goals and objectives. *Int J Integrative Med..* 1999;1:29-34.

38. Venkataramanan R, Ramachandran V, Komoroski BJ, et al. Milk thistle, an herbal supplement, decreases the activity of CYP3A4 and uridine diphosphoglucuronosyl transferase in human hepatocyte cultures. *Drug Metabolism Disposition* 2000;28(11):1270-1273.

39. Arase Y, Ikeda K, Murashima N, et al. The long-term efficacy of glycyrrhizin in chronic hepatitis C patients. *Cancer.* 1997;79(8):1494-1500.

40. Wildhirt E. Experience in Germany with glycyrrhizinic acid for the treatment of chronic viral hepatitis. In: Nishioka K, Suzuki H, Mishiro S. (Eds.). Viral Hepatitis and Liver Disease. Springer-Verlag. Tokyo, Japan. 1994:658-661.

41. Xianshi S, Huiming C, et al. Clinical and laboratory observation on the effect of glycyrrhiza in acute and chronic viral hepatitis. *J Tradit Chin Med.* 1984;4:127-132.

42. Susuki H, Yamamato S, Hirayama C. Cianidanol therapy for HBe-antigen-positive chronic hepatitis :a multicentre, double-blind study. *Liver.* 1986(1);6:35-44.

43. Salama A, Mueller-Eckhardt C. Cianidanol and its metabolites bind tightly to red cells and are responsible for the production of auto- and /or drug-dependant antibodies against these cells. *Br J Haematol.* 1987;66(2):263-266.

44. Iwu M. Dietary botanical supplements with antiviral and anti-inflammatory properties used in the treatment of liver disorders in traditional African medicine. Complementary and Alternative Medicine in Chronic Liver Disease Conference. National Institutes of Health. Bethesda, Maryland. 1999.

45. Ferrea G. In vitro activity of a combretum micranthim extract against herpes simplex virus types 1 and 2. *Antiviral Res.* 1993;21:317-25.

46. Ott M, Thygarajan SP, Gupta S. Phyllanthus amarus suppresses hepatitis B virus by interrupting interactions between HBV enhancer I and cellular transcription factors. *Eur J Clin Invest.* 1997;27(11):908-915.

47. Mehrotra R, Rawat S, Kulshreshta DK, et al. In vitro studies on the effect of certain natural products against heptitis B virus. *Indian J Med Res.* 1990;92:133-138.

48. Forton, DM, Thomas HC, Murphy CA, Allsop, et al. Hepatitis C and cognitive impairment in a cohort of patients with mild liver disease. *Hepatology.* 2002;35:433-439.

49. Viviani B, Corsini E, Binaglia M, et al. Reactive oxygen species generated by glia are responsible for neuron death induced by human immunodeficiency virus-glycoprotein 120 in vitro. *Neuroscience.* 2001;107(1):51-58.

50. Fahn S. The endogenous toxin theory of the etiology of Parkinson's disease and a pilot trial of high-dose sntioxidants in an attempt to slow the progression of illness. *Ann NY Acad Sci.* 1989;570:186-196.

51. Floyd RA, et al. Neuroinflammatory diseases: an hypothesis to explain the increased formation of reactive oxygen and nitrogen species as major factors involved in neurodegenrative disease development. *Free Rad Biol Med.* 1999;26(9/10):1346-1355.

52. Curtis-Prior P, Vere D, Fray P. Therapeutic value of Ginkgo biloba in reducing symptoms of decline in mental function. *J Pharm Pharmacol.* 1999; 51(5):535-41.

53. Ramassamy C, Clostre F, Christen Y, Costentin J. In vivo Gingko biloba extract (EGb 761) protects against neurotoxic effects induced by MPTP: investigations into its mechanisms of action. In: Christen Y, Costentin J, Lacour M (Eds.). Effects of Gingko biloba extract (EGb 761) on the central nervous system. Elsevier. Paris, France. 1992:27-36.

54. Wettstein A. Cholinesterase inhibitors and gingko extracts: are they comparable in the treatment of dementia? Comparison of published placebo-controlled efficacy studies of at least six months duration. *Phytomedicine*. 2000;6(6):393-401.

55. Dwight MM, Kowdley KV, Russo JE, et al. Depression, fatigue, and functional disability in patients with chronic hepatitis C. *J Psychosom Res*. 2000;49(5):311-317.

56. Schubert H, Halama P. Depressive episode primarily unresponsive to therapy in elderly patients: efficacy of Gingko biliba extract (EGB 761) in combination with antidepressants. *Geriatr Forsch*. 1993;3:45-53.

57. Gaby A. Gingko biloba extract: a review. *Altern Med Rev*. 1996;1(4):236-242.

58. Linde K, Ramirez G, Mulrow C, et al. St. John's Wort for depression. An overview and meta-analysis of randomized clinical trials. *BMJ*. 1996; 313(7052):253-258.

59. Schulz V, Hansel R, Tyler VE. Rational Phytotherapy: A Physician's Guide to Herbal Medicine. 4th Ed. Springer. New York, New York. 2000:57-77.

Chapter 14
NUTRITIONAL SUPPLEMENTATION
Lark Lands, PhD and Lyn Patrick, ND

1. Badamaev V, Majeed M, Passwater R. Selenium: a quest for better understanding. *Altern Ther Health Med*. 1996;2(4):59-67.

2. Bernhard MC, Junker E, Hettinger A, et al. Time course of total cysteine, glutathione, and homocysteine in plasma of patients with chronic hepatitis C treated with interferon-alpha with and without supplementation with N-acetylcysteine. *J Hepatol*. 1998;28(5):751-755.

3. Jain SK, Pemberton PW, Smith A, et al. Oxidative stress in chronic hepatitis C: not just a feature of late stage disease. *J Hepatol*. 2002;36(6):805-811.

4. Reeves HL, Burt AD, Wood S, Day CP. Hepatic stellate cell activation occurs in the absence of hepatitis in alcoholic liver disease and correlates with the severity of steatosis. *J Hepatol*. 1996;25(5):677-683.

5. Day CP, James OF. Hepatic steatosis: innocent bystander or guilty party? *Hepatology*. 1998;27(6):1463-6.

6. Bustamante J, Lodge JK, Marcocci L, et al. Alpha-lipoic acid in liver metabolism and disease. *Free Rad Biol Med*. 1998;24(6):1023-1039.

7. Biewenga GP, Haenen GR, Bast A. The pharmacology of the antioxidant lipoic acid. *Gen Pharmacol*. 1997;29(3):315-331.

8. Zeigler D, Hanefeld M, Ruhnau KJ, et al. Treatment of symptomatic diabetic peripheral neuropathy with the anti-oxidant á-lipoic acid. A 3-week multicentre randomized controlled trial (ALADIN Study). *Diabetologia*. 1995;38(12):1425-1433.

9. *Ibid*, ref 6

10. Shabert J, Winslow C, Lacey JM, Wilmore DW. Glutamine-antioxidant supplementation increases body cell mass in AIDS patients with weight loss: a randomized, double-blind controlled trial. *Nutrition*. 1999;15(11-12):860-864.

11. Herzenberg L, DeRosa SC, Dubs JG, et al. Glutathione deficiency is associated with impaired survival in HIV disease. *Proc Nat Acad Sci USA*. 1997;94(5):1967-1972.

12. Beloqui O, Prieto J, Suarez M, et al. N-acetyl cysteine enhances the response to inter-feron-alpha in chronic hepatitis C: a pilot study. *J Interferon Res.* 1993;13(4):279-82.

13. Ideo G, Bellobuono A, Tempini S, et al. Antioxidant drugs combined with alpha-interferon in chronic hepatitis C not responsive to alpha-interferon alone: a random-ized, multicentre study. *Eur J Gastroenterol Hepatol.* 1999;11(11);1203-1207.

14. *Ibid,* ref 2

15. Look MP, Gerard A, Rao GS, et al. Interferon/antioxidant combination therapy for chronic hepatitis C-a controlled pilot trial. *Antiviral Res.* 1999;43(2):113-122.

16. Garland M, Stamper MJ, Willett WC, Hunter DJ. The epidemiology of selenium and human cancer. In: Balz Grei, Balz Frei (Eds.). <u>Natural Antioxidants in Human Health and Disease</u>. Academic Press. San Diego, California. 1994:263-281.

17. Yu MW, Horng IS, Hsu KH, et al. Plasma selenium levels and risk of hepatocellular carcinoma among men with chronic hepatitis virus infection. *Am J Epidemiol.* 1999;150(4):367-374.

18. Yu SY, Zhu YJ, Li WG. Protective role of selenium against hepatitis B virus and primary liver cancer in Qidong. *Biol Trace Elem Res.* 1997;56(1):117-124.

19. Look MP, Rockstroh JK, Rao GS, et al. Serum selenium, plasma glutathione (GSH), and erythrocyte glutathione peroxidase (GSH-Px) levels in asymptomatic versus symptom-atic human immunodeficiency virus-1 (HIV-1) infection. *Eur J Clin Nutr.* 1997;51(4):266-272.

20. Baum MK, Shor-Posner G, Lai S, et al. High risk of HIV-related mortality is associated with selenium deficency. *J Acquir Immune Defic Syndr Hum Retrovirol.* 1997;15(5):370-374.

21. Osman E, Owen JS, Burroughs AK. Review article: S-adenosyl-L-methionine- a new therapeutic agent in liver disease? *Aliment Pharmacol Ther.* 1993;7:21-28.

22. Mato JM, Camara J, Fernandez de Paz J, et al. S-adenosylmethionine in alcoholic liver cirrhosis: a randomized, placebo-controlled, double-blind, multi-center clinical trial. *J Hepatol.* 1999;30(6):1081-1089.

23. Ansorena E, Garcia-Trevijano E, Martinez-Chantar M, et al. S-adenosylmethionine and methylthioadenosine are antiapoptotic in cultured rat hepatocytes but proapoptotic in human hepatoma cells. *Hepatology.* 2002;35(2):274-280.

24. Podymova SD, Nadinskaia MI. Clinical trial of heptral in patients with chronic diffuse liver disease with intrahepatic cholestasis syndrome. *Klin Med (Mosk).* 1998;76(10):45-48.

25. Gorbakov VV, Galik VP, Kirillov SM. Experience in heptral treatment of diffuse liver diseases. *Ter Arkh.* 1998;70(10):82-86.

26. von Herbay A, Stahl W, Niederau C, Sies H. Vitamin E improves the aminotransferase status of patients suffering from viral hepatitis C: a randomized , double-blind, placebo-controlled study. *Free Radic Res.* 1997;27(6):599-605.

27. Houglum K Venkataramani A, Lyche K, Chojkier M. A pilot study of the effects of d-alpha-tocopherol on hepatic stellate cell activation in chronic hepatitis C. *Gastroenterol-ogy.* 1977;113(4):1069-1073.

28. Chojkier M, Houglum K, Lee KS, Buck M. Long- and short-term D-a-tocopherol supplementa-tion inhibits liver collagen a1(I) gene expresion. *Am J Physiol.* 1998;275(6 Pt 1):G1480-1485.

29. Kappus H, Diplock AT. Tolerance and safety of vitamin E: a toxicological position report. *Free Rad Biol Med.* 1992;13(1):55-74.

30. Takagi H, Nagamine T, Abe H, et al. Zinc supplementation enhances the response to interferon therapy in patients with chronic hepatitis C. *J Viral Hepatitis.* 2001;8(5):367-371.

31. Nagamine T, Takagi H, Takayama H, et al. Preliminary study of combination therapy with IFNa and zinc in chronic hepatitis C patients with genotype 1b. *Biol Trace Element Res.* 2000;75(1-3):53-63.

32. Matsukura T, Tanaka H. Review: Applicability of zinc complex of L-Carnosine for medical use. Unpublished data. Research Laboratories, Hamari Chemicals, Osaka, Japan. [Note: At the time of publication, these data were available on the Internet at http://www.protein.bio.msu.su/biokihimiya/contents/v65/full/65070961.htm.]

Berkson B. A triple antioxidant approach to the treatment of hepatitis C using alpha-lipoic acid (thioctic acid), silymarin, selenium and other fundamental nutraceuticals. *Clin Prac Alt Med.* 2000;1(1):27-33.

Chapter 15
PRODUCTS MARKETED TO PEOPLE WITH HEPATITIS C
Lyn Patrick, ND

1. Marcucci MC. Propolis: chemical composition, biological properties and therapeutic activity. *Apidologie.* 1995;26:83-99.

2. Amoros M, Lurton E, Boustie J, et al. Comparison of the anti-herpes simplex virus activities of propolis and 3-methylbut-2-enyl caffeate. *J Nat Prod.* 1994;57(5):644-647.

3. Iwu M, Duncan A, Okunji C. Dietary botanical supplements with antiviral and anti-inflammatory properties used in the treatment of liver disorders in traditional African medicine. Complementary and Alternative Medicine in Chronic Liver Disease Conference. National Institues of Health. Bethesda, Maryland. 1999.

4. Rice-Evans CA, Miller NJ, Paganga G. Stucture-antioxidant relationships of flavonoids and phenolic acids. *Free Radic Biol Med.* 1996;20(7):933-956.

5. Katamaya T. Hypolipemic action of phytic acid (IP6): prevention of fatty liver. *Anticancer Res.* 1999;19(5A):3695-3698.

6. Patney NL, Pachori S. A study of serum glycolytic enzymes and serum B hepatitis in relation to Liv.52 therapy. *The Medicine and Surgery.* 1986(XXVI);4:9.

7. Chawhan, RN, Talib SH, Talib VH, et al.Viral hepatitis in children. *The Medicine and Surgery* 1976; 3, 9. [Note: This information was provided by an herb manufacturer, but is not available through the National Library of Medicine's database PubMed.]

8. Mukerjee AB, Dasgupta M. Cirrhosis of liver. Results of treatment with an indigenous drug Liv.52. *J Ind Med Prof.* 1971; 12:7853.

9. Fleig WW, Morgan MY, Hölzer MA. The ayurvedic drug LIV.52 in patients with alcoholic cirrhosis. Results of a prospective, randomized, double-blind, placebo-controlled clinical trial [Abstract]. a European multicenter study group. *J Hepatol.* 1997;26(Suppl 1):127.

10. Fujisawa K, Suzuki H, Yamamoto S, et al. Therapeutic effects of liver hydrolysate preparation on chronic hepatitis - A double blind, controlled study. *Asian Med J.* 1984;26:497-526.

11. Sanbe K, Murata T, Fujisawa K, et al. Treatment of liver disease - with particular reference to liver hydrolysates. *Jap J Clin Exp Med.* 1973;50:2665-76.

12. Kidd P. Phosphatidylcholine: a superior protectant against liver damage. *Altern Med Rev.* 1996;1(4):258-274.

13. Freidman LS, Martin P, Munoz SJ. Liver function tests and the objective evaluation of the patient with liver disease. In: Zakim D, Boyer TD, (Eds.). Hepatology: A Textbook of Liver Disease. WB Saunders. Phildelphia, Pennsylvania. 1996:791-833.

14. Kahlon JB, Kemp MC, Yawel N, et al. In vitro evaluation of the synergistic antiviral effects of acemannin in combination with azidothymidine and acyclovir. *Mol Biother.*

1991;3(4):214-23.

15. Womble E, et al. The impact of acemannan on the generation and function of cytotoxic T-lymphocytes. *Immunopharm.* 1992;14:3-67.

16. Kelly G. Larch arabinogalactan. Clinical relevance of a novel immune-enhancing polysaccharide. *Altern Med Rev.* 1999;4(2):96-103.

17. Sweeney BF, McDaniel CF. Glyconutritional and phytochemicals in eight HCV-positive patients. *Proceedings of the Fisher Institute for Medical Research.* 1999;1(3):6-7.

18. Ghoneum M, Jewett A. Production of tumor necrosis factor-alpha and interferon-gamma from human peripheral blood lymphocytes by MGN-3, a modified arabinoxylan from rice bran, and its synergy with interleukin-2. *Cancer Detect Prev.* 2000;24(4):314-324.

19. Jacoby HL, Wonorowski G, Sakata K, et al. The effect of MGN-3 on cisplatin and adriamycin induced toxicity in the rat. *Gastroenterology.* 2000;118(4):4962. [Note: This information is not available through the National Library of Medicine's database PubMed, but a synopsis of the article was available at the time of publication at: http://www.jafra.gr.jp/sis-e.html.]

20. Csatary LK, Moss RW, Beuth J, et al. Beneficial treatment of patients with advanced cancer using a Newcastle disease virus vaccine (MTH-68/H). *Anticancer Research.* 1999;19(1B):629-634.

21. Csatary LK, Telegdy L, Gergely P, Bodey B, Bakacs T. Preliminary report of a controlled trial of MTH-68/B virus vaccine treatment in acute B and C hepatitis: a phase II study. *Anticancer Res.* 1998;18(2B):1279-1282.

22. Csatary LK, Schnabel R, Bakacs, T. Successful treatment of decompensated chronic viral hepatitis by bursal disease virus vaccine. *Anticancer Res.* 1999;19(1B):629-633.

23. Stauder G, Kabil S. Oral enzyme therapy in hepatitis C patients. *Int J Immunother.* 1997; XIII (3/4):153-158. [Note: This information was provided by the product manufacturer, but is not available through the National Library of Medicine's database PubMed.]

24. Beardsley T, Hayes SM. Induction of T-cell maturation by a cloned line of thymic epithelium (TEPI). *Proc Nat Acad Sci USA.* 1983;80(19):6005-6009.

25. Riordan NH, Jackson JA, Riordan HD. A pilot study on the effects of thymus protein on elevated Epstein-Barr virus titers in human subjects. Project RECNAC Wichita State University. *Townsend Letter for Doctors.* 1998;175:78-89. [Note: This information was provided by the product manufacturer, but is not available through the National Library of Medicine's database PubMed.]

26. Sherman KE, Sjorem M, Creager RL, et al. Combination therapy with thymosin alpha1 and interferon for the treatment of chronic hepatitis C infection: a randomized, placebo-controlled double-blind trial. *Hepatology.* 1998;27(4):1128-1135.

27. Edelson R, Berger C, Gasparro F, et al. Treatment of cutaneous T-cell lymphoma by extracorporeal photochemotherapy. *N Eng J Med.* 1987;316(6):297-303.

28. Olney RC. Treatment of viral hepatitis with the Knott technic of blood irradiation. *Am J Surgery.* 1959;90:402-409.

Chapter 17
MILITARY VETERANS AND HEPATITIS C
Terry Baker

1. Kizer KW. Hepatitis C standards for provider evaluation and testing. Under Secretary for Health information letter (IL 10-98-013). Department of Veterans Affairs. Veterans Health Administration. Washington, D.C. 1998.

2. Neel S. Medical support of the US army in Vietnam 1965-1970. Department of the Army. CMH Pub. No. 90-16. US Government Printing Office. Washington, DC. 1991.

3. Centers for Disease Control and Prevention. Recommendations for prevention and control of hepatitis C virus (HCV) infection and HCV-related chronic disease. *MMWR.* 1998;47(RR19):1-39. [Note: At the time of publication, this document was available at: http://www.cdc.gov/mmwr/preview/mmwrhtml/00055154.htm.]

4. Kralovic S, Roselle GA, Simbartl L, et al. Hepatitis C virus antibody (HCAb) positivity in Department of Veterans Affairs (VA) facilities. Presented at the Ninth Annual Scientific Meeting of the Society for Healthcare Epidemiology of America (SHEA). San Francisco, California. 1999.

5. Statement of Kenneth W. Wizer, MD, MPH, Under Secretary for Health, US Deptartment of Veterans Affairs before the Committee on Veterans Affairs, United States Senate. April 13, 1999.

6. Projected veteran population as of July 1,1998. Office of the Deputy Assistant Secretary for Policy, Department of Veterans Affairs Document. [Note: The referenced text from this document is also contained in The Maimes Report on Hepatitis C Infection in New Hampshire by Steven Maimes. 2002. This text was available at the time of publication for non-commercial purposes at: http://www.cc-info.net/hepatitis/Hepatitis_C_Report.pdf.]

7. Song P, Duc DD, Hien B, et al. Markers of hepatitis C and B virus infections among blood donors in Ho Chi Minh City and Hanoi, Vietman. *Clin Diag Lab Immunol.* 1994:1(4):413-418.

8. National Institutes of Health, Department of Transfusion Medicine. A controlled prospective study of transfusion-associated hepatitis (TAH). Intramural Research Project Z01 CL-02005-28 DTM. Bethesda, Maryland. 1997.

9. National Center for Veteran Analysis and Statistics. National Survey of Veterans. US Government Printing Office. Washington, D.C. Pub. No. NSV9503. 1995.

10. Pavli P, Bayliss J, Dent O, Lunzer M. The prevalence of serological markers for hepatitis B virus infection in Australian naval personnel. *Med J Aust.* 1989;151(2):71-75.

11. Health status of Vietnam veterans. II. Physical health. The Centers for Disease Control Vietnam Experience Study. JAMA 1988;259(18):2708-2714.

12. Roselle GA, Danko LH, Mendenhall CH. A four-year review of patients with hepatitis C antibody in Department of Veterans Affairs facilities. *Mil Med.* 1997;162(11):711-714.

13. Spolarich AW, Russo B. Hepatitis C and veterans. December 1998/January 1999. *The VVA Veteran®.*

14. United States Department of Veterans Affairs, Board of Veterans' Appeals. Board of Veterans' Appeals Decisions 1994-1996. Pub. No. 98-09166 (CD-ROM). US Government Printing Office. Washington, DC. 1998.

Chapter 18:
HCV/HIV COINFECTION
Section 1:
OVERVIEW
Misha Cohen, OMD, LicAc

1. Cohen M, Gish R. The Hepatitis C Help Book. St. Martin's Press. New York, New York. 2000:68.

2. Clark A. HIV and hepatitis coinfection (oral presentation). XIII International Conference on AIDS. Durban, South Africa. 2000.

3. Nadler JP. HIV and hepatitis C - another perspective. *Infect Med.* 2001;18(6):292-296.

4. Sherman KE, Rouster SD, Chung RT, Rajicic N. Hepatitis C virus prevalence among patients infected with human immunodeficiency virus: a cross-sectional analysis of the US adult AIDS Clinical Trials Group. *Clin Infect Dis.* 2002;34(6):831-837.

5. Thomas D, Vlahov D, Solomon L, et al. Correlates of hepatitis C virus infections among injection drug users. *Medicine.* 1995;74(4):212-20.

6. Ragni MV, Belle SH. Impact of human immunodeficiency virus infection on progression to end-stage liver disease in individuals with hemophilia and hepatitis C virus infection. *J Infect Dis.* 2001;183(7):1112-1115.

7. Poles MA, Dieterich DT. Hepatitis C virus/human immunodeficiency virus coinfection: clinical management issues. *Clin Infect Dis.* 2000;31(1):154-161.

8. Thomas DL, Shih JW, Alter AJ, et al. Effect of human immunodeficiency virus on hepatitis C virus infection among injecting drug users. *J Infect Dis.* 1996;174(4):690-695.

9. Merrik ST, Sepkowitz SA, Boyle BA, Jacobs JL. Seroprevalence of hepatitis C antibody and hepatitis B surface antigenemia in a large urban HIV clinic. Abstract 22263. XII International Conference on AIDS. Geneva, Switzerland. 1998.

10. Proietti F, Caiaffa W, Carneiro-Proietti AB, et al. Seroprevalence correlates of HIV and HCV infection among injection drug users (IDUs) attending an outreach syringe exchange program (SEPs) in five Brazilian cities. Abstract WeOrA530. XIII International Conference on AIDS. Durban, South Africa. 2000.

11. Greub G, Ledergerber B, Grob P, et al. Impact of HCV infection on HIV progression and survival in the Swiss HIV cohort studies. Abstract MoPeB2139. XIII International Conference on AIDS. Durban, South Africa. 2000.

12. Dieterich DT. Coinfection with hepatitis C virus (HCV) and HIV. 37th Annual Meeting of the Infectious Diseases Society of America (IDSA). Philadelphia, Pennsylvania. 1998.

13. Dove LM, Phung Y, Wrock J, et al. HCV quasispecies as a mechanism of rapidly progressive liver disease in patients infected with the human immunodeficiency virus. Abstract 1183. 50th Annual Meeting of the American Association for the Study of Liver Diseases. Dallas, Texas. 1999.

14. Selik RM, Byers RH Jr, Dworkin MS. Trends in diseases reported on U.S. death certificates that mentioned HIV infection, 1987-1999. *J Acquir Immune Defic Syndr.* 2002;29(4):378-387.

15. Saves M, Raffi F, Clevenbergh P, Manchou B. Hepatitis B or hepatitis C virus infection is a risk factor for severe hepatic cytolysis after initiation of a protease inhibitor-containing antiretroviral regimen in human immunodeficiency virus-infected patients. *Antimicro Agents Chemo.* 2000;44(12):3451-3455.

16. Brinkman K, ter Hofstede JM, Burger DM. Adverse effects of reverse transcriptase inhibitors: mitochondrial toxicity as common pathway. *AIDS.* 1998;12:1735-1744.

17. *Ibid*, ref 8

18. Rodriguez-Rosado R, Garcia-Samaniego J, Soriano V. Hepatotoxicity after introduction of highly active antiretroviral therapy. *AIDS.* 1998;12:1256.

19. Barbaro G, DiLorenzo G, Soldini M, et al. Hepatic glutathione deficiency in chronic hepatitis C: Quantitative evalutations in patients who are HIV positive and HIV negative and correlations with plasmatic and lymphocytic concentrations and with the activity of the liver disease. *Am J Gastroenterol.* 1996;91(12):2569-2573.

20. Barbaro G, DiLorenzo G, Asti A, et al. Hepatocellular mitochondrial alterations in patients with chronic hepatitis C: ultrastructural and biochemical findings. *Am J Gastroenterol.* 1999;94:2198-2205.

21. Brinkman K, Kakuda TN. Mitochondrial toxicity of nucleoside analogue reverse

transciptase inhibitors: a looming obstacle for long-term therapy? *Curr Opin Infect Dis.* 2000;13(1):5-11.

22. Kakuda TN, Brinkman K. Mitochondrial toxic effects and ribavirin. *Lancet.* 2001;357(9270):1802-1803.

23. Lafeuillade A, Hittinger G, Chadapaud S. Increased mitochondrial toxicity with ribavirin in HIV/HCV coinfection. *Lancet.* 2001;357(9252):280-281.

24. Wit FW, Weverling GJ, Weel J, Jurriaans S, Lange JM. Incidence of and risk factors for severe hepatotoxicity associated with antiretroviral combination therapy. *J Infect Dis.* 2002;186(1):23-31.

25. Sherman KE, Andreatta C, O'Brien J, et al. Hepatitis C in human immunodeficiency virus-coinfected patients: increased variability in the hypervariable envelope coding domain. *Hepatology.* 1996;23:688-694.

26. Benhamou Y, Bochet M, Di Martino, et al. Liver fibrosis progression in human immuno-deficiency virus and hepatitis C virus coinfected patients. The Multivire Group. *Hepatology.* 1999;30:1054-1058.

27. Poynard T, Bedossa P, Opolon P, et al. Natural history of liver fibrosis progression in patients with chronic hepatitis C. The OBSVIRC, METAVIR, CLINIVIR and DOSVIRC Groups. *Lancet.* 1997;349:825-832.

28. Soto B, Sanchez-Quijano A, Rodrigo L et al. Human immunodefiency virus infection modifies the natural history of chronic parenterally -acquired hepatitis C with an un-usually rapid progression to cirrhosis. *J Hepatol.* 1997;26:1-5.

29. Piroth L, Duong M, Quantin C et al. Does hepatitis C virus coinfection accelerate clini-cal and immunological evolution of HIV-infected patients? *AIDS.* 1998;12(4):381-388.

30. Bonacini M, Govindarajan S, Blatt LM. Patients coinfected with human immunodefi-ciency virus and hepatitis C virus demonstrate higher levels of hepatic HCV RNA. *J Viral Hepatitis.* 1999;6(3):203-208.

31. Zylberberg H, Nalpas B, Pol S. Is there a relationship between hepatitis C virus infec-tion and antiretroviral lipoatrophy? *AIDS.* 2000;14(13):2055-2065.

32. Duong M, Petit JM, Piroth L, et al. Association between insulin resistance and hepatitis C virus chronic infection in HIV-hepatitis C virus coinfected patients undergoing antiretroviral therapy. *J Acquir Immune Defic Syndr.* 2001;27(3):245-250.

33. Manegold C, Hannoun C, Wywiol A, et al. Reactivation of hepatitis B virus replication accompanied by acute hepatitis in patients receiving highly active antiretroviral therapy. *Clin Infect Dis.* 2001;32(1):144-148.

34. Arizcorreta C, Martinez C, Diaz F, et al. Natural history of chronic hepatitis C: Unusually rapid progression to liver fibrosis and cirrhosis in human immunodeficiency virus co-infected patients. Abstract WePeB6036. XIV International Conference on AIDS. Barcelona, Spain. 2002.

35. Stellrecht KA, McKenna B. Risk for the development of HCV-related fibrosis in HIV positive patients. Abstract WePeB6020. XIV International Conference on AIDS. Barcelona, Spain. 2002.

36. Mohsen AH, Taylor C, Portmann B, et al. Progression rate of liver fibrosis in human immunodeficiency virus and hepatitis C virus coinfected patients, UK experience. Ab-stract MoOrB1057. XIV International Conference on AIDS. Barcelona, Spain. 2002.

37. Klausen G, Kolberg J, Niedobitek F, et al. Liver biopsy in HIV/HCV coinfected patients. Abstract WePeB6023. XIV International Conference on AIDS. Barcelona, Spain. 2002.

38. Gyarmathy VA, Neaigus A, Miller M. Increased sexual risk among women who recently initiated drug injecting. Abstract MoPeC3398. XIV International Conference on AIDS. Barcelona, Spain. 2002.

39. Neaigus A, Gyarmathy VA, Miller M, Friedman SR, Des Jarlais DC. Sexual risk and HIV, HBV and HCV seroconversions among non-injecting heroin users. Abstract MoPeC3528. XIV International Conference on AIDS. Barcelona, Spain. 2002.

40. Dakoury C, Eholie S, Aka-Kakou R, Bissagnene E, Konan-Koko R, Kadio A. Role of viral infections HCV and HBV in liver toxicity among patients receiving antiretroviral treatment in HIV drugs access initiative in Cote d'Ivoire. Abstract MoPeB3280. XIV International Conference on AIDS. Barcelona, Spain. 2002.

41. Dorrucci M, Valdarchi C, Castelli F, Zaccarelli M, Pezzotti P, Rezza G. The effect of HIV-HCV coinfection in a cohort of HIV-serconverters before and after the introduction of HAART. Abstract ThPeC7502. XIV International Conference on AIDS. Barcelona, Spain. 2002.

42. Klein MB, Lalonde RG, Suissa S. Hepatitis C (HCV) co-infection is thwarting health improvements associated with highly active antiretroviral therapy (HAART). Abstract ThPeC7515. XIV International Conference on AIDS. Barcelona, Spain. 2002.

43. French MAH, Stone SF, Lee S, Keane NM, Price P. Hepatotoxicity after HAART in HIV/HCV coinfected patients is associated with increased HCV core-specific IgG antibody and sCD26 (DDP IV) enzyme activity. Abstract B10538. XIV International Conference on AIDS. Barcelona, Spain. 2002.

44. Lottero M, Lavarello D, Toledo A, et al. Harm reduction within public health systems: linking intravenous drug users, IDUs, with a primary care health center of Rosario, Argentina. Abstract TuPeF5276. XIV International Conference on AIDS. Barcelona, Spain. 2002.

45. Miller CL, Spittal PM, Laliberte N, Li K, O'Shaughnessy MV, Schechter MT. Risk factors for HIV and HCV prevalence and incidence among young injection drug users in a city coping with an epidemic. Abstract MoPeC3401. XIV International Conference on AIDS. Barcelona, Spain. 2002.

46. Ghauri AK, Rehman N, Azam S, Shah SA. Harm reduction program for injecting drug users (IDUs) in Karachi, Pakistan. Abstract TuPeF5272. XIV International Conference on AIDS. Barcelona, Spain. 2002.

47. Nugraha SAM. Harm reduction in Indonesia. Abstract ThPeE7899. XIV International Conference on AIDS. Barcelona, Spain. 2002.

48. Villarinho L, Gravato N, Barreto AS, Novaes E. Filters for crack users: a new harm reduction strategy in Santos, Brazil. Abstract TuPeF5258. XIV International Conference on AIDS. Barcelona, Spain. 2002.

49. Bolao F, Sanvisens A, Egea JM, Shaw E, Navio M, Muga R. HIV-1 and hepatitis C virus infections among recent injecting drug users. Abstract MoPeC3380. XIV International Conference on AIDS. Barcelona, Spain. 2002.

50. Crum NF, Brodine SK, Grillo M, Wallace MR. Absence of hepatitis C virus (HCV) infection amoung HIV-infected US military members. Abstract ThPeC7504. XIV International Conference of AIDS. Barcelona, Spain. 2002.

51. Reynolds A. The need for harm reduction in US prisons: an activist's view. Abstract WeOrE1320. XIV International Conference on AIDS. Barcelona, Spain. 2002.

52. Taylor LE, Tashima KT, Alt E, Feller ER, Costello T, Flanigan TP. Addiction and mental illness are barriers to hepatitis C treatment among HIV/hepatitis C virus coinfected individuals. Abstract ThPeC7513. XIV International Conference on AIDS. Barcelona, Spain. 2002.

53. Marsh BJ, Rosenberg SD, Butterfield MI, et al. Comorbidity of human immunodeficiency virus, hepatitis B virus and hepatitis C virus in people with severe mental illness. Abstract B10540. XIV International Conference on AIDS. Barcelona, Spain. 2002.

54. Taylor LE, Tashima KT, Alt E, Feller ER, Costello T, Flanigan TP. Addiction and mental illness are barriers to hepatitis C treatment among HIV/hepatitis C virus coinfected

individuals. Abstract ThPeC7513. XIV International Conference on AIDS. Barcelona, Spain. 2002.

55. Calzavara L, Orekhovsky V, Yakovlev A, et al. Fuelling HIV epidemic in Russia: the stigma of IDU and HIV and its impact on treatment access and testing. Abstract ThPpE2153. XIV International Conference on AIDS. Barcelona, Spain. 2002.

56. Schwartzapfel B, Taylor LE, MacLeod C, Feller ER, Rich JD, Tashima KT. A pilot program for treating hepatitis C in HIV/hepatitis C virus coinfected individuals with comorbid psychiatric illness and/or addiction. Abstract ThPeC7512. XIV International Conference on AIDS. Barcelona, Spain. 2002.

Section 2:
WESTERN TREATMENT OPTIONS
Misha Cohen, OMD, LicAc

1. Dieterich DT, et al. Sustained virologic response (SVR) following interferon and ribavirin therapy for hepatitis C patients who are co-infected with HIV. Abstract 17. 38th Annual Meeting of the IDSA (Infectious Diseases Society of America). New Orleans, Louisiana. 2000.

2. Garcia- Samaniego J, Soriano V, Castilla J. Influence of hepatitis C genotypes and HIV infection on histological severity of chronic hepatitis C. The Hepatitis/HIV Spanish Study Group. *Am J Gastroenterol.* 1997;92(7):1130-1134.

3. Torriani FJ. Fabric of the future (satellite symposium). XIII International Conference on AIDS. Durban, South Africa. 2000.

4. Perronne C, Carrat F, Sadr FB, et al. RIBAVIC trial (ANRS HC02): a controlled randomized trial of pegylated-interferon alfa-2b plus ribavirin vs. interferon alfa-2b plus ribavirin for the initial treatment of chronic hepatitis C in HIV coinfected patients: preliminary results. Abstract LbOr16. XIV International Conference on AIDS. Barcelona, Spain. 2002.

5. Smith DM, Puoti M, Sulkowski M, et al. Symptomatic hyperlactatemia during a large hepatitis C treatment trial in HIV/HCV coinfected participants on stable antiretroviral therapy. Abstract MoOrB1059. International Conference on AIDS. Barcelona, Spain. 2002.

6. Stapleton JT, Swindells S, Polgreen PM. Hepatitis C virus infection is associated with a decreased risk of hypercholesterolemia but not hyperglycemia in HIV-infected people. Abstract ThPeC7517. XIV International Conference on AIDS. Barcelona, Spain. 2002.

7. Wunschmann S, Stapleton JT. Hepatitis C virus envelope protein E2 enhances human lipoprotein binding to cells. Abstract WePeB6041. XIV International Conference on AIDS. Barcelona, Spain. 2002.

8. Torriani FJ, Asensi V, Byrnes C, et al. Hepatitis C RNA levels are unchanged after one year of effective antiretroviral therapy. Abstract WePeB6035. XIV International Conference on AIDS. Barcelona, Spain. 2002.

9. Stapleton JT, Polgreen PM, Fultz SL, et al. HCV infection is associated with lower levels of serum LDL cholesterol and total cholesterol in HIV-positive individuals. Abstract ThPeC7519. XIV International Conference on AIDS. Barcelona, Spain. 2002.

10. Schlaak JF et al. Sustained HCV eradication after interleukin-2 therapy in patients with HIV/HCV coinfection. Abstract 431. 50th Annual Meeting of the American Association for the Study of Liver Diseases (AASLD). Dallas, Texas. *Hepatology.* 1999;30(4) Supp2:268A.

Section 3:
ALTERNATIVE EASTERN TREATMENT OPTIONS
Misha Cohen, OMD, LicAc

1. Chen Z, et al. Clinical analysis of chronic hepatitis B treated with TCM compositions Fugan No. 33 by two lots. International Symposium on Viral Hepatitis and AIDS. Beijing, China. Abstract, p 2. 1991.
2. Wang C, He J, Zhu C. Research of repair of liver pathologic damage in 63 cases of hepatitis with severe cholestatis by blood-cooling and circulation-invigorating Chinese herbs. International Symposium on Viral Hepatitis and AIDS. Beijing China. Abstract, p 5. 1991.
3. Zhao R, Shen H. Antifibrogenesis with traditional Chinese herbs. International Symposium on Viral Hepatitis and AIDS. Beijing China. Abstract, p 20. 1991.
4. Ergil K. Fifth Symposium of the Society for Acupuncture Research Conference. Herbal safety and research panel. Society for Acupuncture Research Conference. Palo Alto, California.1998.
5. Batey RG, Benssoussen A, Yang Yifan, Hossain MA, Bollipo S. Chinese herbal medicine lowers ALT in hepatitis C. A randomized placebo controlled trial report. Cathay Herbal Laboratories. Sydney Australia. 1998. [Note: At the time of publication, this unpublished report was available on the Cathay Herbal Laboratories Internet site at: http://www.cathayherbal.com/library/CH100/Clinical_Research/clinical_research.htm.]
6. Li H, et al. *Qingtui fang* applied in treating 128 cases of chronic hepatitis C. *Chinese Journal of Integrated Traditional and Western Medicine for Liver Diseases.* 1994;4(2):40. [Note: This journal is not included in the National Library of Medicine's PubMed database.]
7. Wu C, et al. Thirty-three patients with hepatitis C treated by TCM syndrome differentiation. *Chinese Journal of Integrated Traditional and Western Medicine for Liver Diseases.* 1994;4(1):44-45. [Note: This journal is not included in the National Library of Medicine's PubMed database.]
8. Gish R. California Pacific Medical Center, San Francisco. Personal communication. 1996.
9. Duggan J, Peterson WS, Schutz M, Khuder S, Charkraborty J. Use of complementary and alternative therapies in HIV-infected patients. *AIDS Patient Care STDS.* 2001;15(3):159-167.
   Cohen MR, Wilson CJ, Surasky A. Acupuncture treatment in people with HCV and HIV coinfection and elevated transaminases. XII International Conference on AIDS. Abstract 60211. Geneva, Switzerland. 1998.
11. Cohen MR, Doner K. The HIV Wellness Sourcebook. Henry Holt & Company. New York, New York. 1998.

Section 4:
NATUROPATHIC TREATMENT OPTIONS
Lyn Patrick, ND

1. Muller F, Aukrust P, Svardal AM, et al. The thiols glutathione, cysteine, and homocysteine in human immunodeficiency virus (HIV) infection. In: Watson RR (Ed.). Nutrients and Foods in AIDS. 1st Edition. CRC Press. New York, New York. 1998:35-69.
2. Barbaro G, Di Lorenzo G, Soldini M, et al. Hepatic glutathione deficiency in chronic hepatitis C: quantitative evaluation in patients who are HIV positive and HIV negative and correlations with plasmatic and lymphocytic concentrations and with the activity of the liver disease. *Am J Gastroenterol.* 1996;91(12):2569-2573 .

3. Muller F, Aukrust P, Svardal AM, et al. Thiols to treat AIDS. In: Watson RR (Ed.). Nutrition and AIDS. 2ⁿᵈ Edition. CRC Press. New York, New York. 2001:84.

4. Herzenberg LA, De Rosa SC, Dubs JG, et al. Glutathione deficiency is associated with impaired survival in HIV disease. *Proc Natl Acad Sci USA*. 1977;94(5):1967-1972.

5. Beloqui O, Prieto J, Suarez M, et al. N-acetyl cysteine enhances the response to interferon-alpha in chronic hepatitis C: a pilot study. *J Interferon Res*. 1993;13(4):279-282.

6. Kalayjian RC, Skowron G, Emgushov RT, et al. A phase I/II trial of intravenous L-2 oxothiazone-4-carboxylic acid (procysteine) in asymptomatic HIV-infected subjects. *J Acquir Immune Defic Syndr*. 1994;7(4):369-374.

7. Fuchs J, Schofer H, Milbradt R, et al. Studies on lipoate effects on blood redox state in human immunodeficiency virus infected patients. *Arzneimittelforschung*. 1993;43(12):1359-1362.

8. Packer L, Witt EH, Tritschler HJ. Alpha-lipoic acid as a biological antioxidant. *Free Rad Biol Med*. 1995;19(2):227-250.

9. Kieburtz K, Schifitto G, McDermott M, et al. A randomized, double-blind, placebo-controlled trial of deprenyl and thioctic acid in human immunodeficiency virus-associated cognitive impairment. Dana Consortium on the Therapy of HIV Dementia and Related Cognitive Disorders. *Neurology*. 1998;50(3):645-651.

10. Jayanthi S, Varalakshmi P. Tissue lipids in experimental calcium oxalate lithiasis and the effect of DL alpha-lipoic acid. *Biochem Int*. 1992;26:913-921.

11. Vendemiale G, Altomare E, Trisio T, et al. Effects of oral S-adenosyl-L-methionine on hepatic glutahtione in patients with liver disease. *Scand J Gastroenterol*. 1989;24(4):407-415.

12. Castagna A, Le Grazie C, Accordini A, et al. Cerebrospinal fluid S-adenosylmethionine (SAMe) and glutathione concentrations in HIV infection: effect of parenteral treatment with SAMe. *Neurology*. 1995;45(9):1678-1683.

13. Beach RS, Mantero-Atienza E, Shor-Pozner G. et al. Specific nutrient abnormalities in asymptomatic HIV-1 infection. *AIDS*. 1992;6(7):701-708.

14. Dworkin BD, Wormser GP, Axelrod F, et al. Dietary intake in patients with acquired immunodeficiency syndrome (AIDS), patients with AIDS-related complex, and serologically postive human immunodeficiency virus patients: correlations with nutritional status. *JPEN*. 1990;14(6):605-609.

15. Abrams B, Duncan D, Hertz-Picciotto I. A prospective study of dietary intake and acquired immunodeficiency syndrome in HIV-seropositive homosexual men. *J Acquir Immune Defic Syndr*. 1993;6(8):949-958.

16. Ganser A, Greher J, Volkers B, et al. Azidothymidine in the treatment of AIDS. *N Engl J Med*. 1988;318(4):250-251.

17. Geissler RG, Ganser A, Ottmann OG, et al. In vitro improvement of bone marrow-derived hematopoetic colony formation in HIV-positive patients by alpha-D-tocopherol and erythropoetin. *Eur J Haematol*. 1994;53(4):201-206.

18. Baum MK, Shor-Posner G, Lai S, et al. High risk of HIV-related mortality is associated with selenium deficiency, *J Acquir Immune Defic Syndr Hum Retrovirol*. 1997;15(5):370-374.

19. Look MP, Rockstroh JK, Rao GS, et al. Serum selenium, plasma glutathione (GSH), and erythrocyte glutathione peroxidase (GSH-Px)-levels in asymptomatic versus symptomatic human immunodefiency virus-1 (HIV-1)-infection. *Eur J Clin Nutr*. 1997;51(4):266-272.

20. Delmas-Beauvieux MC, Peuchant E, Couchouron A, et al. The enzymatic antioxidant system in blood and glutathione status in human immunodeficiency virus (HIV)-infected patients: effects of supplementation with selenium or beta-carotene. *Am J Cl Nutr*. 1996;64(1):101-107.

21. Olmstead L, Schrauzer GN, Flores-Arce M, et al. Selenium supplementation of symptomatic human immunodeficiency virus infected patients. *Biol Trace Elem Res.* 1989;29:59-65.

22. Shabert JK, Wilmore DW. Glutamine deficiency as a cause of human immunodeficiency virus wasting. *Med Hypotheses.* 1996;46(3):252-256.

23. Noyer CM, Simon D, Borczuk A, et al. A double-blind placebo-controlled pilot study of glutamine therapy for abnormal intestinal permeability in patients with AIDS. *Am J Gastroenterol.* 1998;93(6):972-975.

24. Clarke RH, Feleke G, Din M, et al. Nutritional treatment for acquired immune deficiency syndrome virus-associated wasting using beta-hydroxy beta-methylbutyrate, glutamine, and arginine: a randomized, placebo-controlled study. *JPE N.* 2000;24:133-139.

25. Shabert J, Winslow C, Lacey JM, Wilmore DW. Glutamine-antioxidant supplementation increases body cell mass in AIDS patients with weight loss: a randomized, double-blind controlled trial. *Nutrition.* 1999;15(11-12):860-864.

26. De Simone C, Tzantzoglou S, Jirillo E, et al. Carnitine deficiency in AIDS patients. *AIDS.* 1992;6(2):203-205.

27. *Ibid*

28. De Simone C, Famularo G, Tzantzoglou S, et al. Carnitine depletion in peripheral blood mononuclear cells from patients with AIDS: effect of oral L-carnitine. *AIDS.* 1994;8(5):655-660.

29. Kuratsune H, Yamaguti K, Lindh G, et al. Low levels of serum acylcarnitine in chronic fatigue syndrome and chronic hepatitis type C, but not seen in other diseases. *Int J Mol Med.* 1998;2(1):51-56.

30. De Simone C, Tzantzoglou S, Famularo G, et al. High-dose L-carnitine improves immunologic and metabolic parameters in AIDS patients. *Immunopharmacol Immunotoxicol.* 1993;15(1):1-12.

31. Campos Y, Huertas R, Lorenzo G, et al. Plasma carnitine insufficiency and effectiveness of L-carnitine therapy in patients with mitochondrial myopathy. *Muscle Nerve.* 1993;16(2):150-153.

32. Dalakas MC, Leon-Monzon ME, Bernardini I, et al. Zidovudine-induced mitochondrial myopathy is associated with muscle carnitine deficiency and lipid storage. *Ann Neurol.* 1994;35(4):482-487.

33. Arnaudo E, Dalakas M, Shanske S, et al. Depletion of muscle mitochondrial DNA in AIDS patients with zidovudine-induced myopathy. *Lancet.* 1991;337(8740):508-510.

34. Davis HJ, Miene LJ, van der Westhuizen N, et al. L-carnitine and magnesium as a supportive supplement with antiviral drugs. Abstract 42384. *Int Conf AIDS* 1998;12:851.

Chapter 19
MY JOURNEY, MY CHOICES
Randy Dietrich

1. Hourigan LF, Macdonald GA, Purdie D, et al. Fibrosis in chronic hepatitis C correlates significantly with body mass index and steatosis. *Hepatology.* 1999;29(4):1215-1219.

Chapter 20
A LOOK TO THE FUTURE
Lorren Sandt

1. National Institues of Health, National Center for Complementary and Alternative Medicine (NCCAM). Expanding horizons of healthcare, five-year strategic plan, 09/25/00. [At the time of publication, this report was available at: http://nccam.nih.gov/about/plans/fiveyear/index.htm.]

2. National Institutes of Health, National Center for Complementary and Alternative Medicine (NCCAM). Hepatitis C: Treatment Alternatives. NCCAM Pub. No. Z-04. Revised July 25, 2001. [At the time of publication, this report was available at http://nccam.nih.gov/health/hepatitisc.]

About the Authors

Terry Baker
Executive Director, Veterans Aimed Toward Awareness
Middletown, DE

Terry Baker is a patient advocate for military veterans and Executive Director of Veterans Aimed Toward Awareness (VATA). Terry and VATA work to educate veterans about the need to be tested for hepatitis. They have recently released a hepatitis C awareness video aimed toward veterans. Terry advocates for veterans' rights regarding hepatitis C related disability. Terry represents a large portion of the hepatitis C population in the United States.

Misha Cohen, OMD, LAc
Clinical Director, Chicken Soup Chinese Medicine
San Francisco, CA

Misha R. Cohen is a doctor of oriental medicine and a licensed acupuncturist. She is an internationally recognized practitioner, lecturer, and leader in the field of traditional Chinese medicine. Dr. Cohen is the author of *The Chinese Way to Healing: Many Paths to Wholeness* (Perigee 1996), *The HIV Wellness Sourcebook* (Holt 1998), and *The Hepatitis C Help Book* (St. Martin's Press 2000, 2001). She has also authored numerous professional articles and book chapters on Chinese medicine and research subjects. Dr. Cohen is Clinical Director of Chicken Soup Chinese Medicine, Research and Education Chair of Quan Yin Healing Arts Center, Research Specialist at the University of California Institute for Health and Aging, and Research Consultant to the University of California, San Francisco School of Medicine Cancer Center. She contributes regular columns to *Hepatitis* magazine and *NuMedx*.com magazine. *POZ Magazine* named her one of the "Top 50 AIDS Researchers in the Country" in 1997.

Randy Dietrich
Patient Advocate
Aurora, CO

Randy Dietrich was diagnosed with hepatitis C in January 1999 following a routine physical examination. Randy is a successful businessman in the finance arena. As a result of his diagnosis, Mr. Dietrich founded the Hepatitis C Caring Ambassadors Program. The purposes of the program are to identify the best possible treatment options for hepatitis C, educate people about those treatments, improve the quality of life of people living with hepatitis C, and provide significant insights towards developing a cure of hepatitis C. Randy's role in the World Class Brainstorming Team is to bring a business perspective.

Gregory Everson, MD
Professor of Medicine, University of Colorado Health Sciences Center
Denver, CO

Dr. Everson received his medical degree from Cornell Medical College, NY, NY. He is currently a Professor of Medicine and the Director of Hepatology in the Division of Gastroenterology and Hepatology, Department of Internal Medicine at the University of Colorado. Dr. Everson is a recipient of both NIH and industry sponsored research grants and contracts to study and treat patients with hepatitis C. He is principal investigator of the HALT C trial in Colorado. Dr. Everson is an author and contributor to many scientific and clinical publications related to hepatitis C and liver disease. He and his coauthor Hedy Weinberg have authored three editions of *Living with Hepatitis C: A Survivor's Guide*, one edition of *My Mom has Hepatitis C*, and the new book, *Living with Hepatitis B: A Survivor's Guide*. Dr. Everson is a fellow of the American College of Physicians, and a member of the American Gastroenterologic Association, the American Association for the Study of Liver Disease, and the American Society of Transplantation. He is the Associate Editor of *Liver Transplantation*, and a reviewer for numerous scientific and medical journals.

Sylvia Flesner, ND

Dr. Sylvia Flesner has maintained a full-time clinical practice in Houston, Texas and Denver, Colorado for the past 23 years. With her relocation to North Carolina, Dr. Flesner has expanded her practice to include the Research Triangle Park area. Dr. Flesner graduated from the Clayton School of Natural Healing, American Holistic College of Nutrition. Her training as a doctor of naturopathy included the study of several alternative medical disciplines including homeopathy, nutrition, pressure points, herbology, massage, acupressure, reflexology, iridology, psychology, degenerative diseases, allergic diseases, immune deficiency problems, and techniques for survival in the 21st century. Dr. Flesner is also certified in psychoneuroimmunology. Dr. Flesner is a member of the American Naturopathic Medical Association, and for the past eight years, a member of the American Holistic Medical Association. Currently, Dr. Flesner is participating in research at the Duke University Rhine Research Center correlating medical records of patients using intuitive diagnostics. She is also working on alternative treatment approaches for cancer and other illnesses. Dr. Flesner has lectured at the School of Public Health and MD Anderson Methodist Hospital in Texas.

Robert Gish, MD
California Pacific Medical Center
San Francisco, CA

Dr. Gish is Medical Director of the Liver Transplant Program at the California Pacific Medical Center in San Francisco, and Associate Professor of Clinical Medicine at the University of California, San Francisco. He is an Associate Clinical Professor of Medicine at the University of Nevada, Reno, and a faculty member at Merced Community Hospital, University of California, Davis. Dr. Gish has conducted extensive research on treatments for hepatitis B and C. He is a corporate consultant for many major pharmaceutical corporations, and lectures internationally. Dr. Gish collaborated with Dr. Misha Cohen to author *The Hepatitis C Helpbook*. The book examines the use of Chinese medicine in combination with conventional western biomedical therapies. *The Hepatitis C Helpbook* is widely available in bookstores.

Robert Gleser, MD
Founder, HealthMark
Denver, CO

Dr. Gleser founded HealthMark in 1985 after overcoming cancer. Born in South Africa, Dr. Gleser completed his medical residency and fellowship at Boston University Medical Center in internal medicine and hematology. Dr. Gleser is also a certified acupuncturist, having completed his certification at University of California, Los Angeles in 1996. Dr. Gleser is a former vice president of Denver's largest health care provider, Columbia. He previously served as the Corporate Medical Director for US West. Dr. Gleser is an author, former radio personality, and former medical director of the Pritikin Longevity Center.

Douglas LaBrecque, MD
Professor and Director of Liver Services, University of Iowa Hospitals and Clinics
Iowa City, IA

Dr. LaBrecque received his medical degree from Stanford Medical School, Stanford, CA. He is currently a Professor in the Department of Internal Medicine at the University of Iowa College of Medicine. Dr. LaBrecque was Chief of Gastroenterology-Hepatology at the Veterans Administration hospital in Iowa City, IA from 1982 to 2001. He has won a number of awards including the Lange Book Award, the J. D. Lane Research Award, and the Medical Residents Teaching Award at the University of Iowa. Dr. LaBrecque is recognized nationally and internationally for his expertise in liver diseases, particularly the field of hepatitis. Dr. LaBrecque has built a nationally recognized program in liver diseases at the University of Iowa with an over 1000% increase in patients over the past 15 years, five full-time faculty members, and a liver transplant program. He has written key chapters on clinical subjects in standard internal medicine and hepatology textbooks, and co-edited a textbook on liver diseases.

Lark Lands, PhD
Patient Advocate
Georgetown, CO

Lark Lands is Science Editor of *POZ Magazine* and Director of Treatment Education for DAAIR. Dr. Lands is also a contributing writer and editor for CATIE, www.AIDSmeds.com, the Boston Buyers Club, and the Houston Buyers Club. Dr. Lands is a long-time HIV treatment activist, journalist, and educator. A former think tank scientist, she was a pioneer in bringing attention to the need for an integrated approach to HIV disease. Her articles, many of which are available at www.larklands.net, have been widely printed and reprinted in AIDS newsletters and on the Internet. She is a frequent speaker at international, national, state, and local HIV/AIDS conferences.

Shri Kant Mishra, ABMS, MD, MS, FAAN, FNAAM
Professor of Neurology and Coordinator of the Integrative Medicine Program
University of Southern California, Check School of Medicine
Los Angeles, CA

Dr. Mishra is a Professor of Neurology and Coordinator of the Integrative Medicine Program at the University of Southern California School of Medicine. He graduated from Banaras Hindu University Ayurveda Charya with an ABMS (bachelor of medicine and surgery) from the Institute of Medical Sciences. He holds an MS degree in anatomy from Queens University, Canada and an MD from the University of Toronto, Canada. He also holds an MBA in Health Systems from the University of Wisconsin. He is a neurologist with a special interest in neuromuscular diseases. He served as medical director at the Veterans Administration Outpatient Clinic and Associate Dean at the University of Southern California. He is a member of many prestigious neuroscience societies and serves on editorial boards of many neurological and integrative medicine journals. Dr. Mishra has been very active in the field of integrative medicine and serves on various committees in this field. He is a practicing Ayurvedist, and yoga teacher and practitioner. Dr. Mishra's goals are to develop evidence-based, cost-effective, quality clinical care education and research in integrative medicine. He is president of the American Academy of Ayurvedic Medicine (AAAM).

Lyn Patrick, ND
Private Naturopathic Physician
Hesperus, CO

Dr. Patrick graduated from Bastyr University in 1984 and was in private practice as a licensed naturopathic physician in Tucson, Arizona for 17 years. She has provided care for HIV positive and HIV/hepatitis C coinfected patients through federally funded programs that incorporated complementary medicine in a primary care treatment model. She is currently an Associate Editor for *Alternative Medicine Review*, a Medline-indexed, peer-reviewed journal and has published over 20 scientific reviews in the field of complementary and alternative medicine. Dr. Patrick has presented information on CAM and hepatitis C at numerous medical meetings and is a longstanding member of the American Association of Naturopathic Physicians.

Peggy McCarthy, MBA
Executive Director, Innovative Medical Education Consortium
Vancouver, WA

Ms. McCarthy received her MBA in health administration at National University in San Diego, CA. She trained as a basic science immunologist, and has published research in leading scientific journals. As an academic researcher at University of California, San Diego, she helped train medical and graduate students, taught a health-care practice survey course for science undergraduates, and developed a comprehensive laboratory-training program. Ms. McCarthy worked in the marketing and medical divisions of a major pharmaceutical company before founding two medical education companies: McCarthy Medical Marketing in 1987 and Innovative Medical Education Consortium in 1992. Ms. McCarthy founded the Alliance for Lung Cancer Advocacy, Support, and Education (ALCASE), a nonprofit patient advocacy organization, in 1995 and served as its Volunteer Executive Director until 2000; she now sits on its Board of Directors. Ms. McCarthy is a founding member of ACORE (Advancing Communication in Oncology through Research and Education), a partner of the National Dialogue on Cancer, a member of the American College of Chest Physicians Task Force on Women, Smoking, & Lung Cancer, and a member of the National Comprehensive Cancer Network Task Force on physician/patient communication.

Sivarama Prasad Vinjamury
Ayurvedic Practitioner
Los Angeles, CA

Dr. Sivarama Prasad Vinjamury graduated from University of Kerala, South India. He is in private practice as a licensed Ayurvedic physician. He is currently studying for his master's degree in acupuncture and oriental medicine at the Southern California University of Health Sciences at Los Angeles. He volunteers and conducts research at the University of Southern California in the Integrative Medicine Program. He is also involved in part-time research at Southern California University of Health Sciences. Dr. Vinjamury is the former Director of Product Development for Venkat Pharma, Hyderabad, South India, and a former consultant Ayurvedic physician at Apollo Hospitals, Hyderabad, South India. For the past eight years, he has been treating various chronic ailments with Ayurvedic medicines at his clinic and at Apollo hospitals. His areas of interest include HIV, hepatitis B and C, and rheumatology. Dr. Vinjamury is a member of the American Association of Alternative Medicine Practitioners.

Lorren Sandt, Patient Advocate
Hepatitis C Caring Ambassador Program
Managing Ambassador
Oregon City, OR

Lorren Sandt has managed the Hepatitis C Caring Ambassadors Program since its inception in 1999. She is responsible for the implementation of the organization's structure and spearheads its ongoing mission. A major focus for Lorren has been to attend cutting-edge medical conferences to gather the most up-to-date information on hepatitis C clinical research and to explore the most promising upcoming therapies. At these conferences and symposiums, Lorren talks with people living with hepatitis C, their families, patient advocates, representatives of hepatitis C organizations, physicians, and other health care workers. Her purpose is to learn those issues that are of most concern to the various disciplines and organizations devoted to hepatitis C, and to determine if there is a way everyone can work together toward a common goal. In August 2001, Lorren was honored with an award from the Hepatitis C Global Foundation in San Francisco, California, The Ronald Eugene Duffy Memorial Award for Patient Activism - for leadership and mentoring of patients, making them advocates for their own health.

Tina St. John, MD
Medical Writer, Editor, and Consultant
Vancouver, WA

Dr. St. John is a graduate of Emory University School of Medicine in Atlanta, Georgia. She is a medical epidemiologist, medical writer, editor, educator, and a clinical research consultant. Dr. St. John is currently a regular medical columnist for *Hepatitis* magazine. Dr. St. John has experience in internal medicine and infectious diseases, and was formerly a senior medical officer with the Centers for Disease Control and Prevention (CDC). At CDC, Dr. St. John designed and conducted epidemiological research and oversaw all continuing medical education activities sponsored by CDC and the Agency for Toxic Substances and Disease Registry (ATSDR). She has extensive experience designing and conducting epidemiological research, and has particular interests in clinical laboratory diagnostics and practice-based research. Dr. St. John is an outspoken patient advocate. She is a member of the American Public Health Association, the American Medical Women's Association, the American Medical Writers Association, and the Alpha Omega Alpha Medical Honor Society.

Qing-Cai Zhang, Lic Ac. MD
Zhang's Clinic
New York, NY

Dr. Qingcai Zhang graduated from Shanghai Second Medical University. He worked as a clinician at Reijing Hospital of the medical university. Dr. Zhang conducted clinical work and research to integrate Chinese and western medicine. In 1980, he was awarded a World Health Organization scholarship, which supported his two-year fellowship at Harvard Medical School and Massachusetts General Hospital. He worked as a research fellow at the Wakai Clinic in Nagoya, Japan. Dr. Zhang received a one-year appointment from the University of California, Davis as a visiting professor. Since 1986, Dr. Zhang has been the primary researcher at the Oriental Healing Arts Institute where he conducts research on treating HIV/AIDS with Chinese medicine. He has published two books on this topic. Dr. Zhang went into private practice in 1990, first in Cypress, California, and now in New York City. He focuses on treating chronic infectious diseases such as viral hepatitis, HIV/AIDS, Lyme disease, and autoimmune diseases. He is the author of *Healing Hepatitis C with Modern Chinese Medicine*.

Hepatitis C: Choices
Order Form

For faster processing of your order, please complete all fields

Person ordering: _____

Title: _____

Organization: _____

Type of organization: _____

E-mail address: _____

Fax number: _____ **Day phone:** _____ **Eve. phone:** _____

ORDER OPTIONS

☐ **$15 x** ____ **= $** _____ (all book(s) shipped to one location)

☐ **$15 + $** _____ (one book shipped to you, additional funds donated to the Caring Ambassadors Program)

☐ **$25** (one book shipped to you, and one shipped to someone of our choice living with hepatitis C)

☐ **$** _____ (I don't need a book, I would like to donate to the Caring Ambassadors Program, Inc.)

(All donations over $15 are tax deductible)

SHIPPING INFORMATION

Recipient:

  Name: _____

  Address: _____

  City: _____ **State:** _____ **Zip:** _____

THANK YOU FOR YOUR ORDER

Please fold this form, enclose your check and affix appropriate postage.
If you have any questions about your order, call 1-877-HCV-CHOICES (877-828-3464)
or to pay by credit card, visit our website: www.hepcchallenge.org
(Allow 3-4 weeks for delivery)

Hepatitis C Caring Ambassadors Program
(A non-for-profit corporation)

Caring Ambassadors Program
P. O. Box 1748
Oregon City, OR 97045